Thrombolysis in Pulmonary Embolism

Carlos Jerjes-Sánchez

Thrombolysis in Pulmonary Embolism

Springer

Carlos Jerjes-Sánchez, MD, FCCP, FACC
Sistema Nacional de Investigadores, Nivel II – Clinical Research Director
Instituto de Cardiología y Medicina Vascular, TEC Salud

Escuela de Medicina, Tecnológico de Monterrey
San Pedro Garza Garcia, Nuevo León, Mexico

Unidad de Investigacion Clinica en Medicina SC
Monterrey, Nuevo León, Mexico

ISBN 978-3-319-19706-7 ISBN 978-3-319-19707-4 (eBook)
DOI 10.1007/978-3-319-19707-4

Library of Congress Control Number: 2015943833

Springer Cham Heidelberg New York Dordrecht London

Printed on acid-free paper

Springer International Publishing AG Switzerland is part of Springer Science+Business Media (www.springer.com)

To my friend, companion, accomplice,
and wife, Alicia, and my two dear children
and friends, Carlos and Alicia,
and to the life we have lived together.

Preface

In spite of all the advances achieved in terms of anticoagulation, antiplatelets, thrombolysis, and pharmaco-invasive and mechanical therapeutic approaches, acute vascular syndromes including acute ischemic syndromes, stroke, and pulmonary embolism are the three major causes of death and disability in developed and developing countries. Pulmonary embolism often does not receive the attention it deserves, in part because the symptoms of this disorder are similar to other more frequent cardiovascular conditions such as acute heart failure and acute coronary syndromes. Recognized cases of pulmonary embolism constitute only a minority of the episodes that occur due to the elusiveness of the diagnosis, with the condition frequently undetected until the patient dies. Therefore, pharmacologic thrombolysis can be considered one of the most important advances in the field of cardiovascular therapeutics. Currently, in ST-elevation myocardial infarction, first-, second-, and third-generation fibrinolytics are the primary therapeutic options in the absence of mechanical reperfusion. However, in 16 randomized control trials conducted between 1970 and 2014, which included 2215 pulmonary embolism patients under thrombolysis use, this therapeutic option is only indicated in the presence of cardiogenic shock or high-risk (troponin expression and right ventricular hypokinesis) pulmonary embolism. Current guidelines developed by the European Society of Cardiology established Class I with Level B recommendations for thrombolysis. In treating a patient with extensive pulmonary thrombus, right ventricular hypokinesis, and clinical stability, physicians need to decide whether to use anticoagulation alone or administer thrombolysis, with the awareness that the latter option can increase bleeding risk.

In this book, we focus specifically on peripheral intravenous thrombolysis because, in our experience, this therapeutic approach can be performed safely and effectively in emergency departments, hospital wards, and intensive critical care units in tertiary and community hospitals. Interventions such as mechanical pulmonary intervention, pharmaco-invasive approach, and thrombolysis driven by ultrasound are outside the scope of this book, as they require specialized training, thus limiting the accessibility of these modalities.

Thrombolysis in Pulmonary Embolism provides a current and comprehensive update on this evolving field. Our contribution is targeted to a broad group of physicians including cardiologists, pulmonologists, internists, angiologists, hematologists, and first-contact physicians involved in pulmonary embolism patient care. In addition, it serves as a valuable resource for medical students, interns, residents, and fellows. The book presents our experience in treating approximately 300 pulmonary embolism patients submitted to first-, second-, and third-generation fibrinolytic regimens successfully used in ST-elevation myocardial infarction patients.

Chapter 1 discusses the complex mechanisms of thrombosis and the relationship between inflammation and thrombosis. In Chapter 2, the pharmacokinetics and pharmacodynamics of the most commonly used fibrinolytics are described. Chapter 3, co-authored by Alicia Ramirez-Rivera, presents a critical analysis of the multicenter trials published in the last 20 years. In Chapter 4, Pedro Gutiérrez-Fajardo, who has made significant contributions in the field of pulmonary embolism, outlines the criteria by which pulmonary embolism patients requiring thrombolysis are identified. Chapter 5 examines one-hour alteplase infusion and the unfractionated heparin regimen used in acute myocardial infarction followed by enoxaparin, a low-molecular-weight heparin. In Chapter 6, the recommendations for thrombolysis use in pulmonary embolism developed by the American Heart Association, the American College of Chest Physicians, and the European Society of Cardiology are presented. Chapter 7 describes our experience in treating patients with extensive pulmonary embolism, right ventricular dysfunction, and clinical stability. Chapter 8, co-authored by Anabel Garcia, reviews the evidence in special situations, such as treating acute pulmonary embolism in cases of in-transit thrombus and in pregnant women.

The co-authors are experts in this field, and we have collaborated for the past 20 years. I wish to thank all of them for their participation in this important project.

We hope that this book enables physicians to make the best decisions for their patients in the field of pulmonary embolism. Finally, thanks to all those patients whom we were able to help, but especially to those whom we could not.

San Pedro Garza Garcia, Mexico Carlos Jerjes-Sánchez, MD, FCCP, FACC

Contents

Contributors

Pedro Gutierrez Fajardo, MD, FASE, MEACI Echocardiography Laboratory, Hospital Bernardette, Instituto Cardiovascular de Guadalajara, Jalisco, Mexico

Anabel Garcia-Sosa, MD Emergency Room Department, Hospital de Cardiologia, Instituto Mexicano del Seguro Social, Monterrey, Nuevo León, Mexico

Carlos Jerjes-Sánchez, MD, FCCP, FACC Sistema Nacional de Investigadores, Nivel II – Clinical Research Director, Instituto de Cardiología y Medicina Vascular, EC Salud

Escuela de Medicina, Tecnológico de Monterrey, San Pedro Garza Garcia, Nuevo León, Mexico

Unidad de Investigacion Clinica en Medicina SC, Monterrey, Nuevo León, Mexico

Alicia Ramirez-Rivera, MD, FCCP Head Pulmonary Physiology Department, Hospital de Cardiologia No 34, Instituto Mexicano del Seguro Social, Monterey, Nuevo León, Mexico

H. David Rodriguez, MD Centro de Investigacion Basica y Transferencia, Hospital Zambrano-Hellion, Escuela de Medicina y Ciencias de la Salud, Tecnológico de Monterrey, Monterrey, Nuevo León, Mexico

Chapter 1
Mechanisms of Thrombosis

Carlos Jerjes-Sánchez

Thrombosis is a critical event in the vascular disorders, associated with considerable morbidity and mortality. Venous thromboembolism (VTE) is the third cause of mortality after myocardial infarction and stroke, and it is the second cause of death in patients with cancer [1]. At first glance, venous thrombosis could be included among thrombosis models of low-pressure segment circulation [2], such as atrial thrombi, and thrombus in-transit or not (left or right heart). The process of thrombosis is a critical protective response that staunches blood loss by generating thrombin and precipitating fibrin and platelet deposits at sites of vascular endothelium or endocardium. In the case of atherosclerosis, this mechanism is driven by vascular injury through molecular and cellular components of the clotting cascade that triggers and propagates inflammatory process. This model highlights how the interface between thrombosis and inflammation can contribute to chronic and acute arterial vascular disease (ischemic heart disease, vascular brain disease, peripheral artery disease, and aortic disease) [3].

Currently, as observed in atrial fibrillation [4] and stent thrombosis [5], multiple clinical and molecular lines of evidence suggest a close link between inflammation, thrombosis, and VTE [6–14]. These data establish a relationship among atherothrombosis risk factors and vein thrombosis, as well as the role of inflammation in triggering clinical events. This review provides an update of mechanisms of thrombosis, Virchow's triad, venous thrombosis, and their links with inflammation mechanisms.

C. Jerjes-Sánchez, M.D., F.C.C.P., F.A.C.C. (✉)
Sistema Nacional de Investigadores, Nivel II – Clinical Research Director,
Instituto de Cardiologia y Medicina Vascular, TEC Salud

Escuela de Medicina, Tecnológico de Monterrey San Pedro Garza Garcia,
Nuevo León, Mexico

Unidad de Investigacion Clinica en Medicina SC Monterrey, Nuevo León, Mexico
e-mail: jerjes@prodigy.net.mx

C. Jerjes-Sánchez, *Thrombolysis in Pulmonary Embolism*,
DOI 10.1007/978-3-319-19707-4_1

Mechanisms of Thrombosis

Hemostasis is the process that maintains the integrity of a closed, low or high-pressure circulatory system; blood coagulation initiated by tissue factor (TF) concludes in the generation of thrombin and fibrin. In the model of arterial thrombosis, vessel-wall injury and the extravasation of blood rapidly start actions in the vessel wall and in the blood that seal the breach. When pathologic processes overcome the regulatory mechanisms of hemostasis, excessive quantities of thrombin form, initiating thrombosis [1]. In this complex process several elements including platelets or high shear stress, have a close relationship in thrombus developing and in the thrombi final structure.

Vascular Endothelium

The vessel wall and its inner lining of endothelium are critical to the maintenance of a patent vasculature. Three thromboregulators (e.g., nitric oxide, prostacyclin, and the ectonucleotidase CD39) [15–17] has been identified in the endothelium as the first defense against thrombosis. After endothelium disruption, collagen and TF are exposed to the flowing blood, starting formation of a thrombus. Exposed collagen triggers the accumulation and activation of platelets, whereas exposed TF initiates the generation of thrombin, converting fibrinogen to fibrin and activating platelets [1].

Collagen in the subendothelial matrix and TF facilitate the maintenance of a closed circulatory system. Endothelial dysfunction can be regarded as the key of the risk factors and a syndrome that exhibits systemic manifestations associated with significant morbidity and mortality [18]. As part of endothelial function, endogenous fibrinolysis is a protective mechanism against length and duration of arterial or venous thrombotic occlusion, which would otherwise lead to permanent tissue damage [19].

The vascular endothelium influences not only the three classically interacting components of hemostasis but also the natural sequels of endothelial dysfunction: inflammation and tissue repair. Two principal modes of endothelial behavior may be differentiated, which are best defined as an anti- and prothrombotic state. The vascular endothelial cell surface is possibly the major site of control of these coagulant and anticoagulant interactions. Under physiological conditions, endothelium mediates vascular vasodilatation, prevents platelet adhesion and activation, blocks thrombin formation, and mitigates fibrin deposition through several pathways. Adhesion and transmigration of inflammatory leukocytes are attenuated, and oxygen radicals are efficiently scavenged. In the elderly, even under physiological conditions, all of these factors are significantly affected [20].

Although classical primary and secondary hemostasis only compromises the sequential formation of the "white" and "red" thrombus, there is growing awareness showing that hemostasis is intimately coupled to fibrinolytic processes, inflammatory reactions, and the initiation of angiogenesis and wound healing. In addition, scientific developments over the last 20 years indicate that the properties of the endothelium may even govern the physiological balance of hemostasis/fibrinolysis and that endothelial derangement can account for numerous pathophysiological disturbances of primary and secondary hemostasis, fibrinolysis, and tissue repair [7].

Tissue Factor

Coagulation is initiated when TF is exposed to plasma, binding coagulation factor F VII/VIIa, and forming a complex on cellular surfaces that triggers the coagulation cascade [21]. TF—a transmembrane glycoprotein—is a member of the class II cytokine receptor superfamily; it is expressed on cells in several anatomical compartments with multiple functions and acts as receptor and essential cofactor for FVII and FVIIa. In the vessel wall, vascular smooth muscle cells, adventitial fibroblasts and pericytes constitutively express TF. The expression of TF can also be induced in monocytes and, to some extent, in endothelial cells in response to various stimuli, including inflammatory cytokines, endotoxin, growth factors, and oxidized/modified low-density lipoproteins. Such expression may lead or contribute to thrombosis under certain pathological conditions, such as inflammatory states (e.g., sepsis, vasculitis) and disseminated intravascular coagulation [21].

At the beginning of blood coagulation, TF mediates intracellular signaling events that are important for angiogenesis, tumor progression, metastasis, and maintenance of the vasculature. Collagen (first line of defense) and TF (second line of defense) associated with the vessel wall provide a hemostatic barrier to maintain the low- or high-pressure circulatory system. Collagen is located in the subendothelial matrix of the endothelium, and it is not exposed to blood under normal conditions. TF located in the smooth muscle (media) and adventitial layers of the vessel wall is exposed to flowing blood when the vessel is disrupted or punctured. Both collagen and thrombin initiate thrombus formation [1].

When coagulation cascade is activated, TF triggers a second pathway that initiates platelet activation. Platelet activation initiated by this pathway does not require endothelium injury and is independent of von Willebrand factor and glycoprotein VI. TF forms a complex with factor VIIa, the enzymatically active form of factor VII, and this TF VIIa complex activates factor IX, thereby initiating a proteolytic cascade that generates thrombin [21].

Thrombin cleaves protease-activated receptor 4 on the platelet surface, thereby activating platelets and causing them to release adenosine diphosphate, serotonin, and thromboxane A_2. These agonists activate other platelets, and amplify the signals for thrombus formation [22]. Platelet activation leads to the release of secondary agonists, thromboxane A_2 and adenosine diphosphate. The first is produced from membrane phospholipids, and the second is released from dense granules. Through autocrine and paracrine mechanisms, both secondary agonists play a critical role in the sustained activation of $\alpha_{IIb}\beta_3$ receptors and stable platelet aggregation [22].

Current Model of Coagulation

Classically, coagulation has been categorized in terms of: (a) extrinsic pathway (initiated by TF/FVIIa), (b) intrinsic pathway (coagulation occurs when plasma is in contact with negatively charged surfaces–contact phase activation), and (c) a common pathway, proceeding after the activation of FX. Currently, the process of coagulation is a cell surface-based model that included three overlapping phases: initiation, amplification, and propagation. The process of coagulation starts on TF-exposing cells, and continues on the surfaces of activated platelets. In the initiation phase, TF-exposing cells and microparticles are exposed to the coagulation factors in the lumen of the vessel. Platelets, activated by vascular injury (plaque rupture) are recruited and adhere to the site of injury [21].

The TF/FVIIa complex activates coagulation factors IX to IXa and X to Xa, and trace amounts of thrombin are generated. In the amplification phase, this small amount of thrombin acts as signal for further platelet activation and aggregation. On the surface of platelets, thrombin activates FV, FVIII, and FXI. In the propagation phase, FVIIIa forms a complex with FIXa (Xase), and FVa forms a complex with FXa (prothrombinase) on the platelet surface, which accelerates the generation of FXa and thrombin, respectively. When FXa associates with FVa, it is protected from TF pathway inhibitor and antithrombin. In the propagation phase, a burst of thrombin is generated, which is sufficient for the clotting of soluble fibrinogen into a fibrin meshwork [21].

Finally, coagulation included a series of enzymatic process; thrombin generation, the last enzyme of coagulation, is the result of an amplifying cascade, with approximately one molecule of FXa generating approximately 1000 molecules of thrombin. Thrombin serves a number of functions in addition to fibrin formation as platelet activation and aggregation, it has proinflammatory actions, amplifies clotting by activating coagulation FXI and the cofactors FV and FVIII into FVa and FVIIIa. In addition thrombin stabilizes clots by activating FXIII and has antifibrinolytic actions, through the activation of thrombin activatable fibrinolysis inhibitor (TAFI) providing a molecular link between coagulation and inhibition of fibrinolysis.

Natural Anticoagulant Mechanisms

Thrombin generation and fibrin formation occur rapidly in the endothelium at sites of vascular injury, in the presence of inflammation states or thrombophilia. Thrombin promotes the activation of protein C and protein S, two natural vitamin K-dependent anticoagulant proteins that contain the coagulation process by inactivating FVa and FVIIIa [23]. To control and localize the thrombus, several inhibitory mechanisms are involved. Antithrombin, protein C and protein S are the most important regulators of coagulation. TAFI and the fibrinolytic system are the main natural anticoagulant and antithrombotic mechanisms.

Thrombomodulin, a transmembrane molecule expressed on endothelial cells, binds thrombin, and the thrombin/thrombomodulin complex activates protein C, a vitamin K-dependent proenzyme, to an active serine protease. The activated protein C anticoagulant system regulates coagulation by modulating the activity of the two cofactors, FVIIIa and FVa. Although, the activation rate of thrombin-mediated protein C activation is slow, it is increased at least 100-fold when thrombin binds to thrombomodulin. The rate increases another 20-fold when protein C binds to endothelial protein C receptor which presents protein C to the thrombin/thrombomodulin complex for efficient activation, highlighting a mechanism for endothelial cell localization of anticoagulation [24].

Virchow's Triad in the Twenty-First Century

In 1856, the German pathologist Rudolf Virchow postulated that a triad of conditions predispose to thrombus formation; these three factors include abnormalities in the vessel wall, blood flow, and the coagulability of blood. The first two components of Rudolf Virchow's triad were based on his meticulous necropsy observations on patients who died secondary to pulmonary embolism (PE); the third reflects Virchow's remarkable insight that is only today—more than 150 years later—being substantiated at a molecular level. While Virchow was referring to venous thrombosis, the same processes have been applied to arterial thrombosis. Nine years ago, in a contemporary viewpoint of Virchow's triad, new elements were considered: inflammation, endothelial dysfunction, and atherosclerosis (e.g., abnormal vessel wall), abnormalities of hemorheology and turbulence at bifurcations and stenotic regions (e.g., abnormal blood flow), abnormalities in platelet function, coagulation, endogenous fibrinolysis, and metabolic factors (e.g., abnormal blood constituents) and finally, polymorphisms driving thrombosis location [7].

Currently, considering the advance on molecular bases, other new elements [22] in the Virchow's triad have to be considered. In Table 1.1 it is possible to identify historic elements of the Virchow's triad and the new components for arterial and venous thrombosis. Metabolic factors remains as other important components. The structure of lipoprotein (a) is similar to plasminogen and tissue plasminogen activator and it competes with plasminogen for its binding site, leading to reduced fibrinolysis. Also, because that lipoprotein (a) stimulates secretion of plasminogen activator inhibitor-1 (PAI-1), it leads to thrombogenesis. Lipoprotein (a) also carries cholesterol and thus contributes to atherosclerosis [25, 26]. Additionally, transports the more atherogenic proinflammatory oxidized phospholipids, which attract inflammatory cells to vessel walls and leads to smooth muscle cell proliferation [27–29].

Another interesting metabolic factor linking with thrombosis is the serum glucose. Elevated levels have a procoagulant effect and decrease fibrinolysis. Hyperglycemia is often accompanied by hyperinsulinemia, which may further inhibit fibrinolysis and increase the prothrombotic effect of hyperglycemia. In addition, it is possible that hyperglycemia acts as marker of increased stress and severity of illness.

Table 1.1 Virchow's triad in the twenty-first century

Abnormal vessel wall[a]	Endothelial dysfunction characterized by endothelial cell activation (due to hypoxia, distension, and neurohormonal activation), increased expression of platelet/monocyte adhesion, tissue factor, von Willebrand factor, and thrombin; decreased expression of nitric oxide, thrombomodulin (due to increase of tumor necrosis factor-α and interleukin-1) and protein C
Abnormal blood flow[a]	Arterial vessels: abnormalities of hemorheology and turbulence at bifurcations and stenotic regions, altered high shear stress and platelet activation. Venous vessels: reduced blood flow secondary to immobility, hypoxia, and reduced clearance of activated coagulation factors
Abnormal blood constituents[a]	Ruptured plaque or endothelium injury induces exposure of prothrombotic factors, enhanced platelet reactivity, increasing expression of fibrinogen and von Willebrand factor. Stasis could induce systemic and local hypercoagulability, tissue factor-bearing microparticles. Endogenous fibrinolysis hypoactivity and metabolic factors as lipoprotein (a) and hyperglycemia

[a]Historic components of Virchow's triad

In acute illnesses, such as PE, stress hormones (i.e., catecholamine, growth hormone, cortisol, and cytokines) are released with increasing hepatic glucose production and insulin resistance [30]. Lipoprotein (a) and hyperglycemia could be the lost link among metabolic and thrombosis disorders.

In Virchow's triad of the twenty-first century, endothelial dysfunction emerges as the most important component. Endothelial dysfunction can be regarded as the key of the risk factors and a syndrome that exhibits systemic manifestations associated with significant morbidity and mortality [18]. As part of endothelial function, endogenous fibrinolysis is a protective mechanism against lasting arterial or venous thrombotic occlusion, which would otherwise lead to permanent tissue damage. Because thrombogenesis is an active, ongoing, and dynamic process, a healthy endogenous fibrinolytic system can prevent the build-up of thrombus before complete occlusion occurs or before breakup of the occlusive thrombus (myocardial infarction, stroke, and limb ischemia or VTE), thus preventing tissue damage [19].

Inflammation

A growing body of evidence links inflammation with an important pathogenic role in several cardiovascular diseases related to thrombosis [4, 5, 31]. Evidence accumulated over the past two decades supports a key role for inflammation in all phases of the atherosclerotic process [10], from endothelial dysfunction and plaque formation through its progression and ultimately to the thrombotic complications that lead to the acute coronary syndrome [4]. Activated inflammatory cells (such as neutrophils, lymphocytes, monocytes, and resident macrophages), proinflammatory cytokines, and activated platelets are important players in this scenario.

Current evidence suggests that historic risk factors for atherothrombosis can instigate production of reactive oxygen species such as hypochlorous acid or superoxide anion; such risk factors often accompany inflammation, promoting proinflammatory cytokines and elevating production of these pro-oxidants. Proinflammatory cytokines such as interleukin-1 or tumor necrosis factor-α as inflammatory mediators can act directly in healthy and disease stages. Cytokines also change the normal anticoagulant and pro-fibrinolytic properties of endothelium to an activated state that fosters thrombus formation and stalls fibrinolysis. The inflammatory mediator CD40 ligand can induce vascular cells and mononuclear phagocytes alike to produce tissue factor, a potent trigger for thrombus formation [10] and finally innate immune system activation.

Proinflammatory cytokines also elicit the acute phase response from the liver, through the intermediary interleukin-6, the "messenger cytokine." The acute phase reactants include proteins involved in the causal pathway of atherothrombosis and vein thrombosis (e.g., fibrinogen or PAI-1) or soluble biomarkers such as C-reactive protein or serum amyloid [14].

Significance of Endogenous Fibrinolysis

The main components of endogenous fibrinolysis are tissue-type plasminogen activator, platelet activator inhibitor-1, plasmin–antiplasmin complex, D-dimer, TAFI, and lipoprotein (a) [19]. The mechanism of the fibrinolytic system at a first glance shows that thrombin converts the inactive proenzyme plasminogen to active plasmin. Plasmin degrades the cross-linked fibrin into soluble degradation products by the tissue-type plasminogen activator and the urokinase type plasminogen activators. It is tissue-type plasminogen activator that is mainly responsible for the dissolution of fibrin formed in the circulation. This fibrinolytic system can be inhibited either by antagonizing plasmin through α_2-antiplasmin or by specific plasminogen activator inhibitors. There are three types of this inhibitor described so far; of these, physiologically, the most important one is the PAI-1 [19].

The thrombin activatable fibrinolysis inhibitor is another important inhibitor of the fibrinolytic system. This inhibitor forms a link between blood coagulation and fibrinolysis. Thrombin forms fibrin to stabilize the platelet thrombus and at the same time produces TAFI to protect the fibrin network. The inhibitor circulates as an inactive proenzyme and becomes activated by thrombin during blood clotting. Its active form inhibits fibrinolysis by cleaving off C-terminal lysine residues from partially degraded fibrin that stimulate the tissue plasminogen activator-mediated conversion of plasminogen to plasmin. Consequently, removal of these lysines leads to less plasmin formation and subsequently to protection of the fibrin clot from breakdown [19].

Although the plasmin-mediated fibrinolytic system is the major physiological mechanism of removing fibrin from the circulation, the plasmin-independent breakdown of fibrin by cellular components of blood also plays a significant role.

An arterial and venous thrombus contains significant amounts of leukocytes (neutrophils and monocytes) covering the thrombus surface or incorporated into it, due to the interaction of activated platelets with leukocytes [10, 11]. Neutrophil membrane proteolytic enzymes (elastase, cathepsin G) can breakdown fibrin directly and also assist the dissolution of thrombus by plasmin. Furthermore, the physical properties of fibrin formed during hemostasis/thrombosis greatly affect the rate and effectiveness of fibrinolysis [18]. In the setting of VTE, the exact mechanism to explain endogenous fibrinolysis hypoactivity is unknown.

Linking Thrombosis with Inflammation

Vein thrombosis has been traditionally associated with red blood cell and fibrin-rich "red clot," whereas arterial thrombi superimposed on atherosclerotic lesions with active inflammation are rich in platelets, giving the appearance of a "white clot." Nevertheless, experimental and morphological studies suggest that inflammation and platelet activation also participate in venous thrombogenesis [7].

A relationship between inflammation and thrombosis has been identified in different clinical scenarios where the inflammatory process and coagulation abnormalities are clearly interlinked (septic shock and disseminated intravascular coagulation, as well as in the context of VTE). The molecular mechanisms that could explain this link are becoming apparent [31]. Inflammation is known to upregulate C-reactive protein expression and to modulate platelet function. Very importantly, it also affects the initiation phase and the fibrinolytic system, enhancing the thrombotic response to vascular injury in-vivo [32]. Evidence suggests that the complement system may serve as a link between inflammation and thrombosis and reveals specific interactions between complement proteins and platelets. The complement system was shown not only to induce platelet activation and aggregation but also to potentiate thrombin-induced platelet secretion and aggregation. At the same time, platelets can activate the complement system via P-selectin [4].

Interleukin-6 induces the expression of tissue factor, fibrinogen, factor VIII, and von Willebrand factor. Coronary and pulmonary vascular release of interleukin-6 and 8 has been observed in some clinical situations [7]. Such enhancements of cytokine and chemokine levels can lead to endothelial activation and endothelial cell damage, as well as increase platelet aggregation, sensitivity to thrombin, and recruitment and activation of leukocytes at the vascular wall. Ultimately, all of these precipitate localized formation of thrombin and fibrin [4, 7]. Moreover, an increased interleukin-6 level lowers the concentration of the natural inhibitors of hemostasis such as antithrombin, protein S [4] and thrombomodulin [22]. This mechanism could explain "unprovoked" or "idiopathic PE" acute index events in high-risk population.

Thrombin has a well-recognized role as a molecular effector at the interface of thrombosis and inflammation and the clotting cascade. Thrombosis can initiate proinflammatory responses central to the pathogenesis of atherosclerosis. Thrombin levels increase at sites of vascular injury and during acute coronary syndromes and has powerful proinflammatory effects on endothelial cells, smooth muscle cell, and platelets that promote the development of vascular disease. It also activates endothelial cells by cleaving and activating endothelial protease-activated receptor-1 and 2, which increase inflammatory gene transcription and stimulate expression of numerous leukocyte adhesion molecules including vascular cell adhesion molecule-1, intracellular adhesion molecule-1, and E-selectin through nuclear factor Kappa-ß and GATA-dependent transcription factor pathways [32].

The nuclear factor Kappa-ß is a pivotal transcription factor that may play a key role in plaque instability by promoting the expression of a cascade of procoagulant and proinflammatory genes in response to a variety of stimuli [33]. It has been identified in monocyte/macrophages, smooth muscle cells, and endothelial cells in human atherosclerotic vessels but not in healthy vessels. Additionally, in coronary plaques from patients with acute coronary syndromes, it exhibits increased expression of several of its genes-including proinflammatory cytokines, growth factors, chemokines, adhesion molecules, and TF [19].

Thrombin promotes endothelial secretion of pro-atherogenic chemokines such as monocyte chemotactic protein-1, platelet-derived growth factor, macrophage migration inhibitory factor, interleukin-6, and interleukin-8 and results in monocyte adhesion. Thus, production of thrombin-induced interleukin-6 by endothelial cells and smooth muscle cells generates a systemic prothrombotic response by increasing levels of circulating PAI-1 and fibrinogen. Thrombin activation induces cell retraction and reorganization of cadherins at endothelial junctions, thereby increasing endothelial permeability and promoting platelet deposition and leukocyte extravasation [31, 32].

CD40 ligand is a member of the tumor necrosis factor superfamily, primarily expressed on activated CD4+ T lymphocytes, but it is also found in a soluble form. CD40 ligand was originally described on T cells, but its expression has since been found on a wide variety of cells, including platelets, mast cells, macrophages, NK cells, B lymphocytes, vascular smooth muscle cells, and endothelial cells. The binding of soluble CD40 ligand to its CD40 receptor on the leukocyte can also induce tissue factor expression [4]. Vascular smooth muscle cells represent a link between inflammation and thrombosis, as the local thrombotic stimulation of smooth muscle cells in the arterial or vein wall can amplify the inflammatory response and increase fibrinogen and PAI-1 levels in the circulation [11, 12].

The behavior of platelets, polymorph nuclear granulocytes, and monocytes in normal human arterial and venous blood, as documented by flow cytometry and direct microscopic visualization, demonstrates the occurrence of platelet–leukocyte microaggregates in whole blood; the analysis of venous thrombi reveals tangled pale strands of aggregated platelets and fibrin within the mass of red blood cells. Induced venous thrombus in the presence of radio-labeled platelets shows early platelet accumulation at the "head" of the thrombus; then, the acquisition of platelets by the thrombi slows, and the clots become "red," being predominantly composed of fibrin and erythrocytes. Another evidence of the participation of platelets in venous thrombosis comes from clinical studies in PE patients showing increased urinary excretion of thromboxane A_2, a marker of platelet activation [7].

Inflammation as a Trigger

From a simple view, inflammation is one of the first responses of the immune system to infection. The symptoms of inflammation include redness and swelling, which are caused by increased blood flow into the tissue. Inflammation is driven by eicosanoids and cytokines, which are released by injured or infected cells. Common cytokines, which regulate inflammatory response, include interleukins (mainly interleukin-6) that are responsible for communication among white blood cells, chemokines that promote chemotaxis, and interferons that have antiviral effects.

Acute infections have been associated with a transient increase in the risk of myocardial infarction and stroke and recently with venous thrombosis as well, supporting the notion that systemic infections increase the risk of thromboembolic events [7]. Among the three precipitants proposed in Virchow's triad, infection could affect venous stasis and increase blood coagulability. Furthermore, parallels with the arterial system suggest that damage to the vessel wall might not be limited to physical damage but could affect endothelial function as well. Inflammation is a key determinant of endothelial activation in arteries and veins (in health and disease states) and a link between infection and venous thrombosis [7, 10, 11].

Acute infections induce white-cell activation, dehydration, and bed rest as collateral thrombosis mechanisms; it is important to recognize that inflammatory and thrombotic pathways share common signaling pathways and that inflammatory responses promote activation of the clotting cascade and stimulate platelet activation [32]. Additionally, several studies have identified an increased risk of VTE in patients with non-infectious inflammatory disorders, such as inflammatory bowel disease and connective tissue disease. Considering the evidence, it is possible that [7] in high-risk populations [12, 14, 32] with atherothrombosis risk factors [3–5], an acute infection could trigger arterial and/or vein thrombosis through endothelial activation [10, 11, 31]. Vaccines to reduce or avoid respiratory infections and early detection of chronic infections (periodontitis, prostatitis, etc.) through office visits and C-reactive protein measurements could be used as new elements in the primary or secondary VTE prevention.

Inflammation directly or indirectly affects the venous endothelium inducing endothelial activity and inflammation-mediated vascular remodeling. In response to inflammatory events, endothelial cells produce inflammatory mediators (chemokines and cytokines), thereby recruiting inflammatory cells (macrophages, dendritic cells, mast cells, B cells, T cells, and T regulatory cells). With the coordination of inflammatory mediators, inflammatory cells might perpetuate the release of cytokines, chemokines, and growth factors [31]. Finally, these processes lead to vascular remodeling and vein thrombosis with or without a thromboembolic event. In any model of endothelial dysfunction the final pathway will be ischemia. In the model of endothelial dysfunction, venous thrombosis and PE complicated with acute pulmonary arterial hypertension (obstruction >30 %), the tissue damage occurs on the right ventricular endocardium, inducing ventricular dysfunction. In all models of pulmonary arterial hypertension, clinical symptoms, signs, and mortality are related to right ventricular dysfunction. Currently, in PE right ventricular dysfunction—with or without acute cellular damage—is a mortality risk marker, identifies submassive or high-risk PE and stratifies patients to fibrinolytic therapy [34–45].

Right Ventricular Myocarditis

Recently Begieneman and colleagues [46] in an elegant necropsy study showed the presence of inflammatory cells and myocytolysis related with intracavitary thrombi in the left and right ventricle of patients who died because of PE as a presumed new source of ventricular dysfunction. Previous evidences showed an increase in the level of CD68-positive macrophages in the right ventricle of PE patients and the influx of macrophages in the heart was attributed to ischemia [47, 48]. In these studies, inflammatory infiltrate and myocarditis were not discussed. Begieneman and colleagues [46] defined myocarditis as aggregation of inflammatory cells in the myocardium coinciding with areas of myocytolysis, conforming to the Dallas criteria for myocarditis. The presence of inflammatory cells in the endocardium of the heart was diagnosed as endocarditis. Compared with controls (no-PE and pulmonary arterial hypertension patients), extravascular foci of aggregates of lymphocytes, neutrophilic granulocytes, and macrophages were found dispersed in the right and left ventricle, coinciding with areas of myocytolysis, indicating myocarditis in acute PE patients.

In the same publication, a significant increase in the number of neutrophilic granulocytes, lymphocytes, and macrophages in the right ventricle ($p=0.012$, $p=0.02$, and $p=0.027$, respectively) and a significant increase in the number of neutrophilic granulocytes and macrophages in the left ventricle ($p=0.034$, $p=0.018$, respectively) was observed. No significant difference was found between the number of neutrophilic granulocytes in the left and right ventricle ($p=0.352$). However, the accumulation of lymphocytes and macrophages was significantly lower in the left ventricle than in the right ventricle in patients with PE ($p<0.001$ and <0.001, respectively). To determine a putative relation between the age of the lung thromboemboli and the accumulation of inflammatory cells in the heart, patients were divided into two groups: thromboemboli <4 days old and thromboemboli >4 days old.

Finally, thrombi in the ventricles were related to the presence of endocarditis. None of the patients without endocarditis of the right ventricle had ventricular thrombi, whereas only one patient without endocarditis of the left ventricle had a thrombus in the left ventricle. In contrast, in patients with endocarditis of the right or left ventricle irrespective of myocarditis ($n=11$ and $n=9$, respectively), thrombi were present in nine patients with right-sided endocarditis and in five patients with left-sided endocarditis. The relation between endocarditis and thrombi was highly significant ($p<0.001$).

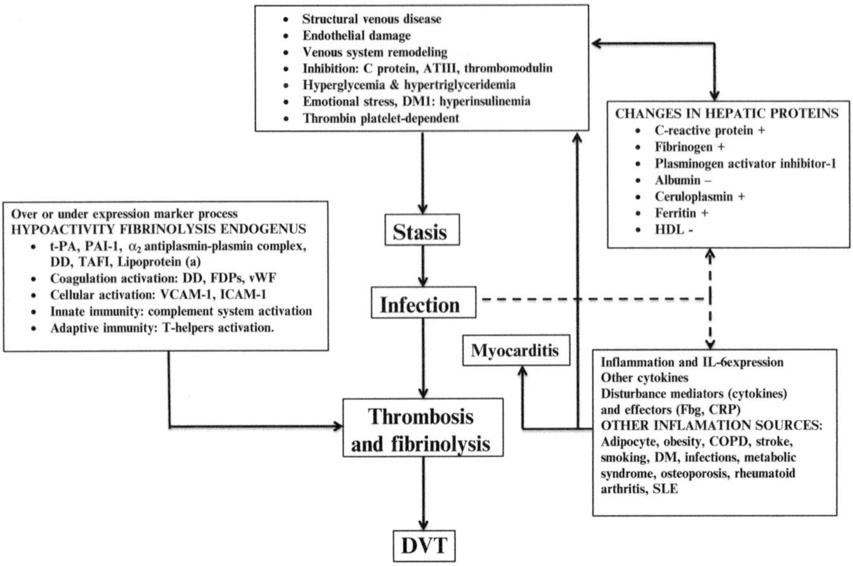

AT= antithrombin III; Fbg= fibrinogen; DM1=diabetes mellitus type 1; CRP= C-reactive protein; PAI-1= plasminogen activator inhibitor-1; t-PA= tissue plasminogen activator; DD= D-dimer; TAFI= thrombin-activable fibrinolysis inhibitor; FDPs= fibrin degradation products; vWF= von Willebrand factor; VCAM-1= vascular cell adhesión protein-1; ICAM-1= intracellular adhesión molecule-1 . Modified from: Jerjes-Sanchez C. Pulmonary Embolism from Molecular Basis to Clinical Practice. Nova Biomedical, 2012

Fig. 1.1 Considering molecular and clinical evidences, complex mechanisms of venous thrombosis are shown. In a high proportion of venous thromboembolism cases, disease starts with structural venous disease, endothelial damage and venous vessel remodeling. Other mechanisms related with hypoactivity of endogenous fibrinolysis, as well as, molecular and clinical inflammation risk factors have important roles. Interleukin-6 overexpression induce inhibition of natural anticoagulant proteins. Emotional stress could induce hyperglycemia and right and left endomyocarditis related with endocardial thrombi. In the middle of this figure, stasis and infection emerge as important triggers for venous thromboembolism

These results could be the first evidence describing the presence of inflammatory cells in the heart of patients who died secondary PE under pathologic and histologic detail. Although the exact mechanism or mechanisms related with right and left ventricular myocarditis/endocarditis is not clear, catecholamine theory could be an explanation, since the infiltrate morphologically could fit with catecholamine myocarditis, so local and/or systemic production of catecholamine, related to the stress of PE, could secondarily result in catecholamine-induced myocarditis. Although endomyocarditis and intracavitary thrombi in the left and right ventricle of PE patients were identified, an open question remains: are these inflammatory changes a cause or consequence.

Because all evidence that we have thrombus is the result of complex mechanisms intimately linked. Figure 1.1 shows all mechanism with active participation in the thrombus process, including inflammation, endogenous fibrinolysis, as well as other important mechanisms.

Molecular Mechanisms of Venous Thrombosis

Currently, with the combination of improved models of VTE and high-resolution microscopy techniques, new evidence linking molecular, cellular mechanisms, platelets and innate immune cells with venous thrombosis have been identified [49].

Historically, the genesis of the thrombus in the venous valvular sinuses has been attributed to stasis and vortices of blood. It is possible that stasis would prevent the efflux and clearance of activated clotting factors from the sinus, which would be sufficient to initiate thrombosis. Stasis is also associated with exaggerated hypoxemia in experimental models [50, 51]. Thrombosis triggered by this systemic hypoxemia is mediated by TF induction in macrophages following activation of the transcription factor early growth response-1 gene. This transcription factor with hypoxia inducible factor-1 is also an important transcription factor mediating adaptive responses to hypoxia in endothelium; in-vitro, these responses include proinflammatory and pro-adhesive changes [49].

New experimental evidence and recent morphologic study of the pro-/anticoagulant phenotype of endothelial cells support this hypothesis. When endothelial cells were exposed to severe hypoxemia in vivo a thrombus-resistant phenotype was observed. This observation suggests that vascular endothelial cells adapt to local hypoxemia in a manner that helps to maintain blood in a fluid, anticoagulated state during health. However, the molecular and cellular events by which impaired venous blood flow evolves into thrombogenesis still require elucidation [49].

Currently, genetic studies identified thrombosis-associated single nucleotide polymorphisms (SNPs) within the human genome. Although very weak VTE predictors in isolated form, in combinations (of five SNPs or more), they may have clinical relevance in the predictive value for VTE. The contribution of individual SNPs in the pathophysiologic mechanism and in the risk of venous thrombosis is unknown [52].

Recently, the participation of innate immune cells insights into the pathogenesis of venous thrombosis has been identified. Additionally; new evidences suggested that systemic inflammatory disorders have a close link with VTE. In addition, acute venous thrombosis is frequently related with clinical symptoms and signs of acute inflammation. The neutrophil extracellular traps (NETs) were described in the year 2012 [53]. These molecules are composed by DNA, histones, and antimicrobial proteins (such as elastase), and are released as a defensive mechanism by activated neutrophils in response to pathogens.

This process is known as NETosis and complements other defensive mechanisms (phagocytosis, production of oxidants, and cytotoxic granule proteins and peptides). NETs trap microbes in their adhesive web-like scaffold, where they are killed by locally concentrated antimicrobial effector molecules [55]. In experimental models it has been observed that TF expressed by circulating monocytes and monocyte-derived microparticles can trigger coagulation during pathological thrombosis [1, 54]. In spite of the current availability of methods for measuring microparticle tissue factor in human blood models, its role in VTE remains unknown [56].

More recently, NETs have been shown to be a second mechanism whereby innate inflammatory cells can activate coagulation in the pathogenesis of venous thrombosis. In experimental models inducing thrombosis by partial occlusion/stenosis of the inferior vena cava, the release of endothelial von Willebrand factor leads to platelets recruitment. P-selectin expression on activated endothelium and platelets then mediates the recruitment and binding of neutrophils. Finally, NETs released by these cells as a result of platelet-induced NETosis promote further platelet as well as, red cell binding and thrombin generation [49].

Recently experimental models show that activated platelets release polyphosphates providing a cofactor for activation of factor XI by thrombin and factor XII-deficient mice appear to be protected from both arterial and venous thrombosis. These studies establish a close link between innate immune cells and in the development of venous thrombosis. In addition the function of neutrophils and monocytes in the mechanisms of venous thrombosis could be different from their participation in the later resolution phase, the success of which may determine whether post thrombotic syndrome develops or not.

In spite of all molecular advances that we have, several issues and questions remain open. Which is the role of erythrocytes, merely generation via activation of factor XII in thrombus propagation? Is depletion of platelets or neutrophils, or the genetic absence of P-selectin, protective against the development of thrombosis? In addition, it is possible that in the future the traditional experimental models including chemical or physical injury in the vessel wall (e.g., application of ferric chloride or laser), complete ligation of the inferior vena cava, or in the case of PE, systemic injection of a procoagulant such as tissue factor or collagen, will be replaced? [49]

References

1. Furie F, Furie BC. Mechanisms of thrombus formation. N Engl J Med. 2008;359:938–49.
2. Steffel J, Braunwald E. Novel oral anticoagulants: focus on stroke prevention and treatment of venous thrombo-embolism. Eur Heart J. 2011;32:1968–76.
3. Kroce K, Libby P. Intertwining of thrombosis and inflammation in atherosclerosis. Curr Opin Hematol. 2007;14:55–61.
4. Kaski JC, Arrebola-Moreno AL. Inflammation and thrombosis in atrial fibrillation. Rev Esp Cardiol. 2011;64:551–3.
5. Inoue T, Croce K, Morooka T, Sakuma M, Node K, Simon DI. Vascular inflammation and repair. J Am Coll Cardiol Intv. 2011;4:1057–66.
6. Smeeth L, Cook C, Thomas S, Hall AJ, Hubbard R, Vallance P. Risk of deep vein thrombosis and pulmonary embolism after acute infection in a community setting. Lancet. 2006;367:1075–9.
7. Jerjes-Sanchez C. Venous and arterial thrombosis. A continuum spectrum of the same disease? Eur Heart J. 2005;26:1–2.
8. Prandoni P, Bilora F, Marchiori A, Bernardi E, Peitrobeli F, Lensing AWA, Prins MH, Girolami A. An association between atherosclerosis and venous thrombosis. N Engl J Med. 2003;348: 1435–41.
9. Becattini C, Agnelli G, Prandoni P, Silingardi M, Salvi R, Taliani MR, Poggio R, de Imberti D, Ageno W, Pogliani E, Porro F, Casazza F. A prospective study on cardiovascular events after acute pulmonary embolism. Eur Heart J. 2005;26:77–83.

10. Libby P, Crea F. Clinical implications of inflammation for cardiovascular primary prevention. Eur Heart J. 2010;31:777–83.
11. Libby P, Ridker PM, Hansson GK, for the Leducq Transatlantic Network on Atherothrombosis. Inflammation in atherosclerosis: from pathophysiology to practice. J Am Coll Cardiol. 2009;54:2129–38.
12. Glynn RJ, Danielson E, Fonseca FA, Genest J, Gotto Jr AM, Kastelein JJ, Koenig W, Libby P, Lorenzatti AJ, Mac Fadyen JG, Nordestgaard BG, Shepherd J, Willerson JT, Ridker PM. A randomized trial of rosuvastatin in the prevention of venous thromboembolism. N Engl J Med. 2009;360:1851–61.
13. Piazza G, Goldhaber ZS. Venous thromboembolism and atherotrombosis. An integrated approach. Circulation. 2010;121:2146–50.
14. Goldhaber ZS. Risk factors for venous thromboembolism. J Am Coll Cardiol. 2010; 56:1–7.
15. Ignarro LJ, Buga GM, Wood KS, Byrns RE, Chaudhuri G. Endothelium-derived relaxing factor produced and released from artery and vein is nitric oxide. Proc Natl Acad Sci U S A. 1987;84:9265–9.
16. Palmer RM, Ferrige AG, Moncada S. Nitric oxide release accounts for the biological activity of endothelium-derived relaxing factor. Nature. 1987;327:524–6.
17. Marcus AJ, Broekman MJ, Pinsky DJ. COX inhibitors and thromboregulation. N Engl J Med. 2002;347:1025–6.
18. Lerman A, Zeiher AM. Endothelial function: cardiac events. Circulation. 2005;111:363–8.
19. Gorog DA. Prognostic value of plasma fibrinolysis activation markers in cardiovascular disease. J Am Coll Cardiol. 2010;55:2701–9.
20. Capodanno D, Angiolillo DJ. Antithrombotic therapy in the elderly. J Am Coll Cardiol. 2010;56:1683–92.
21. De Caterina R, Husted S, Wallentin L, Andreotti F, Arnesen H, Bachmann F, Baigent C, Huber K, Jespersen J, Kristensen SD, Lip GYH, Morais J, Rasmussen LH, Siegbahn A, Verheugt FWA, Weitz JI. General mechanisms of anticoagulation and targets of anticoagulants. Thromb Haemost. 2013;109:569–79.
22. Gurbel PA, Tantry US. Antiplatelet and anticoagulant agents in heart failure. J Am Coll Cardiol. 2014;2:1–14.
23. Dubois C, Panicot-Dubois L, Gainor JF, Furie BC, Furie B. Thrombin-initiated platelet activation in vivo is vWF independent during thrombus formation in a laser injury model. J Clin Invest. 2007;117:953–60.
24. Dahlback B. Blood coagulation. Lancet. 2000;355:1627–32.
25. Schreiner PJ, Morrisett JD, Sharrett AR, Patsch W, Tyroler HA, Wu K, Heiss G. Lipoprotein(a) as a risk factor for preclinical atherosclerosis. Arterioscler Thromb. 1993;3:826–33.
26. Sotiriou SN, Orlova VV, Al-Fakhri N, Ihanus E, Economopoulou M, Isermann B, Bdeir K, Nawroth PP, Preissner KT, Gahmberg CG, Koschinsky ML, Chavakis T. Lipoprotein (a) in atherosclerotic plaques recruits inflammatory cells through interaction with Mac-1 integrin. FASEB J. 2006;20:559–61.
27. Gouni-Berthold I, Berthold HK. Lipoprotein (a): current perspectives. Curr Vasc Pharmacol. 2011;9:682–92.
28. Tsimikas S, Witztum JL. The role of oxidized phospholipids in mediating lipoprotein (a) atherogenicity. Curr Opin Lipidol. 2008;19:369–77.
29. Ichikawa T, Unoki H, Sun H, Shimoyamada H, Marcovina S, Shikama H, Watanabe T, Fan J. Lipoprotein (a) promotes smooth muscle cell proliferation and dedifferentiation in atherosclerotic lesions of human apo (a) transgenic rabbits. Am J Pathol. 2002;160:227–36.
30. Scherz N, Labarére J, Aujesky D, Méan M. Elevated admission glucose and mortality in patients with pulmonary embolism. Diabetes Care. 2012;35:25–31.
31. Schermuly RT, Ghofrani HA, Wilkins MR, Grimminger F. Mechanisms of disease: pulmonary arterial hypertension. Nat Rev Cardiol. 2011;8:443–55.
32. Libby P, Simon DI. Inflammation and thrombosis: the clot thickens. Circulation. 2001;103: 1718–20.

33. Liuzzo G, Santamaria M, Biasucci LM, Narducci M, Colafrancesco V, Porto A, Brugaletta S, Pinnelli M, Rizzello V, Maseri A, Crea F. Persistent activation of nuclear factor kappa-ß signaling pathway in patients with unstable angina and elevated levels of C-reactive protein. J Am Coll Cardiol. 2007;49:185–94.
34. Riveiro A, Lindmarker P, Johnson H, Juhlin-Dannfelt A, Jorfeldt L. Pulmonary embolism: one-year follow-up with echocardiography Doppler and five-year survival analysis. Circulation. 1999;99:1325–30.
35. Goldhaber SZ, Visani L, De Rosa M. Acute pulmonary embolism; clinical outcomes in the International Cooperative Pulmonary Embolism Registry (ICOPER). Lancet. 1999;353:1386–9.
36. Jerjes-Sanchez C, Elizalde GJ, Sandoval JZ, Gutierrez-Fajardo P, Seoane DLM, Ramirez-Rivera A, Pulido T, Beltran M, Santos E, Bautista E, Ibarra-Perez C, Arriaga-Nava R. Diagnostico, estratificacion y tratamiento de la tromboembolia pulmonar aguda. Guias y Recomendaciones del Capitulo de Circulacion Pulmonar de la Sociedad Mexicana de Cardiologia. Arch Cardiol Mex. 2004;74 Suppl 3:S547–85.
37. AHA Scientific Statement from American Heart Association. Management of massive and submassive pulmonary embolism, ileofemoral deep venous thrombosis and chronic thromboembolic pulmonary hypertension. Circulation. 2011;123:1788–830.
38. The Task Force on the diagnosis and management of acute pulmonary embolism of the European Cardiology Society. Guidelines on diagnosis and management of acute pulmonary embolism. Eur Heart J. 2008;29:2276–315.
39. Konstantinides S, Geibel A, Heusel G, Heinrich F, Kasper W. Heparin plus alteplase compared with heparin alone in patients with submassive pulmonary embolism. N Engl J Med. 2002;347:1143–50.
40. Meneveau N, Mingb LP, Seronde MF, Mersina N, Schielea F, Caulfield F, Bernard Y, Bassand JP. In-hospital and long-term outcome after sub-massive and massive pulmonary embolism submitted to thrombolytic therapy. Eur Heart J. 2003;24:1447–54.
41. Goldhaber SZ, Come PC, Lee RT, Brauwald LT, Parker JA, Haire WD, Feldstein ML, Miller M, Toltzis R, Smith JL, Taveira de Silva AM, Mogtader A, McDonough TJ. Alteplase versus heparin in acute pulmonary embolism; randomized trial assessing right-ventricular function and pulmonary perfusion. Lancet. 1993;341:507–511.
42. Jerjes-Sanchez C, Villarreal-Umaña S, Ramirez-Rivera A, Garcia-Sosa A, Canseco LM, Archondo T, Reyes E, Garza A, Arriaga R, Castillo F, Jasso O, Garcia H, Bermudez M, Hernández JM, Garcia J, Martinez P, Rangel F, Gutierrez J, Comparan A. Improving adjunctive treatment in pulmonary embolism and fibrinolytic therapy. The role of enoxaparin and weight-adjusted unfractionated heparin. J Thromb Thrombolysis. 2009;27:154–62.
43. Jerjes-Sanchez C, Ramirez-Rivera A, Arriaga-Nava R, Iglesias-Gonzalez S, Gutierrez P, Ibarra-Perez C, Martinez A, Valencia S, Rosado-Buzzo A, Pierzo JA, Rosas E. High-dose and short-term streptokinase infusion in patients with pulmonary embolism. Prospective with seven-year follow-up trial. J Thromb Thrombolysis. 2001;12:237–47.
44. Jerjes-Sanchez C, Ramirez-Rivera A, Garcia ML, Arriaga-Nava R, Valencia-Sanchez S, Rosado-Buzzo A, Pierzo JA, Rosas ME. Streptokinase and heparin versus heparin alone in massive pulmonary embolism: a randomized controlled trial. J Thromb Thrombolysis. 1995;2:67–9.
45. Lualdi JC, Goldhaber SZ. Right ventricular dysfunction after acute pulmonary embolism: pathophysiologic factors, detection, and therapeutic implications. Am Heart J. 1995;130: 1276–82.
46. Begieneman MVP, Van de Goot FRW, Van der Bilt IAC, Vonk Noordegraaf C, Spreeuwenberg MD, Paulus WJ, Van Hinsbergh VWM, Visser FC, Niessen HWM. Pulmonary embolism causes endomyocarditis in the human heart. Heart. 2008;94:450–6.
47. Iwadate K, Tanno K, Doi M, et al. Two cases of right ventricular ischemic injury due to massive pulmonary embolism. Forensic Sci Int. 2001;116:189–95.
48. Iwadate K, Doi M, Tanno K, et al. Right ventricular damage due to pulmonary embolism: examination of the number of infiltrating macrophages. Forensic Sci Int. 2003;134:147–53.

49. Key NS. Bench to bedside: new developments in our understanding of the pathophysiology of thrombosis. J Thromb Thrombolysis. 2013;35:342–5.
50. Hamer JD, Malone PC, Silver IA. The PO_2 in venous valve pockets: its possible bearing on thrombogenesis. Br J Surg. 1981;68:166–70.
51. Lawson CA, Yan SD, Yan SF, Liao H, Zhou YS, Sobel J, Kisiel W, Stern DM, Pinsky DJ. Monocytes and tissue factor promote thrombosis in a murine model of oxygen deprivation. J Clin Invest. 1997;99:1729–38.
52. Reitsma PH, Rosendaal FR. Past and future of genetic research in thrombosis. J Thromb Haemost. 2007;5 Suppl 1:264–9.
53. Kaplan MJ, Radic M. Neutrophil extracellular traps: double-edged swords of innate immunity. J Immunol. 2012;189:2689–95.
54. Manly DA, Boles J, Mackman N. Role of tissue factor in venous thrombosis. Annu Rev Physiol. 2011;73:515–25.
55. Rautou PE, Mackman N. Microvesicles as risk markers for venous thrombosis. Expert Rev Hematol. 2013;6:91–101.
56. Brooks EG, Trotman W, Wadsworth MP, Taatjes DJ, Evans MF, Ittleman FP, Callas PW, Esmon CT, Bovill EG. Valves of the deep venous system: an overlooked risk factor. Blood. 2009;114:1276–9.

Chapter 2
Pharmacokinetics and Pharmacodynamics of Fibrinolytic Agents

Carlos Jerjes-Sánchez and H. David Rodriguez

Cardiovascular diseases are the number one cause of death, globally. Of the estimated 17.3 million people who died from cardiovascular diseases in 2008 (representing 30 % of all global deaths), an estimated 7.3 million were due to coronary heart disease and 6.2 million to stroke [1]. Pulmonary embolism (PE) is the third cause of cardiovascular mortality, and the second cause of death in patients with cancer [2]. The main pathogenetic event of all of these acute vascular syndromes is a thrombotic occlusion, leading to ischemia and, finally irreversible damage to organ target. Appropriate pharmacologic lysis of the thrombus could preserve the function of the organ, improve survival and quality of life. Fibrinolytic drugs have direct action on fibrinolysis system converting plasminogen to the proteolytic enzyme, which lyses the fibrin of blood clots inducing vessel patency and preserving jeopardized organ.

While the efficacy of thrombolytic therapy has been proven in many clinical trials, finding the optimal dose of therapy is important. There is a narrow "therapeutic window" for fibrinolytic-antithrombotic treatment, and the potential for adverse outcomes is high when an incorrect dose is administered. High doses and long-term infusion of fibrinolytic agents have clearly been models for bleeding complications, such as intracranial hemorrhage; high dose and short-infusion by peripheral vein

C. Jerjes-Sánchez, M.D., F.C.C.P., F.A.C.C. (✉)
Sistema Nacional de Investigadores, Nivel II – Clinical Research Director,
Instituto de Cardiologia y Medicina Vascular, TEC Salud

Escuela de Medicina, Tecnológico de Monterrey San Pedro Garza Garcia,
Nuevo León, Mexico

Unidad de Investigacion Clinica en Medicina SC Monterrey, Nuevo León, Mexico
e-mail: jerjes@prodigy.net.mx

H.D. Rodriguez, M.D.
Research Studies Coordinator, Centro de Investigacion Basica y Transferencia,
Hospital Zambrano-Hellion, Escuela de Medicina y Ciencias de la Salud,
Tecnológico de Monterrey, Monterrey, Nuevo León, Mexico

C. Jerjes-Sánchez, *Thrombolysis in Pulmonary Embolism*,
DOI 10.1007/978-3-319-19707-4_2

reduce mortality and improve the outcome in ST-elevation myocardial infarction and PE in well-selected patients. In the setting of thrombolytic therapy, it is crucial that not only the physician administers the correct dose but also that the labeled potency of the drug is accurate and consistent [1].

In addition, thrombus resistance to fibrinolytic agents is an important issue. Current observations in coronary thrombus suggests that "fresh" thrombi structure have a high proportion of platelets, whereas the proportion of fibrin fibers increases over time, as the level of thrombin increases, leading to "older" fibrin-rich thrombi. The typical composition of "old" fibrin-rich thrombi has been found in patients with an ischemic time >3 h and a "fresh" platelet-rich thrombus has been identified in patients in earlier stages of disease, within the first hour following onset of symptoms. These observations could suggest that thrombus resistance depends specifically on fibrin quality [3]. These findings confirm previous experimental results showing that at very early stages of thrombus formation, just after endothelial injury, when the initial thrombus is primarily composed of activated platelets, it is rapidly stabilized by fibrin fibers with a decreasing proportion of platelets over time.

In this chapter the historical development of thrombolytic therapy will be analyzed, as well as the pharmacokinetics and pharmacological properties of the more frequently used fibrinolytic agents in PE patients, namely streptokinase, alteplase, and tenecteplase. Also, the first PE cases using success thrombolysis will be described.

Fibrinolytic System

The structure of this system has a proenzyme, plasminogen, which can be converted to the active enzyme plasmin by the action of several different types of plasminogen activators (Fig. 2.1). Plasmin is a serine protease, which digests fibrin to soluble degradation products. Natural inhibition of this system occurs simultaneously at the level of plasminogen activator and at the level of plasmin as well [4]. Plasminogen is a single-chain glycoprotein consisting of 790 amino acids, which is converted to plasmin by cleavage of the Arg560-Val561 peptide bond. This molecule contains structures, namely lysine-binding sites, which mediate its binding to fibrin and accelerate the interaction between plasmin and its inhibitor α_2-antiplasmin. This structure has a crucial role in the regulation of fibrinolysis. Plasminogen activators are serine proteases with a high specificity for plasminogen, which hydrolyze the Arg560-Val561 peptide bond, yielding the active enzyme plasmin.

Streptokinase

Historical Development

The history of thrombolysis as therapy for a cardiovascular disease induced by thrombosis began in 1933 when Tillet observed that Lancefield group A beta-hemolytic streptococci isolated from patients produced a fibrinolytic substance that

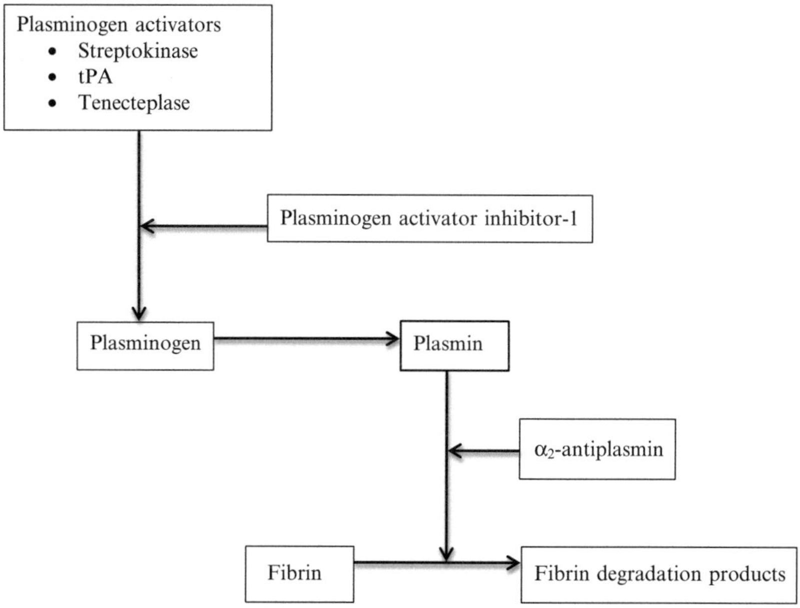

Fig. 2.1 The structure of the fibrinolytic system is shown in this fig. It is possible to observe those plasminogen activators, plasminogen activator inhibitor-1, plasminogen, plasmin, and α_2-antiplasmin role in fibrinogen degradation

Table 2.1 Milestones in historical development of streptokinase

Author and year	Contribution
Tillet (1933)	Streptococcal fibrinolysis
Milestone (1941)	Plasma lysing factor
Christensen (1945)	Plasminogen discovery and streptokinase name
Christensen (1946)	First streptokinase use in a human
Johnson (1952)	Streptokinase lysis experimental venous thrombosis
Sherry (1954)	Two-step reaction with human plasminogen or plasmin
Sherry (1957)	Streptokinase loading dose and prolonged infusion
Johnson (1957)	Streptokinase systemic action
Fletcher (1958)	Streptokinase in ST-elevation myocardial infarction
Browse and James (1964)	First PE patient submitted to successful streptokinase infusion

could be used to dissolve fibrinous exudate (Table 2.1). At this time he did not have biochemical expertise and technology to attempt to isolate and purify the streptococcal fibrinolytic [5].

Eight years later, Milstone observed the necessity of a plasmatic factor for streptococcal-mediated fibrinolysis; this factor was named "plasma lysing factor" [6]. The next advance took place in 1945 when Christensen discovered the mechanism of streptococcal fibrinolysis. His observations showed that plasma contained the precursor of an enzyme system, which he named "plasminogen", while the streptococcal fibrinolysis was renamed as streptokinase. He described an activator in the conversion of plasminogen to the proteolytic and fibrinolytic enzyme, plasmin [7]. Additionally, this researcher observed that plasmin could digest fibrinogen as well as fibrin and that the action of plasmin was buffered by the presence of inhibitors in plasma [8].

In 1946, Christensen provided the first partially purified preparations of streptokinase with the potential for therapeutic use in humans. The clinical model to start the research in humans was hemothorax and empyema, with serial chest X-ray examinations identifying the effect, and sampling of removed fluid for analysis. In 1949, the first in-vivo demonstration of the lysis of clotted human blood was reported in a young man with a loculated hemothorax. Six hour after injecting 400,000 units of streptokinase into the chest [9] (Table 2.1), fluoroscopy revealed the breakdown of all loculations and free mobility of the fluid within the chest. Then, 1300 mL of lysed coagulum were removed and the symptoms and signs of infection disappeared. However, in spite this result, the major interest in the development of streptokinase was for its use in the treatment of ST-elevation myocardial infarction (acute coronary thrombosis) a common medical problem with high in-hospital mortality (≥30 %). Several eminent pathologists in the 1930s had pointed out that the most common cause of ST-elevation myocardial infarction was thrombus superimposed in the surface of atheromatous plaque.

At the beginning of decade of the 50s, Johnson showed that experimental thrombi in rabbit ear veins could be dissolved by the intravenous administration of streptokinase [10]. Soon afterwards, Kline developed a technique, which allowed for a considerable purification of plasminogen [11]. In 1954 the two-step reaction involving streptokinase with human plasminogen or plasmin in the mediation of fibrinolysis was disclosed [12]. This mechanism, is first an immediate and stoichiometric formation of streptokinase-plasminogen or streptokinase-plasmin complex, resulting in the formation of an activator of plasminogen and, second, the kinetic activation of uncomplexed plasminogen to plasmin.

The late 1950s were a very productive period for the development of thrombolytic therapy with streptokinase. An important step was to decide whether to use plasminogen activator like streptokinase or the fibrinolytic enzyme plasmin. Several observations including physiological observations and enzyme specificity, both in-vitro and in-vivo concluded that plasminogen activators would be more successful as thrombolytic agents than the proteolytic enzyme plasmin. A key finding was the demonstration that the primary and most sensitive mechanism for thrombolysis was the activation of the plasminogen, which became bound to fibrin during the clotting process (Fig. 2.2). Additionally, the intravenous infusion of a plasminogen activator like streptokinase would result in two different actions: its diffusion into a thrombus would result in clot lysis, but the streptokinase would also activate plasminogen in the systemic circulation, producing fibrinogenolysis and an impaired hemostatic mechanism.

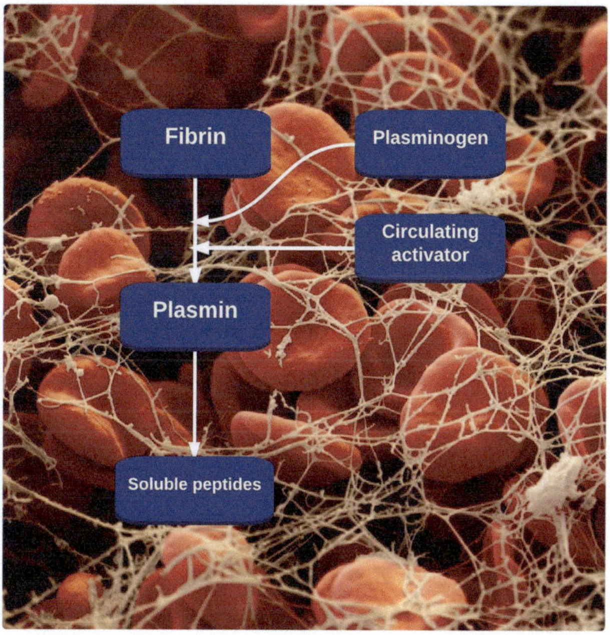

Fig. 2.2 The primary and most sensitive mechanism for thrombolysis is plasminogen activation, which was bound to fibrin during the clotting process

In the meantime, purified preparations of streptokinase were developed. These were well tolerated by patients in the absence of trauma or invasive procedures with few bleeding complications. In 1957, Sherry and colleagues [13] reported the rational approach to thrombolysis with streptokinase, which involved a loading dose and a sustained infusion sufficient to raise the clot-dissolving activity of plasma several hundred fold. Once the plasma plasminogen was exhausted, fibrinogen levels began to rise even though the streptokinase infusion was maintained without changes. The same year, Johnson and colleagues [10] demonstrated a similar system effective in dissolving experimental thrombi in human volunteers. This model included the insertion of a needle into a lower forearm vein with trauma to the intima. Venography showed a thrombus formation which subsequently extended up to the antecubital fossa. An intravenous infusion of streptokinase into the opposite arm mostly resulted in lysis of the clot and the reestablishment of the patency of the vessel.

In 1958, the first study using intravenous streptokinase (30-h infusion) in ST-elevation myocardial infarction was reported [14]. Patients treated within the first 14 h after onset symptoms had a very low in-hospital mortality compared with those treated among 20–72 h. These successful results were reproduced in a three-article series [15–17] and provided the basis for the use of plasminogen activators as thrombolytic agents in cardiovascular and pleural disorders [18].

First PE Patient Submitted to Streptokinase

Browse and James [19], in 1964, published the first cohort of PE patients submitted to thrombolysis with streptokinase. The first case, a 56-year-old man with history of recurrent deep vein thrombosis who was under long-term (9 month) anticoagulation treatment with phenindione and stopped treatment 18 months before of the new acute PE event. A month before admission he had clinical signs of left deep venous thrombosis, breathlessness, and palpitations. Three days before admission breathlessness worsened and he had syncope. When admitted in emergency room with severe chest pain, clinical examination showed respiratory failure, jugular distention, hypotension (80/75 mmHg), and ankle edema. Electrocardiogram had T wave inversion in leads V_1, V_2, and V_3. Clinical diagnosis of PE was established and treatment with heparin, oxygen, and vasopressors was started. On the fourth day, the clinical conditions worsened despite treatment with heparin. On electrocardiogram, right ventricular strain was identified. Streptokinase was given on the fifth, sixth, and seventh days in 8-h intravenous infusion of two mega units each. A maintenance dose about 70,000 units per hour to maintain a reasonably high level of fibrinolytic activity was considered. As adjunctive treatment prednisone 15 mg daily and 10,000 units of heparin was given intravenously between the infusions and during 2 days after treatment. Given the history of recurrent deep venous thrombosis, long-term anticoagulation with phenindione was considered. On the sixth day, blood pressure returned to normal, however the dyspnea was worse and chest pain remained. Twenty-four hours after he has been kept on phenindione, and had good outcome.

This case exemplifies how long-term streptokinase infusion was successful in a massive PE patient. Previous experience in streptokinase development allowed to establish dose and time infusion.

Mechanisms of Action and Challenges of Streptokinase

Streptokinase was the first thrombolytic developed for therapeutic use in the United States, using material purified from culture filtrates of the H46A isolate of Streptococcus equisimilis (Lancefield Group C). All commercial streptokinase currently available for human use is derived from this strain [1]. In the 1960s, European pharmaceutical companies conducted the first clinical trial in humans [20]. At this time, the Committee on Biological Standardization of the World Health Organization identified the need for international standards (IS) for streptokinase potency measurement. Four years later the international unit (IU) for this fibrinolytic was defined as an activity contained in 0.002090 mg of the first IS [1].

Streptokinase is a nonenzyme protein with molecular weight of 47,000 Da produced by β-hemolytic streptococci, which indirectly activates the fibrinolytic system. The drug forms a 1:1 stoichiometric complex with plasminogen which exposes and activates a site in the modified plasminogen moiety, whereby the complex becomes a potent plasminogen activator. The main difference with fibrin-specific fibrinolytics is that streptokinase causes an indirect conformational change in the plasminogen molecule, which then acts as plasmin [1].

Currently, streptokinase remains as the most widely used thrombolytic agent and it is now produced in many developing countries, being an attractive therapeutic option because of its low cost. As a bacterial product, it is immunogenic, which may reduce the effectiveness, and/or cause allergic reactions. Other agents (fibrin-specific) are now generally more used in developed nations. The quality of streptokinase in Europe is maintained and well regulated; however, this could not be the same in developing countries [1] possibly with large discrepancies in activity, purity, and composition. Recently, a wide range of streptokinase products used in India, South Korea, South America, and the Middle East were monitored. The main observation was the poor quality control used to treat ST-elevation myocardial infarction. In this result, deterioration of product during transport was ruled out [21]. Another point to consider is whether patients surviving treatment with suboptimal streptokinase dose will develop antibodies compromising future treatments or poor outcome; this remains as an open question.

Another major source of concern is the standardization of recombinant streptokinase. Several companies are producing recombinant streptokinase engineered in an attempt to reduce immunogenicity, and others are developing new variants of this agent to improve fibrin-specificity. It is known that small changes in the sequence of native streptokinase at the amino and carboxy terminals can significantly impact the activity and fibrin-dependence. Streptokinase in short-dose and long-term peripheral vein infusion have been approved by FDA for the treatment of massive PE patients (Table 2.2). Table shows FDA-approved and non-approved thrombolytic regimens. In the contemporary era, streptokinase in 1,500,000 IU short-term one-hour infusion by peripheral vein was the first regimen that improved in-hospital mortality in severe right ventricular dysfunction PE patients in a controlled-randomized trial [22].

Table 2.2 Thrombolytic regimens

Approved by FDA	
Streptokinase	250,000 IU, bolus in 30 min follow by 100,000 IU/h/24 h
Urokinase	4400 U/kg initial bolus and then 4400 U/kg/12–24 h
Alteplase	100 mg in 2-h infusion
Not approved by FDA	
Urokinase	3,000,000 U in 2-h infusion
Urokinase	15,000 U/kg in 10 min
Streptokinase	1,500,000 IU in 1 or 2-h infusion
Reteplase	10 U double bolus every 30 min
Alteplase	20 mg bolus followed 80 mg in one-hour infusion
Alteplase	50 mg in 1 or 2-h infusion (patients >50 kg)
Tenecteplase	Bolus mg/kg in 5 or 10 s
[a]Ultrasound plus alteplase	17.2–35.1 mg in 14–33.2 h infusion

Modified from Jerjes-Sanchez C, Elizalde GJ, Sandoval ZJ, et al. Arch Cardiol Mex 2004; 74 (supl):S548

[a]Engelberger RP, et al. Eur Heart J 2014; 35:35758

Recombinant Human Tissue-Type Plasminogen Activator

Historical Development

At the beginning of 1947 the first experimental report showing that animal tissues contained an agent—originally named fibrinokinase—that could activate plasminogen was published [23] (Table 2.3). In 1952, Astrup and colleagues [24] obtained a soluble fibrinolytic activator from animal tissues using strong chaotropic agents. Through studies on the human turnover plasminogen performed in the early 70s, it was possible to identify the main physiological plasmin inhibitor: α_2-antiplasmin [25]. In the same decade, the experimental studies of Reich and colleagues [26] revealed that malignant tumors frequently secrete plasminogen activator activity and that their malignancy correlated with the level of malignant protease secreted.

Shortly after that, it was demonstrated that the protease activity could be inhibited by plasma α_2-antiplasmin. The intention was to develop low-molecular weight inhibitor bases on the reactive site sequence of α_2-antiplasmin. The kinetics of inhibition of malignant plasminogen activators source was reviewed and, totally serendipitously, some conditioned culture medium of a melanoma cell line was obtained in 1975, proving to be an excellent source of the *malignant* plasminogen activator. The initial culture medium was developed and 3 years later the cell line was obtained [26]. In 1979, Collen and colleagues observed that the activator, unlike urokinase, had a specific affinity for fibrin.

Many studies have reported the purification and characterization of plasminogen activators from various sources (pig heart and ovaries, human postmortem vascular perfusates, and post exercise blood); in 1979, the first highly purified form of recombinant human tissue-type plasminogen activator (rt-PA) was obtained from uterine tissue [27]. Using an antiserum raised against uterine plasminogen activator, it was

Table 2.3 Milestones in historical development of tissue-type plasminogen activator

Author and year	Contribution
Astrup (1947)	An agent that induces activation of plasminogen was observed: fibrinokinase
Astrup (1952)	Discovery and identification of α_2-antiplasmin
Reich (1970)	Plasminogen discovery and streptokinase name
Reich (1970)	Malignant tumors secrete plasminogen activator activity
Collen (1975)	Malignant plasminogen activator
Collen (1978)	Plasminogen activator obtained from cell line
Collen (1979)	Purify plasminogen activator from melanoma cell culture fluid
Rijken (1979)	Method for purification of plasminogen activator from human uterus
Matsuo (1981)	Effective thrombolysis in experimental model
Bergman (1983)	Selective coronary thrombolysis in dogs
Van de Werf (1984)	Coronary thrombolysis in ST-elevation myocardial infarction
Bounameaux (1985)	First angiographic massive PE patient under recombinant tissue-type plasminogen activator

shown that rt-PA, vascular plasminogen activator and blood plasminogen activator were immunologically identical, but different from urokinase-plasminogen activator [28]. Thus, it was clear that the rt-PA found in blood represents vascular tissue-type plasminogen activator that is released mainly from endothelial cells.

At the end of 1979, professor Rijken developed (Table 2.3) a method for the purification of rt-PA from human uterus. With a simplified version of this procedure was possible to purify melanoma cell culture fluid plasminogen activator, being immunologically identical to the uterine plasminogen activator [29]. This observation clarified the kinetics of plasminogen activation and allowed the development of immunoassays for tissue-type plasminogen activator in plasma [30, 31]. Subsequently, the purification procedure was scaled upward to produce a total amount of approximately 2 g of rt-PA in plasma, sufficient for initial experimental animal and human studies [32].

In 1981, the efficacy of rt-PA was proved in rabbits with jugular thrombosis and PE [33]. In 1983, after isolation and purification of human rt-PA from a Bowes-melanoma—tissue-culture a successful intravenous infusion in dogs with coronary thrombus was published [34]. One year later, Van de Werf showed that coronary and systemic thrombolysis was prompt and occurred without marked depletion of circulating fibrinogen or plasminogen; additionally, the accumulation of fibrinogen degradation products or consumption of circulating α_2-antiplasmin was considered as indicative of a systemic lytic state in seven ST-elevation myocardial infarction patients [35].

First PE Patient Submitted to Recombinant Human Tissue-Type Plasminogen Activator

In 1985, Bounameaux and colleagues [36] published the first successful case with rt-PA in a 63-year-old man with angiographically proved massive PE, hospitalized one-hour after sudden onset of severe dyspnea; patient had a history of renal transplant 5 weeks before onset PE symptoms. On admission, he was cyanotic, polypneic, with blood pressure 145/90 mmHg and heart rate 117/min., and without signs of deep venous thrombosis. Arterial blood gases showed severe hypoxia and hypocapnia. Electrocardiogram was normal, chest X-ray showed atelectasis of the upper lobe of right lung and sequelae of tuberculosis and pulmonary angiography with massive bilateral obstruction of the main pulmonary artery. Non-fractionated heparin infusion was started at the dosage of 30,000 IU/24 h.

rt-PA infusion was started 8 h after onset symptoms through a catheter in right ventricle at a dose of 0.5 mg/kg body weight in 90 min until completing 30 mg. Thirty minutes later patient clinically improved with a progressive increase in arterial PO_2. Pulmonary angiography 24 h after the infusion showed almost complete recanalization of the branch to the right inferior lobe. Patient has transient atrial flutter successfully treated with digital on the second day after thrombolysis. No bleeding events, neither further complication occurred.

The first report of successful thrombolysis using rt-PA confirmed the efficacy of this agent in the setting of angiographic massive PE. Although the infusion was driven by direct catheter in right ventricle, previous clinical experience in ST-elevation myocardial infarction patients was considered. Additionally, this case exemplifies the usefulness of an rt-PA reduced dose as a therapeutic approach in pulmonary artery thrombus.

Mechanisms of Action of Recombinant Human Tissue-Type Plasminogen Activator

This activator is a serine protease in which His 322, Asp 371, and Ser 478 constitute the active site residues; rt-PA is blocked by the active site serine inhibitors diisopropylfluorophosphate (DFP) [37, 38] and chloromethyl ketones, which inhibit the active site histidine. Although Tos-Lys-CH_2Cl (TLCK) weakly inhibits rt-PA, D-Phe-Pro-Arg-CH_2Cl is relatively a strong rt-PA inhibitor [39]. Both one-chain rt-PA and two-chain rt-PA react with DFP. A useful, commercially available tripeptide substrate is H-D-Ile-Pro-Arg-pNA; which is, however, not specific for rt-PA but sensitive to a broad spectrum of serine proteases. Two-chain rt-PA is more active towards low-molecular-weight-substrates [40].

Recombinant human tissue-type plasminogen activator has a specific affinity for fibrin [41]. When rt-PA is present during formation of fibrin clots of increasing density, half-maximal binding occurred at approximately 0–14 g per 1 (0.4 μM) [42]. Experiments on plasminogen activation in the presence of varying amounts of fibrin suggest a dissociation constant of 0.14 μM [30]. Detailed binding studies, however are still lacking, as is the localization of the binding sites, both in the fibrin molecule and in rt-PA.

Recombinant human tissue-type plasminogen activator is a poor enzyme in the absence of fibrin, but fibrin strikingly enhances the activation rate of plasminogen [43, 44]. This has been explained by an increased affinity of fibrin-bound rt-PA for plasminogen without significantly influencing the catalytic efficiency of the enzyme [30]. The kinetic data of Hoylaerts et al. [30] support a mechanism in which rt-PA and plasminogen adsorb to a fibrin clot in a sequential and ordered way, yielding a ternary complex. Fibrin essentially increases the local plasminogen concentration by creating an additional interaction between rt-PA and its substrate. The high affinity of rt-PA for plasminogen in the presence of fibrin thus allows efficient activation on the fibrin clot, although no efficient plasminogen activation by rt-PA occurs in plasma. In another kinetic study Randby [45] observed significantly increased turnover in the presence of fibrin.

Recombinant human tissue-type plasminogen activator-mediated plasminogen activation is also potentiated by fibrin monomer and by cyanogen bromide (CNBr)-digested fibrinogen [46], suggesting that the polymeric fibrin structure is not a prerequisite for the stimulation. It has been reported that the potentiating activity of CNBr-digested fibrinogen resides in the CNBr fragment FCB-2 (Hol-DSK) and more particularly in the fragment consisting of residues 148–207 of the α chain [47]. Stimulation of the activation of plasminogen by rt-PA has also been reported in the presence of denatured proteins, such as fibrinogen, IgG, and ovalbumin [48, 49], and it has been speculated that the ability of rt-PA to recognize misfolded proteins indicates a role in selective catabolism of damaged protein, in general, not solely fibrin clots [48].

A remarkable difference in K_M values in the presence of fibrin was found in two studies from the same laboratory. Hoylaerts et al. [30], using an assay system in which fibrin could be degraded during the experiment, found a K_M of 0.16 μM, whereas Rijken et al. [42], using a system in which lysis of fibrin was inhibited by an excess of aprotinin, found a K_M of 1.1 μM. The difference may be explained by recent results of Suenson et al. [49], who disclosed a strong plasminogen-binding site upon initial fibrin degradation. A K_M value of 1.1 μM [42], close to the physiological plasminogen concentration in plasma, may indicate a regulatory role for histidine-rich glycoprotein, which interacts with plasminogen and thus influences the free plasminogen concentration [50].

Recombinant human tissue-type plasminogen activator occurs either as a one-chain molecule or as a proteolytically degraded two-chain molecule. In contrast to analogous enzyme system, single-chain rt-PA is, however, not an inactive precursor but an active enzyme. Although the single-chain form is less active towards low-molecular-weight-substrates and inhibitors [40], the two forms are almost equally active towards plasminogen [42, 45].

Functional domains responsible for the fibrin-binding and for the catalytic activity of rt-PA have been localized in the rt-PA molecule [51, 52]. Holvoet et al. [51] partially reduced two-chain rt-PA and separated the A chain and the B chain by immune adsorption on monoclonal antibodies reacting with the fibrin-binding site and with the active center of the enzyme, respectively. The purified B chain activated plasminogen following Michaelis-Menten kinetics, with kinetic constants similar to those of intact rt-PA, but fibrin did not stimulate the activation of plasminogen by the B chain. The purified A chain bound to fibrin with an affinity similar to that of intact rt-PA but did not activate plasminogen.

Mechanism of Fibrin-Specific Thrombolysis of Tissue-Type Plasminogen Activator

Plasmin, the proteolytic enzyme of the fibrinolytic system, is a serine protease with relatively low substrate specificity. In purified systems, it will degrade fibrinogen as well as fibrin. When plasmin circulates freely in the blood, it will degrade a number of plasma proteins, including fibrinogen and the blood coagulation factors V and VIII.

Plasma does, however, contain a fast-acting plasmin inhibitor, α_2-antiplasmin, which reacts extremely fast with plasmin [53]. Thus small amounts of plasmin formed in the blood will be inhibited with a $t_{1/2}$ of 0.01 s. The rapidity of this reaction, however, is dependent on the availability of structures in the plasmin molecule called lysine-binding sites and on the availability of a free active site in the enzyme. Plasmin generated on the fibrin surface has both lysine-binding sites and active site occupied and is therefore only slowly inactivated by α_2-antiplasmin. Plasmin generated in the circulating blood will rapidly be neutralized by α_2-antiplasmin, circulating free plasmin activity, and a systemic fibrinolytic state, characterized by degradation of fibrinogen and the blood coagulation factors V and VIII [4]. Clot-specific thrombolysis will have interactions outlined above, that require plasminogen activation at or near the fibrin clot.

The most promising approach to obtaining specific thrombolysis is the use of thrombolytic agents that are stimulated by the presence of fibrin. Indeed, streptokinase and urokinase, which have no specific affinity for the fibrin, activate circulating and fibrin-bound plasminogen in a relatively indiscriminate way. Plasmin formed in the circulation is immediately neutralized by α_2-antiplasmin and, once the inhibitor is exhausted, several plasma proteins are degraded by plasmin (fibrinogen, factors V and VIII, etc.), thereby causing a bleeding tendency. The clot specificity that rt-PA exert in a plasma environment appears to occur via different mechanisms; rt-PA is relatively inactive in the absence of fibrin, but fibrin strikingly enhances the activation rate of plasminogen by rt-PA [30]. This is explained by an increased affinity of fibrin-bound rt-PA for plasminogen and not by alteration of the catalytic efficiency of the enzyme. The high affinity of rt-PA for plasminogen in the presence of fibrin thus allows efficient activation on the fibrin clot without significantly plasminogen activation by rt-PA occurring in plasma.

Based on previous molecular interactions and evidence, the most promising approach to obtain specific thrombolysis seems to be the use of fibrin-specific agents.

Searching for the Ideal Thrombolytic

Thrombolysis has been a major milestone in the management of acute myocardial infarction. In developed countries, first-, second-, and third-generation thrombolytic drugs have proven to reduce mortality and improve the outcome by restoring patency in the infarct-related vessel preserving jeopardized myocardial area [54]. This therapeutic approach prolongs survival and in-hospital outcome in high-risk (troponin expression and right ventricular wall motion abnormalities) PE well-selected patients [55].

However, the available thrombolytic agents have several limitations that could result in less than optimal outcomes, as the risk for systemic and intracranial hemorrhage. Another key issue is their rapid clearance, requiring rt-PA and streptokinase to be administered by continuous peripheral intravenous infusion. In order to decrease these drawbacks in new thrombolytic drugs, specifically mutants of rt-PA have been developed. The main targets for modification have included half-life, fibrin specificity, resistance to plasminogen activator inhibitor-1 and antigenicity. Modification in these factors could offer important clinical benefits [54].

Regarding ST-elevation myocardial infarction patients, 100 % TIMI grade 3 flow reperfusion, it is mandatory. In terms of high-risk PE patients, the main target of thrombolytic therapy is to induce efficient thrombus lysis to reduce pulmonary arterial hypertension leading to the improvement of right ventricular dysfunction to avoid extensive ischemia and right ventricular myocardial infarction [55]. A prolonged half-life permits a single-bolus dosing reducing in-hospital costs and health personnel care.

Enhanced fibrin specificity allows preferential activation of fibrin-bound plasminogen and the clot surface, increasing potency and speed patency. Higher fibrin specificity could limit activation of circulating plasminogen and degradation of fibrinogen. This attribute allows the reduction in the risk of bleeding complications [54]. Considering that rt-PA is inhibited by plasminogen activator inhibitor-1, greater resistance to this inhibitor could promote a more effective thrombolysis. Avoiding deleterious effect on blood pressure improves the quality of patient care. A non-antigenic thrombolytic drug permits repeat administration as rescue thrombolysis or re-thrombolysis. Additionally the ideal agent has to be less procoagulant, a paradoxical effect of several current thrombolytic agents [54].

Tenecteplase-Tissue-Type Plasminogen Activator

Historical Development

In 1987, FDA approved rt-PA (alteplase) for clinical use in ST-elevation myocardial infarction patients [56]; after an elegant randomized controlled trial conducted by Goldhaber, rt-PA was approved in PE [57]. Both conditions had been considered as a landmark in the clinical development of rt-PA. Tenecteplase-tissue-type plasminogen activator (TNK-t-PA) is a novel fibrinolytic protein bioengineered from rt-PA, alteplase for the therapy of ST-elevation myocardial infarction patients. Specific mutations at three sites in the alteplase molecule improved pharmacokinetics and pharmacodynamics properties of TNK-t-PA [56], known worldwide as TNK according to the acronym of the molecular modifications of this fibrinolytic (Table 2.4). Since TNK-t-PA growing is supported by preclinical and clinical rt-PA studies, its historical development is less extensive than streptokinase and rt-PA, alteplase.

Table 2.4 Searching for the ideal thrombolytic

– Intravenous bolus
– No antigenicity
– No effect on blood pressure
– Low incidence of systemic bleeding
– Low incidence of intracranial hemorrhage
– High fibrin specificity
– Rapid thrombolysis and reperfusion
– Low reocclusion and recurrence rate
– Resistant to plasminogen activator inhibitor-1

Modified from Van de Werf FJ. Eur Heart J 1999; 20:1452–1458

TNK-t-PA a faster and more potent form of rt-PA was identified in 1994 [58]. One year later, TNK-t-PA administration produced higher thrombolytic potency against accelerated alteplase in animal models of acute arterial occlusion [4, 59]. In 1997, the pharmacokinetics of TNK-t-PA were elucidated in ST-elevation myocardial infarction patients. The TIMI 10A phase I study included 82 patients randomized to receive 5–50 mg compared with Neuhaus's (90 min) dosing regimen [4, 60]. In 1998, TNK-t-PA established a possible superiority compared with alteplase [4, 61], without significant cost in terms of fibrin-binding or biological activity against fibrin-rich clots. In the same year, De Marco et al. [4, 62] proved that this agent did not induce paradoxical procoagulant effect, one of the most important limitations of thrombolytic agents. Two hours after its infusion, thrombin–antithrombin complex (marker of thrombin generation) determination had same values compared with the controls. In the phase II TIMI 10B in 886 patients under treatment with 30 or 50 mg of TNK-t-PA vs. accelerated alteplase 100 mg resulted in a trend to higher TIMI III flow at 60 min with 40 mg of TNK-t-PA as opposed with alteplase [4, 63] (Table 2.6).

The First PE Patient Submitted to Tenecteplase-Tissue-Type Plasminogen Activator

In 2002 year Caldicott et al. [64] published the first case with TNK-t-PA use in a massive PE patient. A 72-year-old man with previous hypertension and diabetes arrived to emergency department after a collapse episode. Three days ago, had right-sided pleuritic chest pain and severe shortness of breath. On clinical examination he was plethoric and diaphoretic, with tachycardia 118/min, his blood pressure 80/50 mmHg, with respiratory rate 28/min and oxygen saturation of 95 % despite treatment with 10 L/min of oxygen by mask.

Clinical auscultation of lungs and heart was unremarkable. Right lower leg was 3 cm larger in diameter than the left. Arterial blood gases analysis showed pO_2 142.5 mmHg, pCO_2 30.2 mmHg and HCO_3 of 16.7. An electrocardiogram showed sinus tachycardia, anterolateral ST depression, as well as, SI, QIII, TII pattern. Chest X-ray was unremarkable. Ultrasound scan revealed a full thrombus occluding inferior vena cava. A clinical diagnosis of pulmonary embolus was established and bolus of 5000 IU of unfractionated heparin and intravenous infusion was started. CT scan showed massive bilateral pulmonary emboli with right upper, middle, and lower zones of pulmonary infarctions. Thrombolysis with weight-adjusted bolus dose of 45 mg of TNK-t-PA was given. Clinical improvement occurred in 30 min (pulse rate 103/min, respiratory rate 28/min and oxygen saturation 100 % while receiving 10 L/min on mask). Subsequent ultrasonography examination proved a right leg deep vein thrombosis. Patient was discharged on warfarin 6 days after admission without any complications, including systemic or intracranial hemorrhages.

This massive PE patient was successfully treated with intravenous weight-adjusted bolus of TNK-t-PA; the choice of thrombolytic agent was based on pharmacokinetic and pharmacodynamic characteristics and a previous success catheter-directed TNK-t-PA experience in massive PE patient [65]. Data of this case suggest that dose-range used in ST-elevation myocardial patients could be an attractive therapeutic option in PE.

Mechanism of Action of Tenecteplase-Tissue-Type Plasminogen Activator

Extensive basic research leads to specific molecular changes to improve therapeutic performance in alteplase. At the beginning, the modification was directed only to single amino acids or to deletion of entire protein domains. These mutations induced a reduction of plasma clearance against impaired fibrinolytic activity or fibrin specificity [56]. In consequence, a high resolution functional analysis of the alteplase protein sequence to reduce these limitations was done and TNK-t-PA molecule was developed. This third-generation thrombolytic agent is a single-chain glycoprotein with 527 amino acids, 17 disulfide bridges, and 65 kDa molecular mass. It is produced by recombinant DNA technology in Chinese hamster ovary cells.

Properties of native alteplase were modified in three molecular sites. Table 2.4 shows designation and amino acid substitution. Designation T adds a new glycosylation site on kringle-1, which decreases the rate of clearance but decreases fibrin-binding as well; in designation N, the effect removes the existing glycosylation site on kringle-1, which decreases the rate of clearance and restores fibrin-binding in combination with Thr-103 asparagine; finally, designation K increases fibrin specificity and makes the molecule more resistant to the naturally occurring inhibitor plasminogen activator inhibitor-1 [56].

TNK-t-PA shows two classes of glycoforms, namely, type I and type II; the first has three carbohydrate structures at asparagine residues 103, 184, and 448. Type II lacks the carbohydrates at asparagine. The carbohydrates are all complex oligosaccharides without no-high mannose structure. This characteristic in TNK-t-PA avoids fast clearance induced by the hepatic mannose receptor detected for alteplase [66].

Plasminogen activator inhibitor-1, present in high concentrations in platelet-rich thrombus has an important role in non-successful thrombolysis and recurrence. TNK-t-PA was modified to reduce its interaction with plasminogen activator inhibitor-1, obtaining greater fibrinolytic efficacy, as was confirmed in vivo through experimental models. The fibrin specificity of tenecteplase, expressed as the ratio of its catalytic activity in the presence of fibrin as compared to fibrinogen, was 15-fold higher than for alteplase [56]. Additionally, in animal models TNK-t-PA causes less peripheral bleeding compared with alteplase [59].

In terms of pharmacokinetic methods include plasma assays, preclinical efficacy, clot-selectivity measures, data analysis, distribution, biotransformation and elimination (animal studies), and mechanisms of hepatic elimination, TNK-t-PA has been extensively analyzed [56]. Careful clinical pharmacokinetics and pharmacodynamics studies were done, considering that this agent is given as a single dose in an intensive care patient setting, and considering that patients with ST-elevation acute myocardial infarction could have fluctuations in cardiac output and hepatic blood flow increasing intraindividual pharmacokinetic variability [56].

No pharmacokinetic studies were performed with TNK-t-PA in healthy volunteers because of ethical concerns arising from its increased fibrinolytic potency and longer half-life [56]. The clinical pharmacokinetics was studied in 179 ST-elevation myocardial infarction patients. Additionally, comparative data with alteplase were obtained in 53 patients. Two large pharmacokinetic substudies were integrated into the TIMI 10A phase I dose-ranging clinical trial and the TIMI 10B phase II angiographic clinical trial. No pharmacokinetic data were obtained in the phase II safety trial (ASSENT-1) and in the large phase III trial (ASSENT-2), to avoid compromising the clinical objectives of these trials [56]. After approval of the drug, clinical trials have been designed to study TNK-t-PA combined with a low-molecular-weight heparin, enoxaparin or IIb/IIa glycoprotein inhibitor, abciximab in ASSENT-3 study; any pharmacokinetics data has been obtained [56].

In the previously mentioned phase I TIMI 10A trial ST-elevation myocardial infarction patients receive a single-bolus of TNK-t-PA (ranging 5–50 mg). The time courses of the mean immunoreactive TNK-t-PA plasma concentrations were compared with the plasma concentration curve for 100 mg rt-PA (alteplase) in 90 min (accelerated dosing regimen). The estimated peak TNK-t-PA plasma concentrations increased in a dose-dependent fashion. After administration of the bolus injection, the elimination of TNK-t-PA from plasma exhibited a biphasic pattern: the initial phase had a mean half-life ranging from 41 ± 16 to 138 ± 84 min. Across all doses, the mean clearance of TNK-t-PA from plasma was 151 mL/min (range of 216 ± 98 mL/min at the 5 mg dose to 125 ± 25 mL/min at the 50 mg dose), with mean residence time in the body of approximately 1 h. Compared with the data reported for alteplase, the plasma clearance of tenecteplase was approximately two- to four-fold slower [60], suggesting that TNK-t-PA offers important clinical benefits.

Regarding efficacy and safety of TNK-t-PA profile, TIMI-10A trial revealed that at 90 min, a TIMI grade 3 flow was achieved in 59 % and 64 % of patients receiving 30 and 50 mg dose, respectively. In terms of systematic fibrinogen and plasminogen levels (decreased 3 % and 13 % respectively) at 1 h after TNK-t-PA administration, minimal activation of the fibrinolytic system was identified. In terms of safety, among 113 patients enrolled, 6 % had major hemorrhage, 5 % at the vascular access site, and one after bypass surgery. No intracranial hemorrhage or stroke was observed. Mortality at 30 days was 4 % and reinfarction rate 4 %. No antibodies to tenecteplase were evident in any patients at 30 days follow-up. However, the sample size was small to reach statistical significance [54, 60].

In this study TNK-t-PA clearance was not affected by concomitant use of nitrates and beta-blockers. Previously in experimental models, no effect of either aspirin or heparin on the pharmacokinetics of this agent was observed. The substantially reduced hepatic clearance of TNK-T-PA reduces the likelihood for impact by drugs that alter hepatic blood flow. Antibodies were detected in only 1 patient after treatment at 30 days [56].

In TIMI-10B, a phase II security trial, 886 patients were randomized to receive 30 or 50 mg of TNK-t-PA or rt-PA, alteplase 100 mg in 90 min. Due to the increase of bleeding complications, 50 mg dose was early replaced by a 40 mg dose. In terms of coronary reperfusion, similar TIMI grade 3 flow rates (63 %) were achieved at 90 min with 40 mg single-bolus dose of TNK-t-PA compared with accelerated regimen of rt-PA, alteplase. A trend toward a higher rate of TIMI grade 3 flow was evident at 60 min with the 40 mg dose of tenecteplase against alteplase (55 % vs. 48 %). When the patency of vessels was analyzed, a trend toward more rapid reperfusion with 40 mg dose of tenecteplase compared with accelerated rt-PA alteplase was shown [54, 63]. Additionally, antibodies were detected in only 1 out of 364 patients at 30 days after administration; no antibodies were detected in this patient at 90 days. Considering these findings in both, TIMI-10A and TIMI-10B trials, TNK-t-PA is in essence non-antigenic after single administration, and antibody formation can be excluded as a source of pharmacokinetic or pharmacodynamic variability [56].

In TIMI-10B trial patients with intracranial hemorrhage showed high activated partial thromboplastin time levels. For this observation heparin dose was reduced in light-weight patients. A 5000 IU heparin bolus and an initial 1000 U/h infusion was administered to patients who weighed >67 kg, while a 4000 IU bolus plus 800 IU/h infusion was given to those who weighed <67 kg. After this heparin dose modification, the rate of intracranial hemorrhage in all patients decreased significantly, with similar patency rates at 90 min to those in the initial cohorts [54, 63].

ASSENT-1 and ASSENT-II were phase II safety and phase III megatrial, respectively. In ASSENT-1 the rate of intracranial hemorrhage was lower (0.62 %) when a reduced heparin dose combined with 40 mg dose of TNK-t-PA was used. In this study, TIMI grade 3 flow was analyzed by dose: weight ratio. A weight-adjusted dose of 0.50–0.55 mg^{-kg} showed optimal reperfusion and its use was selected in further phase III clinical trial [54]. The phase III ASSENT-2 trial enrolled 16,949 patients randomized to single-bolus TNK-t-PA or accelerated rt-PA, alteplase. In terms of mortality both agents had similar clinical equivalence (6.2 %) at 30 days follow-up. Intracranial hemorrhage rates were also similar; however, in the group of TNK-t-PA, female and older patients had a trend towards fewer cerebral bleedings. Significantly fewer non-cerebral bleedings were noted with TNK-t-PA [54].

The fibrinolytic agent TNK-t-PA is a clear example of the power of rational drug development applied to therapeutic proteins. Through a high resolution structural analysis of the physiological t-PA molecule and combined specific mutagenesis at three sites, a new fibrinolytic drug was developed with better biological properties [56]. Table 2.6 summarizes the main pharmacologic and pharmacokinetic characteristics of the first-, second- and third fibrinolytic agents used in well-selected PE patients. TNK-t-PA is close to be considered as "ideal" (Table 2.5) fibrinolytic agent. TNK-t-PA has been improved in terms of immunogenicity, half-life, fibrin specificity, plasminogen activation, activation of fibrinogen linked to plasminogen, limited activity of fibrinogen and plasminogen; as well as resistance of plasminogen activator inhibitor-1, paradoxical procoagulant effect and no depletion of α_2-antiplasmin compared with streptokinase and alteplase (Table 2.7).

Table 2.5 Molecular modifications in TNK-tissue-plasminogen-activator

Designation	Amino acid substitution
T	Threonine-103 → Asparagine
N	Asparagine-117 → Glycosylation
K	Lysine–His–Arginine–Arginine (296–299) → Alanine–Alanine–Alanine–Alanine

Modified from Tanswell P. Clin Pharmacokinet 2002; 41:1229–1245

Table 2.6 Milestones in historical development of tenecteplase-tissue-type plasminogen activator

Author and year	Contribution
Keit (1994)	Fast and powerful tissue-type plasminogen activator
Benedict (1995)	12-fold greater thrombolytic potency
Cannon (1997)	Pharmacokinetics in ST-elevation myocardial patients vs. alteplase
Modi (1998)	Prolonged half-life, higher fibrin specificity, and resistance to plasminogen activator inhibitor-1
DeMarco (1998)	Does not produce paradoxical procoagulant effect
Cannon (1998)	A trend to better TIMI III flow in ST-elevation myocardial patients vs. accelerated alteplase
Caldicott (2012)	First case of massive pulmonary embolism successfully treated

Table 2.7 Main characteristics of current thrombolytic agents used in pulmonary embolism

Characteristic	Streptokinase	Alteplase	TNK-t-PA
Origin	Streptococcus BH	Recombinant DNA	Recombinant DNA
Molecular weight (Da)	47,000	70,000	70,000
Immunogenicity	Yes	No	No
Plasma half-life (min)	18	4–8	20–25
Fibrin specificity	No	++	+++
Plasminogen activation	Indirect	Direct	Direct
Activation Fbg linked Plg	No	++	+++
Limited activity Fbg and Plg	No	++	+++
PAI-1 resistance	No	No	Yes
Paradoxical procoagulant effect	+++	++	+
No depletion α_2-antiplasmin	+++	++	+
Bolus	No	10–20 mg	Single
Regimen	1,500,000 IU	90 a 80 mg	Weight adjusted
Infusion	2 h/60 min	2 h/1 h	No

Modified from Van de Werf FJ. Eur Heart J 1999; 20:1452–1458
TNK tenecteplase, *Fbg* fibrinogen, *Plg* plasminogen

References

1. Thelwell C. Biological standards for potency assignment to fibrinolytic agents used in thrombolytic therapy. Semin Thromb Hemost. 2014;40:205–13.
2. Furie F, Furie BC. Mechanisms of thrombus formation. N Engl J Med. 2008;359:938–49.
3. Silvain J, Collet JP, Nagaswami C, Beygui F, Edmondson KE, Bellemain-Appaix A, Cayla G, Pena A, Brugier D, Barthelemy O, Montalescot G, Weisel JW. Composition of coronary thrombus in acute myocardial infarction. J Am Coll Cardiol. 2011;57:1359–67.
4. Collen D. On the regulation and control of the fibrinolysis. Thromb Haemost. 1980;43:77–89.
5. Tillet WS, Garner RL. The fibrinolytic activity of hemolytic streptococci. J Exp Med. 1933;58:485–502.
6. Milstone H. A factor in normal human blood which participates in streptococcal fibrinolysis. J Immunol. 1941;42:109–16.

7. Christensen LR. Streptococcal fibrinolysis: a proteolytic reaction due to a serum enzyme activated by streptococcal fibrinolysis. J Gen Physiol. 1945;28:363–83.
8. Christensen LR, MacCleod CM. A proteolytic enzyme of serum: characterization, activation and reaction with inhibitors. J Gen Physiol. 1945;28:559–83.
9. Tillet WS, Sherry S. The effect of streptococcal fibrinolysis (streptokinase) and streptococcal deoxyribonuclease on fibrinous, purulent and sanguinous pleural exudation. J Clin Invest. 1949;28:173–90.
10. Johnson AJ, McCarthy WR. The lysis of artificially induced clots in man by intravenous of streptokinase. J Clin Invest. 1957;38:1627–43.
11. Kline DL. Purification and crystallization of plasminogen (profibrinolysin). J Biol Chem. 1953;2404:949–55.
12. Sherry S. The fibrinolytic activity of streptokinase activated human plasmin. J Clin Invest. 1954;35:1054–63.
13. Sherry S, Fletcher AP, Alkjaersig N, Smyrniotis FE. An approach of intravascular fibrinolysis in the man. Trans Assoc Am Physicians. 1957;70:288–96.
14. Fletcher AP, Alkjaersig N, Smyrniotis FE, Sherry S. The treatment of patients suffering from early myocardial infarction with massive and prolonged streptokinase therapy. Trans Assoc Am Physicians. 1958;71:287–96.
15. Fletcher AP, Alkjaersig N, Sherry S. The maintenance of a sustained thrombolytic state in man. I. Induction and effects. J Clin Invest. 1959;38:1096–110.
16. Fletcher AP, Sherry S, Alkjaersig N, Smyrniotis FE, Jick S. Clinical observations on patients with myocardial infarction and other thromboembolic disorders. J Clin Invest. 1959;38:1111–9.
17. Bett JHN, Castaldi PA, Hale GS, Ibist JP, Mclean KH, O´Sullivan EF, Biggs JC, Chesterman CN, Hirsh J, Mcdonald IG, Morgan JJ, Rosembaum M. Australian multicenter trial of streptokinase in acute myocardial infarction. Med J Aust. 1977;1:553–60.
18. Jerjes-Sanchez C, Ramirez-Rivera A, Elizalde GJ, Delgado R, Cicero R, Ibarra-Perez C, Arroliga AC, Padua A, Portales A, Villarreal A, Perez-Romo A. Intrapleural fibrinolysis with streptokinase as an adjunctive treatment in hemothorax and empyema. A multicenter trial. Chest. 1996;109:1514–9.
19. Browse NL, James DCO. Streptokinase in pulmonary embolism. Lancet. 1964;2:1039–43.
20. Sikri N, Bardia A. A history of streptokinase use in acute myocardial infarction. Tex Heart Inst J. 2007;34:318–27.
21. Longstaf C, Thelwell C, Whitton C. The poor quality of streptokinase products in use in developing countries. Thromb Haemost. 2005;3:1092–3.
22. Jerjes-Sanchez C, Ramirez-Rivera A, Garcia ML, Arriaga-Nava R, Valencia-Sanchez S, Rosado-Buzzo A, Pierzo JA, Rosas ME. Streptokinase and heparin versus heparin alone in massive pulmonary embolism: a randomized controlled trial. J Thromb Thrombolysis. 1995;2:67–9.
23. Astrup T, Permim PM. Fibrinolysis in the animal organism. Nature. 1947;159:681–2.
24. Astrup T, Stage A. Isolation of a soluble fibrinolytic activator from animal tissue. Nature. 1952;170:929.
25. Collen D. Identification and some properties of a new fast-reacting plasmin inhibitor in human plasma. Eur J Biochem. 1976;69:209–16.
26. Collen D, Lijnen HR. History of discovery: the tissue-type plasminogen activator story. Arterioscler Thromb Vasc Biol. 2009;29:1151–5.
27. Rijken DC, Wijngaards G, Zaal-de Jong M, Welbergen J. Purification and partial characterization of plasminogen activator from human uterine tissue. Biochim Biophys Acta. 1979;580:140–53.
28. Rijken DC, Wijngaards G, Welbergen J. Relationship between tissue plasminogen activator and the activators in blood and vascular wall. Thromb Res. 1980;18:815–30.
29. Rijken DC, Collen D. Purification and characterization of the plasminogen activator secreted by human melanoma cells in culture. J Biol Chem. 1981;256:7035–41.

30. Hoylaerts M, Rijken DC, Lijnen HR, Collen D. Kinetics of the activation of plasminogen by human tissue plasminogen activator. Role of fibrin. J Biol Chem. 1982;257:2912–9.
31. Rijken DC, Juhan-Vague I, De Cock F, Collen D. Measurement of human tissue-type plasminogen activator by a two-site immunoradiometric assay. J Lab Clin Med. 1983;101: 274–84.
32. Collen D, Rijken DC, Van Damme J, Billiau A. Purification of human extrinsic (tissue-type) plasminogen activator in centigram quantities from a human melanoma cell culture fluid and its conditioning for use in vivo. Thromb Haemost. 1982;48:294–6.
33. Matsuo O, Rijiken DC, Collen D. Thrombolysis by human tissue plasminogen activator and urokinase in rabbits with experimental pulmonary embolism. Nature. 1981;291:590.
34. Bergman SR, Fox KAA, Ter-Pogossian MM, Sobel BE, Collen D. Clot-selective coronary thrombolysis with tissue-type plasminogen activator. Science. 1983;220:1181.1183.
35. Van de Werf F, Ludbrook PA, Bergmann SR, Tiefenbrunn AJ, Fox KAA, DeGeest H, Verstraete M, Collen D, Sobel BE. Coronary thrombolysis with tissue-type plasminogen activator in patients with evolving myocardial infarction. N Engl J Med. 1984;310:609–13.
36. Bounameaux H, Vermylen H, Collen D. Thrombolytic treatment with recombinant tissue-type recombinant activator in a patient with massive pulmonary embolism. Ann Intern Med. 1985;103:64–5.
37. Binder BR, Spragg J, Austen KF. Purification and characterization of human vascular plasminogen activator derived from blood vessels perfusates. J Biol Chem. 1979;254:1998–2003.
38. Korninger C, Collen D. Neutralization extrinsic (tissue-type) plasminogen activator in human plasma: no evidence for a specific inhibitor. Thromb Haemost. 1981;46:662–5.
39. Ranby M, Bergsdorf N, Nilsson T. Enzymatic properties of one-chain and two-chain forms of tissue plasminogen activator. Thromb Res. 1982;27:175–83.
40. Ranby M, Bergsdorf N, Pohl G, Wallen P. Isolation of two variants of native one-chain tissue plasminogen activator. FEBS Lett. 1982;146:289–92.
41. Thorsen S, Glas-Greenwalt P, Astrup T. Differences in the binding of fibrin to urokinase and tissue plasminogen activator. Thromb Diath Haemorrh. 1972;28:65–74.
42. Rijken DC, Hoylaerts M, Collen D. Fibrinolytic properties of one-chain and two-chain human extrinsic (tissue-type) plasminogen activator. J Biol Chem. 1982;257:2920–5.
43. Camiolo SM, Thorsen D, Astrup T. Fibrinogenolysis and fibrinolysis with tissue plasminogen activator, urokinase, streptokinase-activated human globulin, and plasmin. Proc Soc Exp Biol Med. 1971;138:277–80.
44. Wallen P. Thrombosis and urokinase. In: Paoletti R, Sherry S, editors. Activation of plasminogen with urokinase and tissue activator. London: Academic; 1977. p. 91–102.
45. Ranby M. Studies on the kinetics of plasminogen activation by tissue plasminogen activator. Biochim Biophys Acta. 1982;704:461–9.
46. Nieuwenhuizen W, Verheijen JH, Vermond A, Chang GTG. Plasminogen activation by tissue activator is accelerated in the presence of fibrin(ogen) cyanogen bromide fragment FCB-2. Biochim Biophys Acta. 1983;775:531–3.
47. Nieuwenhuizen W, Vermond A, Voskuilen M, Traas DW. Identification of the site in fibrin(ogen) which is involved in the acceleration of plasminogen activation by tissue-type plasminogen activator. Biochim Biophys Acta. 1983;748:86–92.
48. Radcliffe R, Heinze T. Stimulation of tissue plasminogen activator by denatured proteins and fibrin clot: a possible additional role for plasminogen activator. Arch Biochem Biophys. 1981;211:750–61.
49. Suenson E, Lützen O, Thorsen S. Initial plasmin-degradation of fibrin as the basis of a positive feedback mechanism in fibrinolysis. Eur J Biochem. 1984;140:513–22.
50. Lijnen HR, Hoylaerts M, Collen D. Isolation and characterization of human plasma protein with affinity for the lysine-binding site of plasminogen. Role in the regulation of fibrinolysis and identification as histine-rich glycoprotein. J Biol Chem. 1980;255:10214–22.
51. Holvoet P, Lijnen HR, Collen D. Characterization of functional domains in human tissue-type plasminogen activator with the use of monoclonal antibodies. Eur J Biochem. 1986;158: 173–7.

52. Rijken DC, Groeneveld E. Isolation and functional characterization of the heavy and light chains of human tissue-type plasminogen activator. J Biol Chem. 1986;261:3098–102.
53. Wiman B, Collen D. On the kinetics of the reaction between human antiplasmin and plasmin. Eur J Biochem. 1978;84:573–8.
54. Van de Werf FJ. The ideal fibrinolytic: can drug design improve clinical results? Eur Heart J. 1999;20:1452–8.
55. Jerjes-Sánchez C, Gutiérrez-Fajardo P, Ramírez-Rivera A, García ML, Hernández CHG. Acute right ventricular myocardial infarction secondary to massive pulmonary embolism. Arch Inst Cardiol Mex. 1995;65:65–73.
56. Tanswell P, Modi N, Combs D, Danays T. Pharmacokinetics and pharmacodynamics of tenecteplase in fibrinolytic therapy for acute myocardial infarction. Clin Pharmacokinet. 2002;41:1229–45.
57. Goldhaber SZ, Come PC, Lee RT, Brauwald LT, Parker JA, Haire WD, Feldstein ML, Miller M, Toltzis R, Smith JL, de Silva AM T, Mogtader A, McDonough TJ. Alteplase versus heparin in acute pulmonary embolism; randomized trial assessing right-ventricular function and pulmonary perfusion. Lancet. 1993;341:507–11.
58. Keyt B, Paoni NF, Refino CJ, et al. A faster-acting and more potent form of tissue plasminogen activator. Proc Natl Acad Sci U S A. 1994;91:3670–4.
59. Benedict CR, Refino CJ, Keyt BA, et al. New variant of human tissue plasminogen activator (TPA) with enhanced efficacy and lower incidence of bleeding compared with recombinant human TAP. Circulation. 1995;92:3032–40.
60. Cannon CP, McCabe CH, Gibson CM, et al. and the TIMI 10A Investigators. TNK-tissue plasminogen activator in acute myocardial infarction. Results of the Thrombolysis in Myocardial infarction. Results of the Thrombolysis in Myocardial Infarction (TIMI) 10A Dose-Rangin Trial. Circulation 1997;95:351–6.
61. Modi NB, Eppler S, Breed J, Cannon CP, Braunwald E, Love TW. Pharmacokinetics of a slower clearing tissue plasminogen activator variant, TNK-tPA, in patients with acute myocardial infarction. Thromb Haemost. 1998;79:134–9.
62. DeMarco E, Rebuzzi AG, Quaranta G, et al. Lack of procoagulant effect after TNK-plasminogen activator in patients with acute myocardial infarction. Eur Heart J. 1998;19 (Abstr Suppl):563.
63. Cannon CP, Gibson CM, McCabe CH, et al. TNK-tissue plasminogen activator compared with front-loaded alteplase in acute myocardial infarction. Results of the TIMI 10B trial. Circulation. 1998;98:2805–14.
64. Caldicott D, Parasivam S, Harding J, Edwards N, Bochner F. Tenecteplase for massive pulmonary embolus. Resuscitation. 2002;55:2011–3.
65. Sze DY, Carey MBL, Razavi MK. Treatment of massive pulmonary embolus with catheter-directed tenecteplase. J Vasc Interv Radiol. 2001;12:1456–7.
66. Noorman F, Rijken DC. Regulation of tissue-type plasminogen activator concentrations by clearance via the mannose receptor and other receptors. Fibrinol Proteol. 1997;11:173–86.

Chapter 3
Thrombolytic Therapy: Evidence-Based Results from Multicenter Control Trials

Carlos Jerjes-Sánchez and Alicia Ramirez-Rivera

Pulmonary embolism (PE) is the third most frequent cardiovascular cause of death after myocardial infarction and stroke, and the second cause of mortality in cancer patients. PE is a major cause of mortality and morbidity and hospitalization in Europe, affecting all medical disciplines including pediatric patients. In addition it has an exponential growing in elderly populations, so we are expecting a larger number of patients diagnosed and dying in the next years [1]. Thrombolysis accelerates the dissolution of central thrombi in the pulmonary circulation and it is potentially lifesaving. Despite these potential benefits related with rapid clot lysis, also nonpathologic thrombi are lysed, so thrombolysis could induce serious bleeding complications [2].

Thrombolysis has been available as treatment for acute PE patients in the last 44 years. In spite of decades of clinical research, current recommendations are based on a limited number of randomized control trials. All of them, consistently showed that pharmacologic thrombolysis effectively resolves thromboembolism obstruction and promptly reduces resistances and pulmonary artery pressure increasing cardiac output in PE patients [3]. Currently, there are no head-to-head trials among thrombolytic agent in terms of superiority and efficacy or safety; all randomized control trials generally compared thrombolysis against anticoagulation alone [4]; at the beginning recombinant human urokinase, streptokinase and recombinant human

C. Jerjes-Sánchez, M.D., F.C.C.P., F.A.C.C. (✉)
Sistema Nacional de Investigadores, Nivel II – Clinical Research Director,
Instituto de Cardiologia y Medicina Vascular, TEC Salud

Escuela de Medicina, Tecnológico de Monterrey San Pedro Garza Garcia,
Nuevo León, Mexico

Unidad de Investigacion Clinica en Medicina SC Monterrey, Nuevo León, Mexico
e-mail: jerjes@prodigy.net.mx

A. Ramirez-Rivera, M.D., F.C.C.P.
Head Pulmonary Physiology Department, Hospital de Cardiologia No 34,
Instituto Mexicano del Seguro Social, Monterey, Nuevo Leon, Mexico
e-mail: aliramirez@prodigy.com.mx

C. Jerjes-Sánchez, *Thrombolysis in Pulmonary Embolism*,
DOI 10.1007/978-3-319-19707-4_3

Table 3.1 Randomized control trials in thrombolysis and PE

Years	Author	Number of patients
1970–2000	UPETSG (1970)	160
	Tibbutt et al. (1974)	30
	Ly et al. (1978)	25
	Marini et al. (1988)	30
	Levine et al. (1990)	58
	PIOPED (1990)	13
	Dalla-Volta et al. (1992)	36
	Goldhaber et al. (1993)	101
	Jerjes-Sanchez et al. (1995)	8
Studies	Nine	461
2000–2014	MAPET-3 (2002)	256
	TIPES (2010)	58
	Fasullo et al. (2011)	72
	MOPETT (2012)	121
	ULTIMA (2013)	59
	PEITHO (2014)	1005
	TOPCOAT (2014)	83
Studies	Seven	1654
1970–2014	16 studies	2115

tissue plasminogen activator (rt-PA), alteplase were the best studied thrombolytic agents. Currently a third-generation thrombolytic agent, tenecteplase-tissue-type plasminogen activator (TNK-t-PA) is under intensive clinical research.

Streptokinase is less expensive, but it is frequently associated with collateral effects as allergic reactions and hypotension. In the modern era, alteplase has been approved for FDA in 2-h infusion regimen; additionally, TNK-t-PA, a new agent proved in ST-elevation myocardial infarction, has not been approved for use in PE, but has been extensibly studied. The main randomized control trials in the last 40 years are shown in Table 3.1. From 1970 to 2014 sixteen studies including 2115 PE patients have been conducted. Randomized control trials could be included in two periods, from 1970 to 2000 and from 2000 to 2014. The evidence coming for these randomized control trials support thrombolysis treatment in well-selected PE patients. Through these data, guidelines have been written, modified and new one has been published in the last decade [2].

Randomized Controlled Trials from 1970 to 2000 Years: Urokinase Pulmonary Embolism Trial Phase 1 (UPET)

Background

At the end of the decade of 60s, thrombolytic agents had a significant development and were considered as important therapeutic options. Two plasminogen activators, streptokinase and urokinase were considered therapeutically effective. Streptokinase was under extensive clinical experience in patients with thromboembolic disorders. Pyrogenicity of the early streptokinase preparations led to the searching a non-antigenic and nontoxic plasminogen activator, a research promoted by National Heart and Lung Institute in 1964. Urokinase meanwhile, had been identified as a promising agent with high specific activity, free from thromboplastic contamination and adventitious virus and nontoxic and nonpyrogenic reactions in animals. Additionally, the dissolution of de novo intravascular human thromboembolism founded the path for clinical trials [5].

Acute PE was considered as an ideal clinical entity for the initial evaluations of thrombolytic agents for several reasons: (a) it is a common and important disease; (b) objective methods for diagnosis and course of thrombus in pulmonary arterial circulation were available; (c) these methods allow evaluation of the thrombolytic agent effect on thrombus; (d) in PE, a fresh thrombus consisting mainly of fibrin and red blood cells is lodged in normal pulmonary vessels perfused by a large blood flow. This feature could allow thrombus dissolution by thrombolytic agents [3]. Several preliminary clinical observations established in 1966 that urokinase induced an active fibrinolytic state well tolerated even in critically ill patients. Additionally, the evidence suggested that thrombolysis dissolved thrombus from the pulmonary circulation restoring normal hemodynamics [5].

Methodology

UPET, a controlled, multi-institutional study, had as primary target to determine whether PE abnormalities, produced by obstructive thrombus, and measured by V/Q lung scan, pulmonary angiography, and pulmonary hemodynamic, would return toward normal more rapidly with a urokinase regimen when compared to heparin alone [5].

Two independent analysis panels for pulmonary angiography and V/Q lung scans reviewed data. Pre-infusion and post-infusion blood samples included fibrinogen, plasminogen, bilirubin, and various enzyme levels. Pulmonary angiography was the basis for inclusion. The minimal angiographic eligibility criterion was occlusion of at least one segmental artery [5].

Patients were considered in: Class 1, without shock at the time of inclusion; Class 2 with persistent shock; Subclass S, with submassive embolism (i.e., less than the equivalent of two lobar arteries with significant filling defects or completely obstructed); subclass M included massive PE patients (i.e., obstructions or significant filling defects present in two or more lobar arteries or the equivalent).

Lung scans with anterior and posterior views were also required in all patients except in those in shock; here the lung scan was optional, in order not to delay therapy and not to decrease the accession of critically ill patients into the trial. Right heart catheterization with pressure measurements was performed immediately before angiography. Fick cardiac output measurements were also made except when patients were receiving oxygen therapy. A well-documented clinical episode suggesting that PE had occurred within 5 days of the institution of therapy was necessary for patient eligibility. Patients with recent operations or with the usual contraindications for the use of anticoagulant or thrombolytic therapy were excluded from the trial [5].

After randomization, 12 h intravenous infusion of urokinase or heparin was started. Patients in urokinase group received a loading dose of 2000 CTA units/lb of body weight followed by 2000 CTA units/lb/h; patients in heparin group had a loading dose of 75 units of heparin/lb of body weight followed by 10 U/lb/h. After infusion, all patients received heparin intravenously for 5 days at least, followed by oral anticoagulation. Heparin was given in to obtain Lee-White clotting time to 30–45 min within 1 h before the next dose. In the follow-up right heart catheterization, V/Q lung scan and pulmonary arteriography were performed [5].

Recurrence was considered if both lung scan and clinical evidence data were obtained. An episode was considered probable if either lung scan evidence or characteristic clinical signs were present. Bleeding complications were classified as: moderate, defined as an estimate of blood loss of 500–1500 mL with an associated hematocrit reading fall of 5–10 points or a blood transfusion of 2 units or less, or severe, defined as one in which any of these limits was exceeded [5].

Results

From October 1968 to August 1970, 160 patients were included; 78 in heparin group and 82 in urokinase group. Regarding demographic characteristics the balance between treatment groups was appropriate. However, patients in urokinase group tended to be younger and with more severe thrombosis. Both factors could be associated with treatment response. To adjust for these imbalances, all data on response to treatment were adjusted by the direct method for imbalances in age and baseline severity [5].

Dyspnea, pleuritic pain, apprehension, and cough, as well as, tachycardia, rales, an increased pulmonary component of the second heart sound, and gallop rhythm were the most common symptoms and physical findings. Peripheral thrombophlebitis was present in only one-third of patients upon entry into the trial. Most patients did not have persistent shock, for only 5 patients given heparin and 9 patients given urokinase were in the class 2 category. The class 1 patients, 73 in each treatment group, had equally distribution between the submassive and massive embolism subclasses [5].

The most common causes for exclusion were normal V/Q lung scan and pulmonary arteriography which did not satisfy diagnostic criteria for the study. A minority of patients were excluded secondary of contraindications to thrombolytic agent. Patients in heparin group did not have any significant change in plasminogen and fibrinogen compared to those in urokinase group in whose a significative fall in both biomarkers was observed [5].

Regarding pulmonary arteriography, the baseline averages for the heparin- and urokinase-treated patients corresponded closely to an average severity class of "moderate." With heparin, a small improvement in the arteriograms occurred; this amounted to 0.68 on the seven-point scale, lying between "no improvement" and "minimal improvement." With urokinase, the mean improvement was larger, amounting to 1.56, positioned halfway between "minimal" and "moderate" improvement. The difference in mean change between urokinase and heparin-treated groups was 0.88 grades with a standard error of only 0.17. The critical ratio, i.e., the difference in mean change divided by the standard error, was 5.2, highly significant. While arteriographic improvement after urokinase was only occasionally dramatic, distinct improvement did occur much more frequently after urokinase than after heparin infusion [5].

Only 5 of 57 (9 %) in the heparin group showed "moderate" or greater improvement, while among the urokinase patients 30 of 57 (53 %) showed this improvement. It is of some interest that in no case for patients in either group did an arteriogram worsen sufficiently for a shift to a higher severity class. In patients receiving urokinase, baseline angiography severity appeared to influence treatment response, showing greater improvement patients with more severe baseline findings. Patients given heparin gave no evidence of this trend [5].

Complete hemodynamic measurements were obtained in 71 % and pressures alone in 92 % of patients. Elevated right ventricular systolic pressure (>25 mmHg) and low arterial oxygen tension (PO_2) (<90 mmHg), present in 96 % and 94 %, respectively, were the most common baseline hemodynamic abnormalities. The baseline mean right ventricular systolic pressure of 45 mmHg was moderately high but only 15 % of patients had a baseline value greater than 60 mmHg. The mean 24-h changes were significantly better for urokinase group than for heparin-treated patient [5].

Concerning V/Q lung scans, the baseline mean defect in both groups was 25 % which corresponds to a perfusion defect of one half of one lung. The first day heparin group improved 8.1 % and urokinase group 22.1 %. The greatest effect of urokinase on the lung scans appeared within the first 24 h. It interesting to note that 1-year follow-up lung scan data were available in 59 patients without any evidence of the effect of urokinase [5].

Patients in urokinase group had better response when they were younger (<50 years) and embolus age was <48 h. In addition, patients with PE and cardiogenic shock had greater response [5].

In terms of non-antigenic and nontoxic effects, urokinase was a safe plasminogen activator. The most common complication was overt bleeding or an unexplained fall in hematocrit reading. Some bleedings were expected since patients were under venous cutdowns, arterial punction, and venipunctures. Twenty-one or 27 % of the heparin group and 37 or 45 % of the urokinase group were classified as having a moderate or severe bleeding complication at some time during the 2-week period of hospitalization. The main difference between the two groups was related to severe bleeding complications. Patients receiving urokinase suffer twice as frequently from such episodes as those receiving heparin. The increase in bleeding attributed to urokinase occurred in the first 24 h coinciding with urokinase infusion [5].

Urokinase patients showed no evidence of increased bleeding after the first 24 h. Unexplained hematocrit falls occurred in 26 % of patients given heparin and in 24 % of patients given urokinase. These hematocrit drops usually occurred in the first few days of therapy, were rarely severe, and did not necessitate transfusion. Bleeding from venous cutdowns site for the pulmonary arteriogram catheter was much more troublesome than from arterial sites. Extensive dissection necessary to perform venous cutdowns in obese arms was the most common predisposing factor. Spontaneous bleeding occurred with nearly equal incidence in both treatment groups. In urokinase group one patient with 1-month history of stroke had intracerebral bleeding. The protocol was modified to exclude patients with this characteristics. One patient with chronic alcoholism, died of hemorrhage from multiple gastric stress ulcers approximately 12-h after the completion of the urokinase infusion. This patient had several baseline hemostatic abnormalities including a prothrombin time twice the control [5].

Recurrence of PE occurred in 19 % in heparin group and 15 % in urokinase group in the first 2 weeks. While these episodes were usually well tolerated by the patient, one was fatal for a patient who had received urokinase 10 days earlier. The class-2-M patients (massive PE patients in shock) had a 2-week case fatality rate of 18 %. The surprisingly low mortality in this subgroup emphasizes an interesting observation in which most massive PE, even those desperately ill, had a high rate of spontaneous improvement. On the other hand, all three of the class 2-S patients (submassive embolism in shock) died within the 2-week follow-up period. Each of these latter patients was critically ill prior to pulmonary embolization and this most likely explains the mortality and the fact that these patients with submassive PE presented in shock [5].

The results of this study showed: angiography evidence of clot lysis, reversion toward normal of the hemodynamic abnormalities, and pulmonary capillary perfusion scanning, were significantly different in favor of urokinase treatment. In addition, established that urokinase is capable of dissolving thromboembolism at least in part and that such dissolution is associated with an improvement in the physiological abnormalities created by the occlusive lesion. Pulmonary angiography was the earliest and most consistent indicator of pulmonary reperfusion [5].

This study concluded that pharmacological thrombolysis therapy may well become the preferred treatment for patients in shock with massive embolism, especially for those with borderline cardiac reserve, as surgical embolectomy in this group is associated with a very high mortality. During the study 11 patients underwent pulmonary embolectomy had an operative mortality of 73 %. The complete evaluation of the therapeutic benefit of thrombolysis therapy in PE will be difficult. This trial established that urokinase significantly improved quantitative measurements of cardiopulmonary dysfunction, but the invasive procedures for necessity-enhanced bleeding risk. Furthermore, an attempt to demonstrate a significant improvement in mortality with urokinase in PE would have required limiting the study to a large number of class 2-M, high-risk patients, who are relatively rare (note that only 7 % of patients were in this category) or conducting a trial studying all patients with PE, in addition a sample 20–40 times the size of the study.

Lessons Learned from This Study

In spite of theses results several unmet answers remained: establishing the thrombolytic effects of urokinase, this trial incorporated only one treatment regimen. While clot resolution was unequivocal, nevertheless it was not dramatic in terms of lysis of the entire pulmonary occlusion and, presumably, of resolution of the original venous thrombosis, remembering that recurrent PE was not uncommon. Under these circumstances a reasonable question is whether longer regimens of urokinase therapy can more readily achieve maximum pulmonary and venous thrombolysis without further increasing the risk of hemorrhage. Urokinase proved clot-lysing capacity but, as with all potent drugs, it can be dangerous if used outside strictly prescribed limits. Clearly, further evaluation was required before it can be recommended as a proven clinical pharmaceutical [5].

Streptokinase and Heparin Alone in Treatment of Life-Threatening Pulmonary Embolism

Background

Pulmonary embolism is very common cardiovascular disease, in the acute phase patients have two possibilities: recover spontaneously or die before treatment can be given. Several previous reports suggesting that streptokinase is superior to heparin. However, these studies were uncontrolled. The necessity to assess the role of streptokinase in a comparative randomized control in this situation was mandatory. This report included 30 patients with life-threatening PE allocated at random to streptokinase plus heparin or heparin alone [6].

Methodology

Any patient presenting with clinical symptoms and signs of acute or progressive life-threatening PE was considered for inclusion. Patients were excluded at the discretion of the physician in charge if they had: recent surgery, gastrointestinal disease, malignant hypertension, a recent cerebrovascular episode, pregnancy, or recent delivery. In all patients 12-lead electrocardiogram, chest X-ray, full blood count, plasma thrombin clotting time, fibrinogen, serum glutamic oxaloacetic and glutamic pyruvate transaminase, lactic dehydrogenase, and bilirubin was performed [6].

Assessment of the severity of the thrombus and progress after treatment were based mainly on information gained from pulmonary angiography. Hemodynamic measurements were right atrial, right ventricular, and pulmonary arterial phasic and mean pressure; additionally oxygen difference, arterial oxygen saturation, cardiac index calculated by Fick principle from measurement or assumed, oxygen consumption, total pulmonary resistance and brachial arterial oxygen and carbon dioxide tensions, pH, and bicarbonate estimations were obtained. Right heart catheterization was carried out using standard method [6].

Angiographic and hemodynamic studies were repeated at 72-h, after which the cardiac catheter was removed. Six months later patients were clinically reassessed and, if agreed, further pulmonary angiographic and hemodynamic studies were performed. All pulmonary angiographs were subsequently reviewed by two independent radiologists who had no knowledge of the clinical state of the patients or the response to treatment. Miller classification was used to know the severity of the pulmonary arterial occlusion. This system provides a score from 0 to 34, made up of a maximum of 16 for the thrombus itself and 18 for peripheral perfusion as assessed by opacification of the peripheral vessels by contrast medium [6].

Heparin or streptokinase was allocated according to random lists, each center using a separate list. A loading dose of 100 mL of normal saline or 5 % glucose containing 600,000 units of streptokinase or 5000 units heparin, each with 100 mg of hydrocortisone added, was infused through the catheter in the pulmonary artery over 30-min. This was followed by an hourly infusion of either 100,000 units of streptokinase or 2500 units of heparin for 72-h. Sixty-hours after infusion warfarin was prescribed at an initial dose of 25 mg and continued with laboratory control for 6 months. Treatment was monitored as follows: in patients treated with heparin if the protamine heparin titration exceeded 1–5 mg/100 mL the maintenance dose was reduced by 500 U/h and the test repeated in 6 h. In the streptokinase group if the observed fibrinogen titer (in saline) fell below 1 in 4 the dose of streptokinase could be increased by 50,000 U/h and the test repeated in 6 h. Subsequent oral anticoagulation was controlled by the one-stage prothrombin time [6].

Results

Thirty patients entered the trial. Twenty-three patients completed the 72-h trial regimen, 12 in heparin group and 11 in streptokinase group. The 7 patients who failed to complete were excluded from the overall analysis of results. The ages and clinical features were similar in both treatment groups, but there were more men than women in the heparin group and more women than men in the streptokinase group. The severity of illness, as judged by hemodynamic measurements and angiography, was similar in both groups [6].

Of the 8 patients treated with heparin and who had an initial angiographic score greater than 16, none had a score of less than 16 at 72-h. In contrast, in 10 patients of streptokinase group with an initial score above 16, it fell to below this figure in all except 2. Additionally, angiographic findings in 4 heparin group patients showed no change or deteriorated. The mean angiographic score in the streptokinase group fell by 61 %, whereas the score in the heparin group fell by only 15 %. Improvement during the 72 h of treatment, assessed by the two group *t* test, was significantly greater in the streptokinase group for the angiographic score ($p<0.001$), the pulmonary arterial systolic pressure ($p<005$), and the mean pulmonary arterial pressure ($p<0.02$) [6].

Seven patients failed to complete 72 h of the trial treatment. One patient having made satisfactory clinical progress suddenly died 18 h after starting heparin treatment. The angiography had shown complete occlusion of the right pulmonary artery. At necropsy there was fresh thrombus in the left pulmonary artery and it was concluded, therefore, that the patient had died from a PE recurrence. The clinical condition of the other 6 patients deteriorated, hypotension persisted, therefore they were withdrawn from the trial so that in accordance with the trial, protocol alternative treatment could be instituted. Successful pulmonary embolectomy was carried out on 4 patients (2 from each group). The treatment was changed from heparin to streptokinase in 2 patients: in one the angiographic score fell from 26-0 to 20-5 at 72-h, but in the other the score rose from 24-0 to 27-0 [6].

Four heparin group patients and 7 in streptokinase group had 6-months follow-up. Two patients, one from each group, had mild dyspnea on exertion. In one case pulmonary hypertension remained with a mean pulmonary arterial pressure of 40 mmHg and an angiographic score of 16. Another patient from the streptokinase group had a loud pulmonary valve closure sound. Seven patients agreed to have a third pulmonary angiogram carried out after the purpose of the study had been explained to them. Two had been treated with heparin and 5 with streptokinase. There was a tendency towards further improvement; unfortunately, the pulmonary arterial pressure data was not completed for all three examinations in each case [6].

Eighteen (78 %) of the 23 patients completing 72 h of the trial suffered one or more side effects; 10 in heparin group and 8 in streptokinase group. One patient became severely hypotensive with peripheral vasoconstriction during the loading dose of streptokinase; this responded well to additional intravenous hydrocortisone and chlorpheniramine. Another patient developed a widespread erythematous irritating rash on the third day of streptokinase treatment, which rapidly cleared within 48-h. A rise in temperature was frequent in streptokinase group. Bleeding was not a serious problem, though one patient in each group required blood transfusion.

Lessons Learned from This Study

The results of this trial provide clear evidence that streptokinase was superior to heparin in terms of the early clearance of PE and in the reduction of the pulmonary hypertension. There was significantly evidence in favor of thrombolysis with streptokinase compared with heparin group ($p<0.001$). The reduction of systolic and mean pulmonary arterial pressures was also significantly greater ($p<0.05$ and $p<0.02$ respectively) in the streptokinase group. Seven patients failed to complete 72 h of the trial treatment: five successfully underwent pulmonary embolectomy. Six of these "failures" had initial pulmonary angiographic scores of 24 of more and systemic systolic blood pressure recordings of 100 mmHg or less. Patients with these features should probably be considered for pulmonary embolectomy as the initial treatment. A febrile reaction commonly occurred in the streptokinase group: otherwise side effects were no more common than in the heparin group [6].

Regarding deaths related to PE, about 50 % of them occurred within 2 h. All except 1 of the patients in this trial began treatment more than 6 h after the major episode, raising the need for a trial including larger samples of patients in order to show a significant difference based specifically on mortality between heparin and streptokinase treatment.

Given the clinical deterioration observed in several patients, pulmonary embolectomy with cardiopulmonary bypass was considered as therapeutic option, and authors analyzed indications of these approaches. As has been previously published patients under thrombolysis with streptokinase and poor peripheral lung perfusion seem to have poor outcome. Six out of 10 patients with perfusion indices of 10 or more failed to complete allocated trial therapy. Also, a systemic systolic blood pressure of ≤100 mmHg with an angiographic score of ≥24 was associated with a 70 % chance of death or the need for pulmonary embolectomy. Considering the results a question still remains as to whether the initial accelerated thrombolysis by streptokinase is of value in terms of long-term resolution and survival [6].

In the 6-month follow-up study, 5 patients from streptokinase group had lower scores than the two in heparin group, but these numbers are too small for definitive answers. Side effects of treatment with streptokinase were no more severe than those of heparin. A final consideration was that with an initial pulmonary angiographic score ≥24 or more and systemic systolic arterial blood pressure ≤100 mmHg, pulmonary embolectomy is probably the treatment of choice.

Streptokinase and Heparin in the Treatment of Major Pulmonary Embolism

Background

Pulmonary embolism is a common disease in medical and surgical patients. At that time several studies claimed that fibrinolytic treatment with streptokinase or urokinase was superior to heparin. However, only two prospective randomized, controlled trials compared the effect of fibrinolytic treatment and heparin in major PE patients. In UPET trial [5], urokinase compared with heparin alone, significantly accelerated the resolution rate of pulmonary thromboemboli at 24 h. In the trial conducted by Tibutt et al. [6], significantly greater evidence of thrombolysis was reported in streptokinase group (72-h) than in heparin group for the same period. It was not yet settled, however, whether the increased rate of thrombolysis following fibrinolytic treatment reduced the mortality in patients with massive pulmonary embolism. This report concerns a controlled trial in which patients with proven major PE were randomized to heparin alone or streptokinase in standard dose plus heparin [7].

Methodology

Patients with symptoms of acute major PE were considered. Diagnosis was established by pulmonary angiography in all cases. Angiography was done in the acute stage on admission and repeated after 3 or 4 days of treatment (72 h as a mean). Severity of the pulmonary artery occlusion was assessed by Miller score, which provides a score from 0 to 34, made up of a maximum of 16 for the thrombus itself and 18 for peripheral perfusion as assessed by opacification of the peripheral vessels by contrast medium. Exclusion criteria were known bleeding tendency or recent gastrointestinal or urogenital tract bleeding, major surgery within the last 10 days, recent stroke, severe hypertension (diastolic pressure ≥120 mmHg), hypertensive retinopathy grade 3–4, severe renal or hepatic insufficiency, pregnancy, recent delivery or known malignant disease. An arbitrary upper age limit was set at 70 years [7].

In patients with less severe symptoms, lung VQ scan was performed prior to pulmonary angiography. Additionally blood samples were taken for quantification of hemoglobin, thrombocyte count, activated partial thromboplastin time, fibrinogen, thrombin clotting time, serum creatinine, serum glutamic oxaloacetic and glutamic pyruvate transaminase. Clinical features were noted daily during the first 10 days after the start of treatment, including any sign of bleeding. When possible, a daily electrocardiogram was recorded. Special care was taken to record any sign of deep vein thrombosis or recurrent PE [7].

Streptokinase was given in standard doses. After a loading dose of 250,000 IU I.V. in 20 min, a maintenance dose of 100,000 IU/h was given by continuous I.V. infusion. Infusion was continued until control pulmonary angiography after 72 h was done. Streptokinase was then discontinued and oral anticoagulation with warfarin was started. To avoid anaphylactic reactions, 100 mg of soluble hydrocortisone were given I.V. before the loading dose of streptokinase, where after prednisone, 10 mg three times daily, was given until discontinuation of streptokinase.

Heparin was given in an initial dose of 15,000 IU I.V., followed by a maintenance dose of 30,000 IU/day as a continuous i.v. infusion. The dose of heparin was subsequently adjusted according to the thrombin clotting time. Warfarin was started after control angiography and heparin was discontinued when therapeutic values of thrombotest were obtained. As a mean, heparin was given for 7 days, but was continued for 70 days in one patient with symptoms of persistent massive embolism. Intramuscular injections were avoided in both treatment groups [7].

Results

Twenty-five patients entered the trial and all except 5 were allocated to treatment groups by using sealed envelopes. The demographic characteristics were similar in both treatment groups, excepting higher age and more frequent female gender in heparin group. Only one patient in each group had a systolic blood pressure <90 mmHg and 3 patients in each group had electrocardiogram signs of acute right ventricular strain. The interval from onset of symptoms to initiation of treatment was similar in both groups, excepting 2 patients in the streptokinase group who have had symptoms for more than 5 days. In terms of angiographic scores streptokinase was more severe than heparin group. There was only one patient in each group with an angiographic score >30 and these patients were both in shock on admission [7].

The mean angiographic score fell 52.3 % in the streptokinase group compared with 20.6 % in heparin group. Of the 10 patients treated with streptokinase and who had an initial angiographic score >20, 8 had a score <16 at 72 h. Angiographic deterioration (rise in score from 15 to 24) occurred in one patient treated with heparin. After discontinuation of heparin, this patient experienced clinical and angiographic improvement (fall in score from 24 to 12) following treatment with streptokinase for 3 days. The clinical progress during the treatment period of 72 h was satisfactory in all patients with marked angiographic improvement, regardless of the type of treatment. It should be noted, however, that 8 of the 10 patients in this category had been treated with streptokinase. It is also important to note that clinical improvement might occur in spite of unchanged or even worse angiographic appearance and that the clinical features might be moderate in patients with massive embolism [7].

One patient in heparin group, a 66-year-old woman, failed to complete the 72-h trial. She presented with severe hypotension and an angiographic score of 34, deteriorated and died 15 h after starting heparin treatment. Necropsy demonstrated large, occluding thrombi in both the right and the left pulmonary artery. The other heparin-treated patient who died was a 49-year-old man. Five weeks prior to embolization he was under neurological surgery by a meningioma. He developed severe dyspnea and cyanosis and was also moderately hypotensive. Pulmonary angiography demonstrated central bilateral thrombus with no change in the next 72-h with heparin treatment. Intravenous infusion was continued for 70 with slight clinical improvement until she died. Necropsy revealed multiple partially occluding and organized thrombus in several lobar arteries. A glioblastoma was found in the right hemisphere. As judged form the clinical course, persistent PE contributed to the fatal outcome [7].

In streptokinase group there was one late dead a 66-year-old woman with an undiagnosed pulmonary adenocarcinoma. She had a 1-week history of deep vein thrombosis of the right leg and had complained of dyspnea during the last 2 days. Phlebography demonstrated deep vein thrombosis on both sides, probably affecting the iliac veins. Bilateral major pulmonary embolism was shown by angiography and the angiographic appearance was only slightly improved following streptokinase. Patient died 3 weeks later from phlegmasia cerulea dolens with gangrene of both feet. Necropsy disclosed occluding thrombi in vena cava inferior and in the iliacal and femoral veins on both sides but no evidence of thrombotic occlusion of the arteries. Pulmonary emboli could not be demonstrated. An undifferentiated adenocarcinoma was found in the right lung and metastases were demonstrated in the pancreas, kidneys and adrenals [7].

Major bleeding was more frequent in streptokinase group (4 patients) than in heparin group (2 patients). This complication was most often related to punction or cutdown sites in streptokinase group. Spontaneous bleeding occurred more frequently in heparin patients. A rise in temperature was more frequent in the streptokinase group but more serious anaphylactic reactions were not seen. In no case did streptokinase have to be withdrawn because of side effects [7].

Lessons Learned from This Study

Previous evidence suggesting that in man substantial resolution of PE may occur spontaneously within days or weeks as demonstrated by pulmonary angiography. However, the early resolution rate of major PE is slow, as judged by angiography or lung scanning and significant resolution of major emboli does not seem to occur during the first week. Contrasting with these observation of slow PE resolution during treatment with heparin there are reports of rapid lysis after streptokinase or urokinase. When comparing heparin and streptokinase effects in PE patients, each group needs to be comparable in terms of prognostic factors and factors known to affect resolution as severity and duration of the PE and coexisting cardiorespiratory disease. In this study both groups were comparable, with the exception that the angiographic obstruction was more severe in the streptokinase group than in heparin group and PE duration was longer than 1-week in 2 streptokinase-treated patients. This, however, would be expected to disfavor the spontaneous thrombolysis in the streptokinase group [7].

Angiographic evidence of thrombolysis was significantly greater ($p<0.01$) in the 14 patients treated with streptokinase than in the 1 treated with heparin. In streptokinase group the mean angiographic score fell by 52.3 % compared with heparin group 20.6 %. These observations were similar to those obtained by Tibutt et al. [6]. Right-sided pressure measurements were performed in only 4 patients in streptokinase group. Three of them had normal pulmonary arterial pressures. This finding was in accordance with previous observations in which the enhanced thrombolysis obtained with fibrinolytic agent was accompanied by a reduction of systolic and mean pulmonary arterial pressures. One patient deteriorated during treatment with heparin, but was subsequently successfully treated with streptokinase, thus serving as his own control. The systemic fibrinolytic effect was sufficient in all streptokinase groups, as judged from the coagulation assays. Hence, the failure to obtain significant thrombolysis in 2 of the streptokinase-treated patients remains obscure and possibly related with age of the thrombus [7].

Considering that in the present study only one patient in heparin group, suffered early death attributed to massive PE, and based on previous evidence, the authors considered that the only survival chance would probably have been embolectomy. However, its best indications remain unknown. An important contribution in this study was that in critically ill patients with severe hypotension and an angiographic score of 3, streptokinase was a successful therapeutic approach. However, the important question of whether the accelerated thrombolysis obtained with fibrinolytic agent might reduce mortality in massive PE remains unknown. As stressed by several authors, a trial including larger sample was mandatory [7].

Major bleeding complications were more frequently seen in streptokinase group than in those treated with heparin alone. Its higher frequency was closely related to punction or cutdown sites in connection with diagnostic procedures. Three patients developed inguinal hematoma following pulmonary angiography. To avoid this complication, it is advisable that catheterization for pulmonary angiography in patients with suspected PE should be performed via the cubital vein. Also, authors established that acute life-threatening PE patients had three treatment options: heparin, streptokinase or emergency embolectomy [7]. According to Tibutt et al. [6] embolectomy should be restricted to patients with sustained hypotension and an initial angiographic score of ≥24. The final conclusion was that streptokinase is the treatment of choice for most patients with acute life-threatening PE, provided that a careful screening for bleeding tendencies is carried out before treatment is started. It is also important that the number of invasive diagnostic procedures should be kept as low as possible [7].

Fibrinolytic Effects of Urokinase and Heparin in Acute Pulmonary Embolism

Background

Despite previous randomized control trials [5–7], several limitations were identified specifically in UPET trial [5], where heparin infusion in therapeutic doses was given also during the diagnostic evaluation before randomization. In addition, the anticoagulant mechanism of heparin was not fully understood. Aditionally, heparin had proved value in the treatment of PE, even in severely ill patients. Furthermore, thrombus resolution reported in the literature as spontaneous, occurred after heparin treatment. So, a fibrinolytic effect of heparin cannot be ruled out. The main target of this study was to compare the effect of heparin infusion with that of urokinase administered alone in acute PE patients [8].

Methodology

From September 1979 to August 1983, 792 patients were screened for PE by V/Q lung scan. Inclusion criteria were: (a) >9 unperfused lung segments, computed for both lungs on the lateral projections of perfusion lung scans; (b) age <72 years; (c) clinically identified PE not older than 7 days; (d) fibrinogen and plasminogen plasma concentration within the normal plasma level; (e) Lee-White clotting time, platelet count, prothrombin time, also within the normal range. Exclusion criteria included thrombolytic therapy contraindications as and/or angiographic procedure: recent cerebrovascular episodes, severe hypertension, history of occurrence of bleeding, trauma or major surgery within 7 days, pregnancy, and shock.

Thirty patients were submitted to confirmatory pulmonary arteriography. None of them had significant cardiac or pulmonary diseases. Mean pulmonary artery pressure was measured [8].

Patients were randomly allocated to the treatment groups: (A) urokinase 800,000 CTA units (IU) infusion for 12 h a day for 3 days (total dose 2,400,000 IU) followed by oral anticoagulants: (B) heparin infusion at a mean daily dose of 30,000 IU for 7 days followed by oral anticoagulants; heparin was adjusted to Lee-White clotting time between 20 and 30; (C) infusion of 3,300,000 IU of urokinase in 12 h followed by oral anticoagulants. The dosages used in A and C of urokinase groups were lower than those employed in the UPET [5] study. The oral anticoagulant treatment was continued in all patients for 1 year [8].

Perfusion V/Q lung scans and arterial blood gas determinations were obtained at 24-h, 3, 7, and 30 days, 6 and 12 months after the start of treatment in all patients. Pulmonary arteriography and mean pulmonary artery pressure were obtained again at day 7 in all the patients. Venous blood samples were drawn in all patients before randomization and at 6, 12, 24, 48, and 60 h of treatment to assess fibrinogen and plasminogen. Oral anticoagulants were given then to keep the prothrombin activity between 20 and 40 % of the normal value. Impairment of pulmonary perfusion was assessed from: (1) the number of unperfused lung segments; (2) the PaO_2, standard value (PaO_2 standard deviation), i.e., the PaO_2 in mmHg corrected to a $PaCO_2$ of 40 mmHg [8].

Results

In all patients pulmonary arteriography showed massive PE. Pulmonary perfusion impairment was extensive and related with the index of angiographic severity. The number of unperfused lung segments was 13.6, 13.0, and 13.8 in the treatment groups A, B, and C at the moment of admission. No significant difference was found in the pretreatment values for the three groups. Patients in heparin group (B) showed less impairment of some pretreatment values, the difference from the pretreatment values of groups A and C was small and statistically nonsignificant [8].

Multiple comparisons among groups showed a difference of group C vs. groups A and heparin (B), but not between groups A and B.

Simple main effects for time were significant in treatments A and C. In the former, plasminogen was lower at 48 and 60 h than at 6 h and at 60 h than at 12 h. In the latter, plasminogen at 6 h was higher than at all the other times and at 48 h than at 12 h. Regarding the number of unperfused lung segments observed between 24 h and 1-year follow-up, no differences with treatment in spite of significant time reduction. In one patient of group C, bleeding of the urinary tract was observed. This complication did not require any therapeutic measure. In 12 months follow-up no PE recurrence was identified. As to the clinical outcome, no patient showed recurrence of PE after up to 12 months of observation. Moreover, none of total of patients enrolled had mortality [8].

Lessons Learned from This Study

Previously, several reports indicated a possible apparent fibrinolytic effect of heparin due to inhibition of deposition of fresh fibrin onto an established thrombus which facilitates the natural lysis and resolution of the thrombus. In vitro studies failed to show any influence of heparin on the euglobulin lysis time and on the diluted clot lysis time suggesting a lack of effect of heparin on the fibrinolytic mechanisms. However, in other studies heparin was found to have a dual effect on fibrinolysis: high concentrations inhibited lysis of preformed fibrin while low concentrations enhanced it. Additionally, several authors reported enhancement of fibrinolysis after intravenous administration of heparin. A main finding in this study indicates that before treatment, at about 3 days from the episode of PE, the fibrinogen plasma level is within normal limits, whereas, after 6 h of treatment, it falls to the same level in the various treatment groups. After 12 h, groups A and B showed the same plasma level of fibrinogen while group C had a lower level [8].

These data suggest that heparin may induce fibrinogenolysis, and shows the differences with urokinase depending of the respective dose. The behavior of plasminogen showed that its plasma level, up to 24 h of treatment, is reduced to the same extent in groups A and B, and even more in group C, suggesting that heparin has the same effect on plasminogen as urokinase in group A and may determine a systemic lytic state. After the initial decrease and up to 48 h, fibrinogen did not show any significant difference of plasma concentration between the various treatments. At 60 h, group C shows a plasma level of fibrinogen higher than that of group A and group B a level lower than that at 6 h. These results appear to be directly related to the timing of administration and to the amount of urokinase and heparin administered [8].

The authors considered that the stable decrease in the plasma concentration of fibrinogen in group B suggests that, under continuous heparin infusion, a new equilibrium is reached within a few hours between fibrinogen destruction and production. Similar results were observed at 48 and 60 h, for the plasma level of plasminogen with the exception that group B at 60 h shows a plasminogen concentrate on less reduced than group A. Authors commented that fibrinogen and plasminogen plasma levels provide a consistent picture of the fibrinolytic changes induced by the treatments. And also established that decreasing plasminogen and fibrinogen are considered sufficient to define a lytic state [8].

Regarding the mechanism of enhanced fibrinolysis by heparin it has been suggested that this effect is attained through the release of tissue plasminogen activator. Authors observed that fibrinogen level fell by 23, 26, and 27 % after 6 h of treatment in groups A, B, and C, respectively. Induction of a lytic state by heparin might also be the result of the activation by the drug of Hageman factor and prekallikrein. This intrinsic pathway of plasminogen activation qualitatively acts with a urokinase-like mechanism but seems weaker than urokinase. The characteristics of both of these mechanisms might then explain the observation that plasminogen level in group B is less reduced than in group A at 60 h [8].

Another interesting finding was the agreement between angiographic score and the number of unperfused lung segments at the time of diagnosis and after 7 days. While in each group of treatment a significant reduction ($p<0.001$) of the number of unperfused lung segments throughout all the period of observation up to 12 months was obtained, no statistical differences between groups were found at any time. The results of the study agree only in part with those reported in the UPET study [5]; in fact, even in this study, after the first 24 h and up to 12 months, no statistically significant difference between heparin and urokinase treatments was found in mean absolute and percentage resolution at perfusion lung scanning [8].

However, the results after the first 24 h, showed a significantly greater angiographic and scintigraphic improvement in urokinase groups than heparin group. Heparin infusion during the diagnostic evaluation of all patients before their random allocation to treatment groups may account for the differences observed in the UPET study [5] after 24 h. The observation of a fibrinolytic activity of heparin infusion alone in this study could be related in some way to this effect observed in human and experimental studies [8].

Regarding bleeding complications, only one patient in this trial (group C) had marked bleeding from the urinary tract. It was an interesting finding compared with 45 % in urokinase group and 27 % in heparin group of bleeding complications in the early phase treatment in UPET [5]. For the authors, this significative differences may be attributed to heparin infusion. In UPET [5] infusion was performed before and immediately after urokinase infusion inducing plasma fibrinogen level reduction and increasing fibrin degradation products. In turn, these products could have impaired the coagulation systems [8].

Considering that different treatments, including tissue plasminogen activator, induce significant decrease in fibrinogen plasma level in PE patients, it may be convenient to use this parameter as an index of a systemic lytic state to compare the dosages of different drugs, especially with reference to bleeding complications. Changes in angiographic and scintigraphic severity and bleeding complications appear correlated with the reduction in fibrinogen levels [8].

A Randomized Trial of a Single Bolus Dosage Regimen of Recombinant Tissue Plasminogen Activator in Patients with Acute Pulmonary Embolism

Background

Treatment of thrombosis by activation of the plasma fibrinolytic enzyme system provides a nonsurgical method for relieving thrombus in pulmonary arterial circulation. Urokinase and streptokinase, the plasminogen activators approved for the treatment of PE induce early lysis of pulmonary thrombus administered over long-term 12–24 h infusion. These agents are not fibrin specific and convert circulating plasminogen to plasmin inducing systemic lytic state leading to a generalized coagulation defect which could contribute to the increased risk of bleeding complications [9].

Recombinant human tissue-type plasminogen activator (rt-PA), a new plasminogen activator, preferentially activates plasminogen in the presence of fibrin, produce effective thrombolysis in experimental models and because of its relative fibrin specificity induce thrombolysis without generalized coagulopathy; rt-PA has been evaluated in clinical trials in myocardial infarction, PE, and venous thrombosis patients. In all of these studies, rt-PA was administered in short-term (90 min) and long-term (8 h) continuous infusion. These regimens were associated with a systemic lytic state, less fibrinogenolysis than streptokinase, for an equivalent thrombolytic effect, and excessive bleeding [9].

Experimental studies suggesting the effectiveness of rt-PA in inducing lysis of venous thrombus and PE is increased using high concentrations infused over a short interval. In previous studies, a 15-min infusion regimen produced less plasma proteolysis and less experimental bleeding than an identical dose infused over 1 or 4 h. For these results a clinical trial was conducted to determine whether a bolus injection of rt-PA is effective in producing accelerated thrombolysis in patients with acute PE [9].

Methodology

PE patients proved by either pulmonary angiography or a high probability VQ lung scan (segmental or greater perfusion defect with ventilation mismatch), plus deep venous thrombosis confirmed by venography or ultrasound were included. Exclusion: active bleeding process, active peptic ulcer disease, acquired bleeding diathesis, abnormal platelet count, recent (2 months) stroke or active intracranial process; also recent major surgery, major trauma, obstetric delivery, organ biopsy, severe systolic or diastolic hypertension, pregnancy patients, PE >2 weeks or had under parenteral heparin >72 h. Considering that the experimental bolus regimen was not used in humans, massive PE patients were excluded [9].

All patients were under 5000 IU intravenous heparin bolus followed by continuous infusion at a starting dose of 30,000 units for the first 24-h. The heparin dose was adjusted daily to maintain activated partial thromboplastin time between 55 and 75 s. Patients were randomly assigned to receive either rt-PA or saline solution placebo. They were stratified according pulmonary angiography or not and the time since onset symptoms of PE (<48 or ≥48 h). Patients in rt-PA group received 0.6 mkg ideal body weight reconstituted in 50 mL sterile water by bolus injection over 2 min. Heparin was interrupted only for the duration of the study drug infusion. The same procedure was followed for patients who received placebo [9].

The effectiveness of the regimens for producing lysis of pulmonary thrombus was assessed by comparing the baseline perfusion VQ lung scan with the scan performed at 24-h and 7 days after treatment. The primary outcome measure was relative improvement in perfusion of more than 50 % from the baseline VQ perfusion scan.

Three physicians, experienced in the interpretation of lung scans, reviewed the scans. A perfusion defect was defined as an area of absent perfusion or hypoperfusion. The results of lung scanning were interpreted without knowledge of the clinical findings or the treatment group to which the patient had been, randomized. Any disagreement in size of the perfusion abnormality was resolved by consensus [9].

To determine the improvement in pulmonary perfusion between pretreatment and 24 h and 7 days, the change in the total perfusion defect in the anterior and posterior views was used as was described [5]. Patients were examined daily during the 10-day study period for evidence of bleeding. Major bleeding: if it was overt and associated with either a fall in hemoglobin level of 20 g/L or more, or a need for transfusion of two or more units of blood, or if it was retroperitoneal or intracranial. Minor bleeding: if it was overt, but did not meet the other criteria for major bleeding. Daily hemoglobin determination was performed. Mortality and recurrent PE were not primary outcome measures, however, were documented during the first 10 days post-randomization [9].

Results

Fifty-eight patients with proved PE were enrolled, 33 patients were randomized to rt-PA and 25 to placebo. Patients in rt-PA group had chest pain in 20 cases (60.6 %), dyspnea in 27 (81.8 %), hemoptysis in five (15 %), while six (18 %) had syncope. In placebo group, chest pain was experienced by 23 patients (92 %), dyspnea in 22 (88 %), hemoptysis in seven (28 %), and five (20 %) presented with syncope. In rt-PA group 22 patients (67 %) had diagnosis confirmed by pulmonary angiography, 6 (18 %) by a high probability VQ lung scan associated with a positive venogram, and 5 (15 %) by high probability VQ lung scan plus positive duplex ultrasonography. In placebo group, 18 (72 %) had diagnosis by pulmonary angiography, 4 (16 %) by high probability VQ lung scan associated with a positive venogram, and three (12 %) by a VQ high probability lung scan associated with positive duplex ultrasonography. In terms of baseline characteristics age, gender, underlying presence of malignancy, previous history of venous thromboembolic disease, duration of symptoms prior to randomization, and duration of heparin therapy prior to study, both groups were reasonably comparable [9].

Perfusion lung scan assessment: In rt-PA group, the mean baseline perfusion defect was 27.4 and 21.3 % in the control group. Repeated VQ lung scans were available for 57 patients (98 %): 32 patients in rt-PA group, and 25 in those receiving placebo. Eleven (34.4 %) rt-PA patients experienced a greater than 50 % improvement in the lung scan at 24 h compared to 3 (12 %) placebo patients ($p=0.026$). Neither age, gender, cancer history, previous venous thromboembolism, duration of symptoms and magnitude of the baseline perfusion defect were significantly different in the rt-PA patients with >50 % improvement in perfusion at 24 h compared to those with <50 % improvement.

At 24 h, mean absolute improvement in the perfusion defect was 9.7 % in rt-PA group compared to 5 % in placebo group ($p = 0.07$) and the mean relative improvement in perfusion was 37 % compared to 19 % ($p = 0.01$) respectively. At 7 days, no statistically significant difference was detected for absolute improvement in the perfusion defect, 16 % rt-PA group compared to 11 % placebo group, and mean relative improvement, 58 % compared to 49 % respectively [9]. In this 10-day study period, in rt-PA group 1 patient died compared with no mortality in placebo group. Patient died 10 h post-rt-PA injection and necropsy showed saddle PE. None recurrence in both groups were observed [9].

In this study rt-PA bolus infusion was reasonably well tolerated, however, 3 patients had allergic reactions. One patient felt hot and diaphoretic within 10 min of the infusion; a second patient felt hot and developed mild hypotension within 2 min of the infusion, and a third patient experienced mild hypotension associated with urticaria which resolved within 15 min of injection. In placebo group, one patient experienced hypotension shortly after administration of placebo.

No major bleeding complications were identified in both groups. Three patients in each group required transfusions during the 10-day study period. None of these patients had an overt site of hemorrhage and in all 6 patients who required transfusion it was secondary to medical conditions unrelated with study drug administration. In rt-PA group 9 patients had bruising either in the groin and/or at antecubital fossa venipuncture site used for study laboratory tests [9]. An additional 4 patients who received rt-PA had oozing at either one or both of these sites. One patient in each group experienced epistaxis and one patient who received rt-PA had increased serosanguineous drainage from an abdominal wound site. So, 15 rt-PA patients (45 %) experienced minor bleeding compared to placebo group ($p = 0.0005$) [9].

Lessons Learned from This Study

Previous evidences with rt-PA in doses between 50 and 100 mg over of 2–7 h infusion were related with a systemic lytic state and high proportion of major bleeding complications. In this study, rt-PA bolus over 2 min in patients fully heparinized showed: (a) significative increase of proportion of patients who achieved >50 % improvement in perfusion defects at 24 h; (b) was associated with a mean absolute improvement in perfusion defect (9.7 %) and a mean relative improvement (37 %). This relative improvement in lung scan perfusion was of the same order of magnitude with rt-PA in higher dose in longer period infusion was used. The improvement in lung perfusion is also comparable with UPET study. In addition, the results were similar when urokinase was given over 12 h period [5]. By 7 days there was no longer any difference in the resolution seen in both groups, similar findings to those reported in UPET trial [5]. Another important apportation was the use of lung scan, a noninvasive and reliable index of pulmonary arterial obstruction as a surrogate outcome [9].

This study introduced for first time in the history of thrombolysis and PE the concept of bolus infusion for patient treatment. The thrombolytic regimen was chosen based on three observations coming from experimental models: (1) thrombolysis was improved when rt-PA was administered in a high concentration over a short period of time; (2) rt-PA produced continuing thrombolysis after cleared from the circulation; and (3) bleeding was reduced when the same dose of the drug was administered over a short period of time. Although a 15-min infusion was used in the experimental models, another clinical observation using a bolus regimen over 2 min was chosen because of its simplicity amid convenience [9].

In spite of the results, the optimal regimen for rt-PA has not been established. Short infusion in high concentration regimens induces more rapid thrombolysis than similar doses infused over a longer time interval in experimental PE and in ST-elevation myocardial infarction patients. The bolus dose regimen, was effective in achieving accelerated thrombolysis, was well tolerated, and easy to administer to PE patients who are also being treated with heparin. Although, rt-PA bolus regimen was safety in terms of major bleeding, invasive procedures and/or venous punction were related with an increase of minor bleedings. The relatively small sample size inducing type two error could explain the absence of major bleeding complications. Finally, the study was not designed to determinate mortality, it is well known that this kind of design requires larger sample size [9].

Tissue Plasminogen Activator for the Treatment of Acute Pulmonary Embolism: A Collaborative Study by the PIOPED Investigators

Background

Considering its pharmacokinetic and pharmacodynamic characteristics, rt-PA has great potential for the treatment of acute PE; however, the experience with this thrombolytic agent is limited, and no comparisons to placebo have been published. The main target of this study was to evaluate the efficacy of rt-PA in combination with heparin compared to placebo plus heparin in patients with acute PE. The thrombolytic effects of rt-PA may be enhanced when administered in combination with heparin because the addition of new fibrin to the thrombus is prevented by heparin during lytic therapy [10].

Methodology

Between November 30, 1986, and June 30, 1987, 13 patients were studied; group rt-PA included 9 patients and heparin group 4 patients. Among those who received rt-PA, 8 of 9 patients received heparin simultaneously. All patients received either rt-PA or placebo in a randomized double-blind fashion; twice as many patients were randomly assigned to the treatment group as to the control group.

All patients had PE onset symptoms within 7 days of the angiogram. Patients were eligible if they had occlusion of a lobar artery or at least two segmental arteries on pulmonary angiography. Nine patients were men and 4 women with an age range from 20 to 78 years. Patients with shock or clinical instability were excluded. A large number of exclusion criteria were similar to previous studies to enhance safety. Although, six clinical centers with approximately 5500 hospital beds were included, the rate of patient accession was slow. Therefore, the independent Study Policy and Data Safety Monitoring Board recommended that the investigators discontinued recruitment, although the initial study design called for 50 patients [10].

Patients received rt-PA intravenously at a rate of approximately 1 mg/mm. Initially, a dose of 80 mg was selected on the basis of experience with ST-elevation myocardial infarction. After one major hemorrhage, the dose was reduced to 40 mg. Five patients received rt-PA 40 mg, one patient received 64 mg (hemorrhage interrupting an intended 80 mg treatment), and 3 patients received rt-PA 80 mg. The 40 mg dose of rt-PA was administered over 40 min. The 80 mg dose was administered over 90 min. During the infusion of rt-PA, heparin was administered to all but one patient in an open fashion; doses were determined by the attending physician. In one patient, heparin was discontinued during the double-blind administration of rt-PA [10].

Pulmonary angiographies were obtained before the administration of rt-PA and 2 h following the double-blind therapy. Pretreatment pulmonary angiography was bilateral in 12 of 13 patients. Posttreatment pulmonary angiography was obtained in 12 patients and was bilateral in 8. No posttreatment study was obtained in the one patient who hemorrhaged while receiving rt-PA. Pulmonary angiography was obtained in the anterior–posterior projection. Radiologist who interpreted pulmonary angiography was blinded to treatment [10].

Pulmonary angiographies were scored according to the size and number of pulmonary arterial branches that contained intraluminal filling defects. Each vessel, irrespective of its size, received a vessel occlusion score as follows: Size grades entered in each column were added and multiplied by the occlusion grade assigned to the vessel. The total clot size score was then obtained by adding the clot size scores for each vessel. If the entire pulmonary arterial tree were filled with clots, a total of 102 units would be obtained for clot size. The total clot size, therefore, approximated the percentage of obstructed vascular volume in the two lungs [10].

V/Q lung scans and chest X-ray were obtained before the pulmonary angiography; perfusion scans were performed again after double-blind treatment at intervals of 24 h, 48 h, and 7 days; V/Q lung scans were graded by two blinded readers to therapy. Baseline mismatched perfusion defects were assessed as follows: Each segment of the lung was assumed to constitute 11 % of the involved lung. The number of mismatched segments in each lung, therefore, was multiplied by 11 % to determine the percentage of the involved lung that showed a mismatched perfusion defect [10].

Pressures in the right atrium, right ventricle, and pulmonary artery were measured in triplicate with fluid-filled catheters prior to the injection of contrast material. Cardiac output was measured in triplicate by the indicator dilution technique. Total pulmonary resistance was calculated as the fraction of pulmonary arterial mean pressure (mmHg) divided by cardiac output (L/min) times 80. Hemodynamic measurements were repeated 90 min after the onset of therapy. Heart rate, respiratory rate, and blood pressure were recorded during these intervals as well as after 24 h, 48 h, and 7 days. Fragmented dimers were measured prior to thrombolytic therapy and after therapy at intervals of 90 min, 3 h, 24 h, and 7 days. Fibrinogen also was measured [10].

Results

Fragment-D dimers in the blood at one and half and 3 h after beginning therapy indicated the in vivo occurrence of clot lysis. Higher levels of fragment-D dimers were present 3 h after the onset of therapy in the blood of rt-PA group than in heparin-alone group (40 ± 29 vs. 4 ± 3 pg/mL, $p < 0.01$). At 3 h after the start of treatment among heparin-alone group, plasma fibrinogen was 388 ± 126 mg/dL as compared to 222 ± 182 among group rt-PA and heparin patients ($p = 0.14$). Among patients under 80 mg of rt-PA, plasma fibrinogen at 3 h was 74 ± 51 mg/dL. The mean angiographic scores were evaluated for patients who had angiographies both before and 2 h after treatment. Among patients who received rt-PA, the angiographic scores of the left lung were 12.2 ± 5.6 before treatment and 12.5 ± 7.4 after treatment. The angiographic scores of the right lung among patients treated with rt-PA were 10.0 ± 4.4 before treatment and 8.2 ± 3.8 after treatment [10].

Among patients in heparin-alone group, the angiographic scores of the left lung were 12.9 ± 2.2 before treatment and 12.8 ± 4.1 after treatment. The angiographic scores of the right lung among patients treated only with heparin were 15.5 ± 6.3 before and 18.0 ± 10.0 after. Changes of the angiographic score with treatment were not significantly different compared rt-PA group with heparin-alone group. A trend suggested improvement over time of mismatched perfusion defects among patients treated with rt-PA plus heparin. The pretreatment, 1, 2 and 7 days mismatched scan deficits respectively were 39 ± 18, 29 ± 21, 28 ± 22, and 19 ± 14 %. Among heparin-alone group, mismatched perfusion defects were unchanged during the first 2 days and decreased only slightly by day 7. Values before treatment, at 1, 2, and 7 days respectively were 41 ± 15, 41 ± 18, 40 ± 16, and 34 ± 18 %. The trend toward improvement among patients treated with rt-PA and heparin did not achieve statistical significance in comparison to the small number of patients in heparin-alone group [10].

In rt-PA group, total pulmonary resistance after one and half hours decreased from 550 ± 220 to 360 ± 180 dyn/cm [5]. Pulmonary arterial mean pressure showed no significant change in these patients (28 ± 9 vs. 25 ± 8 mmHg). The total pulmonary resistance did not change after one and half hours in patients treated with heparin (770 ± 710 vs. 760 ± 700 dyn/s/cm^5). Pulmonary arterial mean pressure remained unchanged (33 ± 13 vs. 33 ± 13 mmHg) among heparin-alone group. The reduction of total pulmonary resistance among rt-PA group was greater than the reduction among patients treated with heparin alone ($p = 0.03$). No prominent changes were noted either in the respiratory rate or the heart rate over the 7 days of the investigation [10].

Among the 9 patients who received rt-PA, one major bleeding (upper gastrointestinal tract, sites of catheter insertions and needle punction) episode occurred in an 81-year-old woman who received 64 mg of rt-PA in combination with heparin. Eight units of packed red blood cells were required. Gastroscopy showed oozing from mild superficial mucosal ulcerations. Coagulopathy was corrected and a Greenfield filter was inserted. However, patient continued with clinical instability, developed a ST-elevation myocardial infarction, and died of an arrhythmia 19 days after treatment with rt-PA. Serious bleeding was not observed among the patients included in rt-PA or heparin-alone groups [10].

Lessons Learned from This Study

Fibrinolysis occurred within one and half hours after receiving rt-PA, based upon the prompt elevation of fragment D-dimers. The assay used was specific for fibrin and did not detect fibrinogen degradation products. The observed reduction of fibrinogen levels in each of 3 patients receiving 80 mg of rt-PA was consistent with a fibrinogen systemic lysis. In spite of the prompt onset of fibrinolysis, there was only a limited change of the pulmonary vascular resistance and no significant improvement of the angiograms at 2 h [10].

Perfusion scans, however, showed trends toward more rapid improvement by 24 h than patients treated with placebo. Massive bleeding occurred in one patient. The observations in this study suggest that rt-PA has little effect in 2 h on angiographic clot burden, but may produce some improvement in hemodynamics. The treatment, however, is not without risk. Reported experience using rt-PA for venous thromboemboli in patients is limited, and there are no placebo-controlled studies.

Alteplase Combined with Heparin vs. Heparin in the Treatment of Acute Pulmonary Embolism: Plasminogen Activator Italian Multicenter Study 2 (PAIMS-2)

Background

At the beginning of 90s decade the evidence of effectiveness of recombinant human tissue-type plasminogen activator, rt-PA (alteplase) for the treatment of acute massive PE was coming from noncontrolled and controlled trials in comparison with urokinase and heparin. Alteplase was given as a slow infusion or intravenous bolus in doses ranging from 50 to 100 mg. In all clinical situations, rt-PA showed effective clot lysis. Therefore PAIMS-2 trial was carried out to compare the efficacy and safety of rt-PA, alteplase followed by heparin with those patients under heparin alone [11].

Methodology

PAIMS-2 was an open, parallel, multicenter randomized trial undertaken from October 1988 to November 1990 in eight participating centers. As interesting observation the Committee suggested that informed consent should not be required, considering that patients will have critical condition for a satisfactory application of the procedure. Nevertheless, medical staff were ready to provide explanations to the patient and family upon request.

Inclusion criteria were: age 18–80 years, acute PE within 10 days of onset, pulmonary angiography showing vascular obstruction >30 %, corresponding to a Miller index score >11. Exclusion criteria: cardiogenic shock (systolic pressure <90 mmHg and urinary output <20 mL/h), surgical procedure or organ biopsy in the previous 7 days, gastrointestinal or genitourinary bleeding in last 3 months; stroke or transient ischemic attack in previous 3 months, punction of noncompressible vessels, uncontrolled hypertension (diastolic blood pressure >120 mmHg, systolic blood pressure >200 mmHg) hematologic disorders and contraindication for heparin use, severe hepatic or renal failure and pregnancy or lactation [11].

On admission all patients with clinical symptoms suggesting acute PE were under electrocardiography, chest X-ray, lung scan (optional), plus selective pulmonary angiography of the right and left pulmonary arteries. Also, pulmonary artery pressure and measurement of pulmonary artery oxygen were obtained [11].

All patients received heparin bolus 10,000 IU, and then were randomized in two groups: (1) 2-h infusion of alteplase 100 mg, 10 mg bolus plus 50 mg in hour 1 and 40 mg in hour 2 through a peripheral vein followed by intravenous heparin; or (2) heparin infusion 1750 IU/h for 7–10 days, adjustment of the rate of heparin infusion was though activated partial thromboplastin time two to three times the mean normal.

A second pulmonary angiography with measurement of pulmonary artery pressures, was performed at the end of the 2-h infusion of alteplase or heparin. Pulmonary angiography was evaluated by the Miller index. This index yields score of 0–34 (34 represents the sum of a maximal score of 16 for the thrombus and of 18 for the peripheral perfusion defects). Angiographies were evaluated separately by three investigators who had no knowledge of treatment allocation and were not aware of the chronologic sequence of the two angiographic studies. When possible, perfusion lung scans were performed by conventional methods at 7 and 30 days. Anterior, posterior, lateral, and oblique projections were obtained. Lung scan was evaluated by two physicians who did not know the angiographic results. Perfusion impairment was assessed by giving score of 1 to each unperfused segment and 0.5 to each poorly or partially perfused segment [11].

Major bleeding definition: intracerebral hemorrhage confirmed by computed tomography, or bleeding requiring transfusion of one or more units of blood. Also, partial thromboplastin time, prothrombin time, platelet count, D-dimer and, plasminogen, and fibrinogen were obtained.

Results

A total of 36 patients had full inclusion criteria, 20 were assigned to rt-PA group and 16 to heparin group. Demographic data, distribution of risk factors and the time from the onset of symptoms of PE to the beginning of treatment were homogeneous in both groups. Pulmonary angiographic index and mean pulmonary artery pressure values were greater in the rt-PA group, but only the basal pulmonary artery pressure was significantly ($p<0.05$) higher in this group. In patients who underwent fibrinolytic treatment, at the end of the 2-h infusion, the Miller total score decreased (from 28.3 ± 2.9 to 24.8 ± 5.2) in the heparin group this value did not change (from 25.3 ± 5.3 to 25.2 ± 5.4) [11].

Nested analysis of variance showed significant differences between the treatments in right, left and total lung scores. In rt-PA group 17 of 20 patients had a decrease in the index of vascular obstruction; in heparin group, angiograms indicated clot lysis in 4 of 16 patients; the mean pulmonary artery pressure decreased significantly in the rt-PA group ($p<0.01$) whereas it increased significantly in the heparin group ($p<0.01$). Cardiac index increased in the rt-PA group from 2.1 to 2.4 L/min ($p<0.01$) but remained without any changes (2.9 L/min) in heparin group. Although the increase in pulmonary artery oxygen was more evident after thrombolysis, there was no significant difference between the two groups [11].

Regarding bleeding episodes, 14 patients in group rt-PA had bleeding complications; 3 of them were major bleeding (2 with hemoglobin decreases 25 g/dL); in heparin group 6 of 16 patients had a bleeding episode that was classified as a major complication in two. No significant difference between the two groups was found in the number of patients with bleeding events. Minor bleeding events: Hematomas at the site of catheter insertion were the most frequent in both groups (9 in alteplase and 4 in heparin group) [11].

Two women in rt-PA group died. The first was a 71 year-old diabetic patient with hypertension who died on day 6 of cardiac arrest after an intracerebral hemorrhage. The second was a 62 year-old woman who had cardiac tamponade due to right ventricular perforation during angiography; 19 days later, she died of acute renal failure. The pericardial hemorrhage that occurred in 3 of 36 patients (0 rt-PA group and 3 in the heparin group) was secondary to the use of stiff catheters 7 F. In heparin group, a 74-year-old woman died of recurrent PE 2-days after randomization, she had no-therapeutic heparin effect. Two additional patients in heparin group had PE recurrence after 6 h and on day 8, respectively. One had a partial heparin effect before the episode. The second had a lung scan on day 8 without any change in perfusion from baseline; this patient also had nontherapeutic anticoagulant effect despite the administration of oral anticoagulant agents [11].

On day 13, one patient in rt-PA group had PE recurrence documented by a positive lung scan. The secondary prevention anticoagulation at that time was inadequate according the prothrombin time (63 %). In one woman treated with alteplase, thrombosis involving femoral veins bilaterally and extending to the inferior vena cava was diagnosed by Doppler echocardiography. On the same day, she had disseminated intravascular coagulation. Standard therapy with intravenous antithrombin III was started; patient recovered and was discharged 2 months later [11]. Although in both groups, hematocrit significantly decreased 24 h after the start of treatment, no difference was observed between two groups. In rt-PA group, 2 patients had decrease of hemoglobin >5 g/dL [11].

Activated partial thromboplastin time increased significantly in both groups 2 h after rt-PA or heparin infusion, and was still higher at 24 h. At 2 h, by the end of the lytic infusion, prothrombin time had a statistically significant decrease in comparison with baseline values, and then rose to the previous levels 24 h after treatment. In heparin group no major changes in this variable were observed. Plasma fibrinogen decreased significantly (56 %) at the end of alteplase infusion, but no decrease was observed after 2 h of heparin infusion. Plasma fragment D-dimers, indicators of the occurrence of a clot lysis, doubled after alteplase treatment, but did not change in patients allocated to heparin. In contrast to heparin, alteplase induced a significant decrease in free circulating plasminogen (70 %) [11].

Lessons Learned from This Study

The results confirm that alteplase leads to greater lysis of pulmonary clots compared to heparin, as indicated by changes in the Miller score index. On admission, patients allocated to thrombolysis were in more critical condition than those assigned to heparin. In rt-PA group, the baseline pulmonary angiograms showed greater involvement of pulmonary vessels, responsible for a higher Miller index score, and greater hemodynamic impairment evidenced by the higher pulmonary artery pressure. Alteplase induced rapid lysis of the thrombi, confirmed by the 2-h pulmonary angiograms and by hemocoagulative variables. However, the differences between two groups tended to narrow during the first week, as indicated by the perfusion lung scans, probably as consequence of the endogenous fibrinolysis. The 12 % decrease of the Miller angiographic index after 2-h infusion of 100 mg of alteplase in this trial is comparable with the 12 % decrease observed in previous evidence after a 2-h infusion of 50 mg of alteplase [11].

In terms of bleeding complications, the frequency was higher in the rt-PA plus heparin group than in heparin-alone group. However, high dose of intravenous heparin adopted in this study (10,000 IU bolus and 1750 IU/h) together with the invasive procedure might have increased the risk of frequency of bleeding episodes. Major bleeding occurred in 15 % of the cases in rt-PA group. Considering the small number of PE patients in this study, the real risk of intracranial hemorrhage has still to be determinated. Considerations for futures studies with alteplase regimen for PE treatment included the need to optimize dose, whether fixed or adjusted for body weight, and the rate of infusion [11].

Although the risk of bleeding complications during and after treatment with alteplase should not be minimized, alteplase did result in more effective reperfusion. Therefore, a fibrinolytic treatment should be considered for the more compromised PE patients. The less critically ill patients should probably receive standard heparin therapy until new dosage regimens of thromboembolytic agents prove safety. Eventually, large prospective trials comparing alteplase and heparin are required to balance mortality, PE recurrence and other adverse clinical events against the hemorrhagic risk. Finally, alteplase resulted in a greater and faster improvement of the angiographic and hemodynamic variables compared with heparin. However, the high frequency of bleeding observed in rt-PA group suggests that patients should be carefully selected before thrombolytic therapy [11].

Alteplase vs. Heparin in Acute Pulmonary Embolism: Randomized Trial Assessing Right Ventricular Function and Pulmonary Perfusion

Background

In 1986, these group of clinical investigators reported that 2–6 h recombinant human tissue-type plasminogen activator (rt-PA) infusion was rapidly effective and relatively safe in achieving angiographically proven clot lysis in acute PE. Seven PE patients—for the first time in the setting of PE and thrombolysis—were evaluated echocardiographically before and, on average, 9 h after thrombolysis, with evidence of substantial and rapid improvement in right ventricular function. However, this observation was coming from a nonrandomized study, so the improvement observed in right ventricular function might have occurred with heparin alone.

Considering this evidence, randomized trial was designed to determinate, whether thrombolysis followed by anticoagulation could be superior to anticoagulation alone in reversing echocardiographic evidence of right ventricular dysfunction associated with PE. Two subsidiary questions were: does thrombolysis improve pulmonary tissue perfusion more rapidly than does heparin alone? and does it more effectively lower the incidence of clinically suspected recurrent PE? [12].

Methodology

Study included patients aged 18 years or more who presented with symptoms or signs of PE within 14 days. PE was proved by high probability V/Q lung scans and/or pulmonary angiograms within 24 h of randomization. High probability lung scans definition: two or more segmental or greater perfusion defects in the presence of normal ventilation. The decision of high probability V/Q lung scan was made locally at the participating hospital. Patients with abnormal but not high probability scans were also eligible to be screened for the trial if angiograms demonstrated pulmonary arterial thrombus. All patients had a baseline echocardiogram that was considered technically adequate at the local participating hospital [12].

Exclusion criteria: major internal bleeding within previous 6 months; intracranial or intraspinal disease; operation or biopsy in the preceding 10 days (or open heart surgery within 14 days); occult blood in stool; hematocrit <28 % or platelet count <100,000/μL; blood pressure >200 mmHg systolic or >110 mmHg diastolic; severe impairment of hepatic function; pregnancy; active infective endocarditis; hemorrhagic retinopathy; or any concurrent condition considered to limit survival to within 1 month. Follow-up echocardiography was at 3 and 24 h and follow-up perfusion lung scans were done 24 h after the start of therapy [12].

One hundred and one patients were included, and rt-PA dose was infused at doses of 100 mg by peripheral vein over 2 h (50 mg/h). Heparin was administered at a concentration of 1000 IU when the thrombin time or partial thromboplastin time (PTT) was less than twice control. Subsequently, continuous intravenous heparin was administered to achieve a target PTT of 1 1/2 to 2 1/2 times the upper limit of normal. For heparin group patients, the initial dose was 5000 units as a bolus followed by 1000 units/in as a continuous peripheral intravenous infusion; 4 h after randomization a PTT was obtained. Subsequent heparin doses were administered to achieve a target PTT of 1 1/2–2 1/2 times the upper limit of normal [12].

After the 24 h echocardiogram and perfusion lung scan were obtained. Patients received heparin for at least 5 days and were placed on oral anticoagulants. Regulation of oral anticoagulation was undertaken at local laboratories, and the target prothrombin time was 16–20 s, corresponding to an international normalized ratio of 2.0–4.0. Patients were educated about symptoms and signs of recurrent PE and were assessed between days 14 and 21 for possible recurrent PE by a physician visit or follow-up telephone call [12].

Echocardiogram and Lung Scan

Baseline, 3 and 24 h echocardiograms were performed and then were assessed by two expert echocardiographers. Echocardiographic study was acceptable when it was possible to obtain right and left ventricular sizes measurement, as well as, assessment of right ventricular wall motion from at least two views (parasternal long axis, apical four-chamber, subcostal four-chamber). Right wall motion abnormalities were classified by qualitative evaluation: (a) normal, (b) mildly (1+), (c) moderately (2+), or (d) severely (3+) hypokinetic. Tricuspid regurgitation was assessed qualitatively, by visual inspection of the size of the largest color doppler jet, as: (a) absent, (b) mild (1+), (c) moderate (2+), or (d) severe (3+). Quantitative assessment of the right ventricular cavity was by planimetry of the right ventricular end-diastolic endocardial area from the apical four clamber view. Two nuclear medicine specialists scored each lung scan with a segmental method that accounts for anterior, posterior, lateral, and oblique views [12].

Follow-up for adverse outcomes (death, recurrence, and major bleeding) included 14 days, or longer if they remained in hospital. Major hemorrhage definition: bleeding that required surgery (e.g., laparotomy for retroperitoneal bleeding) or any intracranial bleeding. Also, a decrement in hematocrit of more than 0.1 between baseline and 72 h was considered.

Results

Between November, 1988 and July, 1991, 101 patients were randomized to rt-PA plus heparin (46 patients) or heparin alone (55 patients). No difference in baseline characteristics was identified between both groups. PE was established by lung scan alone in 80 patients. Most patients had normal right ventricular function at baseline and no patient had a systolic arterial pressure less than 90 mmHg at the time of randomization; 89 patients had sets of three technically adequate echocardiograms. In 2 patients echocardiograms were not adequate or not accesibles [12].

When baseline and 24 h echocardiographic qualitative assessment of right ventricular wall movement were subsequently compared, 39 % in rt-PA group improved and 2 % had worsened, compared with 17 % improvement and 17 % worsening among those in heparin-alone group ($p=0.005$). With a general linear model procedure, rt-PA group had a decrease in right ventricular end-diastolic area during the 24 h after randomization whereas those in heparin-alone group had none ($p=0.01$). In the majority of rt-PA group a decrease in right ventricular end-diastolic area occurred during the first 3 h; 36 patients (18 rt-PA, 18 heparin alone) with baseline right ventricular hypokinesis had three serial echocardiograms that were technically adequate [12].

Among this subgroup, 89 % of the rt-PA group improved and 6 % worsened, compared with 44 % improvement and 28 % worsening among heparin-alone group ($p=0.03$). Paired perfusion lung scans in 95 patients demonstrated that, on average, more than one-third of the lung tissue was not perfused at baseline. The proportion of the lung that lacked perfusion at baseline was similar in the two groups. However, at the follow-up scan, rt-PA group had an absolute improvement in pulmonary perfusion of 14.6 % (95 % CI for difference 10.2–19.0 %) compared with 15 % (95 % CI 0–4.3 %) improvement among heparin-alone group ($p<0.0001$).

There were no fatalities other than 2 attributed to recurrent PE. No PE recurrence occurred among rt-PA group plus heparin but 5 (9 %) recurrent PE (2 fatal, 3 non-fatal) occurred within 14 days in heparin-alone group ($p=0.06$). All 5 patients presented with impaired right ventricular wall motion. They had, on average, a greater proportion of nonperfused lung (0.50) than the other patients assigned to heparin alone (0.35), but the difference was not significant ($p=0.12$). A 66-year-old woman had a nonfatal intracranial bleed as well as a fatal recurrent PE. She had fallen on her head when she initially presented with syncope; she had been randomized to receive heparin alone but was given rt-PA off protocol when syncope recurred with jugular venous distention ascribed to recurrent PE. Because of the head injury she should have been excluded from the trial and should have been considered to have a contraindication to rt-PA [12].

Four patients received blood transfusions, 3 in rt-PA group, one had a hematocrit decrement of more than 0.1 within 72 h of randomization; this was ascribed to bleeding at the groin punction site. The indication for transfusion in the other patients was for augmentation of the hematocrit, and both received 2 units of packed red blood cells. One patient in heparin-alone group had a hematocrit decrement of more than 0.1 ascribed to blood loss per rectum; this patient was not transfused [12].

Lessons Learned from This Study

The results of this important study in the field of PE and thrombolysis suggested that rt-PA regimen approved by FDA followed by heparin was associated with a greater 24 h improvement in right ventricular wall motion abnormalities than heparin alone among a population of clinical stable of PE patients [12].

Another important observation was that the changes in right ventricular wall motion abnormalities over time were very different in the two treatment groups. An unexpected finding was the worsening of right ventricular wall motion between baseline and 24 h in 17 % of heparin-alone group and 28 % of the heparin alone subgroup that presented with right ventricular hypokinesis. In terms of pulmonary perfusion differences, it substantially improved (15 %) in rt-PA patients plus heparin compared with heparin group (2 %). During the first 14 days after randomization, 5 patients assigned to heparin alone had clinically suspected recurrent PE compared with none in the rt-PA group [12].

Two recurrences were fatal and 3 nonfatal. Three of these 5 patients received thrombolysis off protocol (2 rt-PA, 1 urokinase) in an effort to improve their clinical outcome after recurrent PE. All 5 had presented initially with right ventricular hypokinesis on echocardiogram. Possibly, echocardiography can help to identify a subgroup of PE patients at high risk of adverse clinical outcomes if treated with heparin alone. Such patients would appear to be excellent candidates for thrombolysis, in the absence of contraindications. This sentence changes the concept of clinical stability in PE patients.

Additionally, in terms of pulmonary perfusion, this study was suggestive of a difference favouring rt-PA group ($p=0.06$) for this endpoint. Another important contribution was that high probability scans, in the presence of PE symptoms, could confirm PE diagnosis in patients considered to thrombolysis. And so, 80 % were treated more quickly than in UPET study [5] because angiography was needed only for abnormal but not high probability lung scans [12].

Compared with previous evidences patients recluted in this study had fewer hemorrhagic complications. This can be attributed to the fact that shorter infusion by peripheral vein was as effective and safe as infusion through a pulmonary arterial catheter, thus decreasing the time, technological requirements, and expense of utilizing thrombolysis for PE and noninvasive diagnosis. Also, this findings suggest that rapid improvement of right ventricular function and pulmonary perfusion, accomplished with thrombolytic therapy followed by heparin, can lead to a lower rate of death and recurrent PE, especially among patients who present with right ventricular hypokinesis [12].

Three possible mechanisms may be operative: thrombolysis may prevent the downhill spiral of right heart failure by "medical embolectomy," with lysis of massive pulmonary arterial thrombus; among patients with anatomically smaller PE, thrombolysis may prevent the continued release of serotonin and other neurohumoral factors which might otherwise lead to worsening pulmonary hypertension; and in theory, thrombolysis may dissolve much of the source of the thrombus in the pelvic or deep leg veins, thereby decreasing the likelihood of recurrent PE [12].

A final consideration of professor Goldhaber was the necessity to have a large randomized trial of PE thrombolysis vs. heparin alone with clinically meaningful endpoints such as death or clinically suspected recurrent PE. The study will have to include massive PE and also clinical stable patients with smaller PE for they are also at risk of recurrent PE and chronic pulmonary hypertension. After this study a new age in PE and thrombolysis starts: short alteplase infusion by peripheral vein, noninvasive diagnosis and fast workup through perfusion lung scan. Finally, considering that PE symptoms and signs, as well as mortality are closely related with right ventricular dysfunction, an echocardiographic stratification is mandatory to identify a risk subgroup: namely patients with regional o global right ventricular wall motion abnormalities in clinical stable PE patients.

Streptokinase and Heparin vs. Heparin Alone in Massive Pulmonary Embolism: A Randomized Controlled Trial

Background

In 1977, streptokinase, a first generation thrombolytic agent, was approved by the FDA in long-term peripheral vein infusion (250,000 IU/30 min and then 100,000 IU/h/24 h) for the treatment of PE. Previously, we successful use 1,500,000 IU of streptokinase over 1 h in one patient with massive PE and cardiogenic shock. We use the same streptokinase regimen successfully proved in hundred of thousand ST-elevation myocardial infarction patients to induce a fast "pharmacological embolectomy" to improve right ventricular dysfunction [13].

Also a noninvasive and fast workup was established [12]. So we undertook a randomized, controlled open-label trial to prove the efficacy and safety of high dose, short-infusion streptokinase followed by heparin vs. heparin alone in PE patients. When all four heparin-alone patients died compared with none in the streptokinase group, we terminated the trial for ethical reasons [13].

Methodology

Inclusion criteria: (a) age >15 years, (b) previously healthy patients, (c) PE diagnosis sustained by high clinical suspicion (one or more major risk factors and clinical, ECG, chest X-ray, blood gas findings), (d) PE proven by high probability V/Q lung scan, suggestive echocardiogram, or deep venous thrombosis by radiovenogram, (e) massive PE, defined as >9 obstructed segments on V/Q lung scan with or without cardiogenic shock (systolic BP <90 mmHg), (f) <9 obstructed segments on V/Q lung scan but with right ventricular dysfunction and/or extensive deep venous thrombosis, and (g) symptoms or signs of PE within 14 days after the onset of symptoms [13].

Exclusion criteria (a) previous PE, (b) patients with <3 segmental defects on V/Q lung scan, with normal echocardiogram and without deep venous thrombosis, and (c) absolute contraindication for thrombolytic therapy: active or recent hemorrhage, intracranial disease, head trauma, neurologic or major surgery within previous 6 weeks, or any concurrent condition considered to limit survival to a few months. Patients were randomized to streptokinase followed by heparin or to heparin alone [13].

Streptokinase group received 1,500,000 IU of SK over 1 h by peripheral vein, followed by a bolus of 10,000 U of heparin and then a constant infusion of 1000 U/h of heparin titrated to obtain a partial thromboplastin time of 2–2.5 times control. The heparin group followed the same regimen, but without streptokinase. In the survivors of the acute phase, on the fifth day heparin was overlapped with coumadin and was stopped on day 7. Patients were kept on coumadin, aiming for an INR of 2.0–3.0 for 3 months or more, depending on the presence of major risk factors [13].

V/Q lung scans, echocardiograms, and radionuclide venograms V/Q lung scans were performed in the anterior, posterior, lateral, and oblique views. Echocardiograms required measurements of right and left ventricular size and motion, ejection fraction, abnormal septal position, paradoxical systolic motion, and tricuspid and/ or pulmonary regurgitation. Parasternal long axis, apical four-chamber, and subcostal four-chamber views were performed. Pulmonary arterial pressure was determined with the modified Bernoulli formula. Static and dynamic venograms with 99 technetium labeled albumin macroaggregates were performed [13].

Results

At the beginning of the study 8 patients were enrolled, 4 in each group, all with massive PE and cardiogenic shock. The mortality in the streptokinase group was 0 % compared with 100 % ($p=0.02$) in the heparin group. Therefore, after discussion with the ethics committee the trial was terminated. These 8 patients had similar baseline characteristics, except in time elapsed from onset of symptoms of the first event of PE before randomization, which occurred by chance. Patients in the streptokinase group arrived at the Emergency Department from 1 to 4 h after the onset of symptoms of PE, whereas patients in the heparin group had a first PE in other hospitals. In this first pulmonary event, they had minor PE in one, two, two and three occluded segments on V/Q lung scan, with hemodynamic stability, without any evidence of acute pulmonary arterial hypertension, and with therapeutic PTTs, respectively. They were asymptomatic and suddenly had recurrences of massive PE, with severe respiratory failure, and were transferred to our hospital at 2–4 h after the onset of symptoms of a new event. The time that elapsed from the onset of cardiogenic shock was comparable in both groups [13].

All patients had similar clinical characteristics and echocardiographic abnormalities. Patients who were randomized to receive streptokinase plus heparin improved their clinical and echocardiographic findings in the first hour after treatment.

The V/Q lung scans post-thrombolytic therapy showed three, four, four, and five segment perfusion defects, respectively, and DVT was proved. All patients in the heparin group died despite endotracheal intubation, mechanical ventilation, and Swan-Ganz catheterization. Necropsy was performed in 3 patients; all had massive PE, and in both macroscopically and histologically right ventricle myocardial infarction was found; 2 were subendocardial and one was transmural myocardial infarction, in all cases without significant coronary arterial obstruction. All the 4 patients who lived were discharged in good condition. After a 2 year follow-up, all were in functional class I, without pulmonary arterial hypertension and without recurrent PE [13].

Lessons Learned from This Study

We present the first randomized clinical trial that demonstrated a decreased mortality rate with thrombolysis compared with heparin alone among patients with massive PE and cardiogenic shock. Because of their severely ill clinical condition, the diagnosis of PE in the acute phase was sustained by high clinical suspicion and only a bedside echocardiogram. Later on, diagnosis of PE was confirmed by means of high probability V/Q lung scans and proven deep venous thrombosis in the streptokinase group and through a high probability V/Q lung scan in 2 patients of the heparin group and by necropsy in three of them [13].

On admission, the baseline clinical and echocardiographic data showed severe right ventricular dysfunction and cardiogenic shock. However, after treatment patients who received streptokinase plus heparin had earlier reversal of hemodynamic disturbances than patients who received only heparin, who deteriorated and died. We did not observe major or minor hemorrhagic complications, possibly due to the patients' young age, because the streptokinase was administered through a peripheral vein, and because of a diagnostic strategy that avoided vascular punction [13].

In our cases, the role of echocardiography was to establish a bedside diagnosis of massive PE, to ascertain the severity of pulmonary arterial hypertension, and to document abnormalities of motion and geometry of the right ventricle. The findings in the necropsy studies have been previously reported and suggest that right ventricular myocardial infarction could cause irreversible right ventricular dysfunction and mortality. The patients who received thrombolysis had reductions in pulmonary arterial hypertension, right ventricular dysfunction, and preservation of ventricular myocardial viability [13].

Rapid reversal of right ventricular failure, previously noted in rt-PA patients when compared with heparin-alone patients [12], is the likely mechanism that prevented death from acute PE. There were two limitations of this study: (1) the small sample size and (2) the gross imbalance in the onset of the first PE; however, at that moment patients in the heparin group did not have right ventricular dysfunction. Previously to massive PE, patients had minor PE. The observations from this randomized, controlled clinical trial indicate that among patients with massive PE and cardiogenic shock, prompt administration of thrombolytic therapy can be lifesaving when compared with heparin alone. Our results reproduced previous observations from professor Goldhaber [12] as noninvasive and fast-track diagnosis reducing bleeding complications through avoid major venous punctions. In addition, identifying right ventricular dysfunction by echocardiography marks the beginning of a new stratification era in PE [13].

Randomized Control Trials from 2000 to 2014 Years: Heparin Plus Alteplase Compared with Heparin Alone in Patients with Submassive Pulmonary Embolism—MAPET-3 Trial

Background

Considering previous evidences thrombolysis was recognized as therapeutic option for patients with acute massive PE and hemodynamic instability or cardiogenic shock [13]. In contrast, the effect of thrombolytic agents on the outcome of clinically stable patients with submassive pulmonary embolism had been debated for decades. Professor Konstantinides considered several factors contributing the ongoing controversy: first, the lack of a large, randomized study assessing clinical end points, second, the risk of serious hemorrhage associated with thrombolytic therapy, and finally, the fact that patients with clinical stability may gradually improve with heparin alone [14].

The clinical data available in this time underscore the need to identify patients in whom thrombolysis may have a favorable risk–benefit ratio. Two large, multicenter registries reported that patients with right ventricular dysfunction secondary to PE had increased rates of in-hospital death, even in the absence of arterial hypotension or shock. These registries also suggested that early thrombolytic therapy might favorably affect the prognosis of these patients. Under these evidence, authors conducted a randomized, placebo-controlled trial to compare the effects of rt-PA, alteplase plus heparin with heparin alone on the outcome of acute submassive PE patients. Although, patients with pulmonary hypertension, right ventricular dysfunction, or both, were considered, those with clinical instability were excluded [14].

Methodology

The study was designed as a prospective, randomized, double-blind, placebo-controlled trial. Patients with PE had to fulfill at least one of the following criteria; right ventricular dysfunction detected by echocardiogram defined as right ventricular enlargement combined with loss of inspiratory collapse of the inferior vena cava, without left ventricular or mitral-valve disease; pulmonary artery hypertension, defined as a tricuspid regurgitant jet velocity greater than 2.8 m/s, followed by confirmation of PE (V/Q lung scan, spiral computed tomography or pulmonary angiography); precapillary pulmonary hypertension diagnosed based on catheterization of the right side of the heart, defined as a mean pulmonary artery pressure above 20 mmHg and a pulmonary capillary wedge pressure below 18 mmHg, followed by confirmation of PE; or new electrocardiographic signs of right ventricular strain (defined as complete or incomplete right bundle-branch block, S waves in lead I combined with Q waves in lead III, or inverted T waves in precordial leads V1, V2, and V3), followed by confirmation of PE [14].

Exclusion criteria: one or more of the following: age >80 years; clinical instability, defined as persistent arterial hypotension (i.e., systolic pressure <90 mmHg), with or without signs of cardiogenic shock; onset of symptoms more than 96 h before diagnosis; thrombolytic treatment, major surgery, or biopsy within the preceding 7 days; major trauma within the preceding 10 days; stroke, transient ischemic attack, craniocerebral trauma, or neurologic surgery within the preceding 6 months; gastrointestinal bleeding within the preceding 3 months; uncontrolled hypertension; a known bleeding disorder; known inability to tolerate alteplase; known diabetic retinopathy; current therapy with an oral anticoagulant; current pregnancy or lactation; a life expectancy of less than 6 months because of underlying disease; or planned use of thrombolytic agents for extensive deep vein thrombosis [14].

Patients with high clinical suspicion to have acute submassive PE received an intravenous bolus of 5000 U of unfractionated heparin before undergoing further diagnostic workup. Patients enrolled in the study were randomized to receive 100 mg of rtPA, alteplase as a 10 mg bolus, followed by a 90 mg intravenous infusion over a period of 2 h plus heparin or placebo plus heparin alone. Both groups received an intravenous infusion of unfractionated heparin, starting at a rate of 1000 U/h, with infusion doses adjusted to maintain partial thromboplastin time at 2.0–2.5 times upper limit of normal. Measurements of the activated partial thromboplastin time were performed at 6-h intervals on day 1 after randomization and at 12-h intervals thereafter for at least 4 days. Overlapping oral anticoagulant therapy was started on day 3 after randomization, and the dosage was adjusted to maintain an INR 2.5–3.5 [14].

Patients were evaluated at the end of their hospital stay or on day 30 after randomization, whichever occurred first. The primary end point was in-hospital death or clinical deterioration that required an escalation of treatment after the infusion of alteplase or placebo was terminated. Escalation definition: infusion of a catecholamine by persistent arterial hypotension or shock (except for dopamine infused at a rate no more than 5 μg per kilogram of body weight per minute); secondary, or "rescue," thrombolysis (for one of the following indications: worsening clinical symptoms, particularly dyspnea, or worsening respiratory failure due to PE; arterial hypotension or shock; and persistent or worsening pulmonary hypertension or right ventricular dysfunction detected by echocardiography or right heart catheterization); endotracheal intubation; cardiopulmonary resuscitation; and emergency surgical embolectomy or thrombus fragmentation by catheter [14].

Secondary end points: recurrent PE, major bleeding, and ischemic stroke. Recurrence of PE was confirmed by V/Q lung scan, spiral CT, or pulmonary angiography. Major bleeding was defined as fatal bleeding, hemorrhagic stroke, or a drop in the hemoglobin concentration by at least 4 g/dL, with or without the need for red-cell transfusion. Hemorrhagic or ischemic stroke was confirmed by CT or magnetic resonance imaging [14].

Results

Between September 1997 and August 2001 at 49 centers in Germany 256 patients were randomized; 118 were assigned to the alteplase plus heparin group and 138 to the placebo plus heparin group. Both groups were well matched in relation to major clinical characteristics at base line. There were no significant differences in systolic or diastolic blood pressure, heart rate, or the severity of dyspnea or arterial hypoxemia. Right heart catheterization was performed in 43 patients, 19 (16 %) in the alteplase plus heparin and 24 (17 %) in the placebo plus heparin group [14].

There were no significant differences between both groups regarding pulmonary artery pressures (systolic: 55.2 ± 14.0 mmHg in alteplase plus heparin group and 60.42 ± 15.9 mmHg in placebo plus heparin group; diastolic: 21.9 ± 8.0 and 23.9 ± 8.9 mmHg, and mean: 34.0 ± 8.5 and 36.1 ± 10.6 mmHg, respectively). Echocardiography was performed in 106 of alteplase plus heparin group (90 %), and 129 of those assigned to receive placebo plus heparin (94 %). The incidence of right ventricular dysfunction was almost identical in both. Doppler echocardiography showed that the mean tricuspid regurgitant jet velocity was elevated in the two groups (3.23 ± 0.66 m/s in the alteplase plus heparin group, and 3.31 ± 0.78 m/s in placebo plus heparin group) [14].

In-hospital stay was 16.7 ± 8.4 days (range, 2–70), and the mortality rate was low in both treatment groups: 4 patients died in alteplase plus heparin group, 2 from PE and 2 from underlying disease. In placebo plus heparin group, 3 patients died, 2 from PE and 1 from a bleeding complication. But despite this similarity in mortality, the rate of treatment escalation due to clinical deterioration was much higher in the placebo plus heparin group compared with alteplase plus heparin group [14].

Rescue thrombolysis was performed roughly three times in both groups. In placebo plus heparin group, this indication was driven by cardiogenic shock (4 patients), by arterial hypotension requiring catecholamine infusion (4 patients), and due to worsening symptoms and respiratory failure (in 24 patients, 3 of whom underwent endotracheal intubation and mechanical ventilation). In alteplase plus heparin group, 9 patients required additional thrombolysis, one because of arterial hypotension and the remaining 8 because worsening symptoms; one of these latter patients underwent endotracheal intubation [14].

Overall, the incidence of death or treatment escalation was significantly greater in placebo plus heparin group (34 patients, 25 %) compared to alteplase plus heparin group (13 patients, 11 %, $p = 0.006$). Additionally, the probability of 30-day event-free survival was significantly higher in alteplase plus heparin group than in those in placebo plus heparin treatment ($p = 0.005$). Further analysis using proportional-hazards model confirmed that treatment with placebo plus heparin predicted an unfavorable in-hospital outcome: the relative risk of the primary end point with placebo plus heparin as compared with alteplase plus heparin was 2.63 ($p=0.006$) [14].

The incidence of recurrent PE was low in both treatment groups. However, its incidence may have been underestimated because of the relatively strict criteria for confirmation of recurrent thromboembolic events. Bleeding complications were uncommon, and the incidence of bleeding was not higher in the alteplase plus heparin group compared with placebo plus heparin treatment. In particular, there was only one fatal bleeding episode in the placebo plus heparin group, and there were no hemorrhagic strokes. Minor symptoms that may have been related to the study medication were reported in 72 patients in alteplase plus heparin group (61 %) and in 78 patients in the placebo plus heparin group (57 %) ($p=0.55$), and they did not result in discontinuation of treatment or breaking of the randomization code [14].

Lessons Learned from This Study

Previous results to this study had convincingly demonstrated the efficacy of thrombolytic agents to resolve pulmonary emboli improving pulmonary perfusion and right ventricular function. Therefore, thrombolytic agents were recommended for the treatment of massive PE. However, the efficacy of thrombolytic agents in the treatment of submassive PE had remained unclear. The most important issue was to identify PE patients in whose the benefit of thrombolysis may outweigh risks of bleeding complications; a large-scale clinical trial was an unmet task. MAPET-3 study was designed to address these issues directly. The results indicated that alteplase plus heparin, improved the clinical course of clinically stable patients with acute submassive PE, with a low incidence of major hemorrhagic complications [14].

Another important observation was that clinical course and prognosis of acute PE patients widely vary, depending on their clinical and hemodynamic status at the time of diagnosis. Considering that right ventricular dysfunction have been identified as a predictor of poor outcome, investigators in MAPET-3 trial focused on patients with evidence of pulmonary hypertension, right ventricular dysfunction, or both conditions. Patients with persistent arterial hypotension or shock resulting from overt right ventricular failure were excluded since investigators considered that withholding thrombolytic therapy would be unethical in this subset [14].

Survival analysis showed that the probability of event-free survival during in-hospital stay was significantly lower in placebo plus heparin group compared with alteplase plus heparin group. Although in-hospital mortality rate was similar in the both groups, the incidence of clinical deterioration requiring escalation of treatment was higher in the placebo plus heparin group. Secondary or rescue thrombolysis was needed three times more frequently in placebo plus heparin group. This higher incidence may be explained by bias since investigators favored thrombolytic therapy [14].

Therefore, it seems reasonable to assume that delayed resolution or lack of resolution or recurrence of PE with heparin alone resulted in persistence or deterioration of pulmonary hypertension and right-sided heart failure. Another interesting observation was the low in-hospital mortality rate in both groups, a finding maybe explained by a closer monitoring and higher alertness in a randomized controlled trial, leading to prompt response to early signs of clinical deterioration. The very low rates of major bleeding complications could be explained by the noninvasive diagnosis approach. Finally, this randomized, double-blind, placebo-controlled trial showed that treatment with alteplase plus heparin may improve the clinical course of patients with acute submassive PE, in particular, that such treatment may prevent further clinical or hemodynamic deterioration requiring the escalation of treatment during the hospital stay. On the basis of these data, authors considered that indications for thrombolysis, which are currently limited to massive PE, can be extended to include submassive PE characterized by right ventricular dysfunction in a clinically stable patient [14].

Bolus Tenecteplase for Right Ventricle Dysfunction in Hemodynamically Stable Patients with Pulmonary Embolism: TIPES Study

Background

Right ventricular dysfunction assessed by echocardiography has close relationship with adverse in-hospital outcome in patients with acute PE, reaching hospital mortality ranges from 5 to 17 %, significantly higher than in patients without right ventricular dysfunction. Then right ventricular dysfunction maintains its prognostic value in clinically stable PE patients. Thrombolytic treatment was recommended for PE patients with shock or sustained hypotension. Clinical benefit of thrombolytic treatment in clinically stable patients with PE and right ventricular dysfunction remains to be defined [15].

In TIPES study, a new fibrinolytic agent, tenecteplase, or TNK-t-PA, with better pharmacokinetic characteristics was used. This genetically engineered variant of the alteplase (recombinant tissue-type plasminogen activator) molecule offers a number of pharmacological advantages such as an increased plasma half-life, improved resistance to plasminogen activator inhibitor-1, and high thrombolytic potency. Additionally, it can be delivered as a single intravenous bolus injection, with a more practical administration compared to the 2-h alteplase infusion [15].

In ASSENT-2, a large randomized trial which included 16,949 ST-elevation myocardial infarction patients, tenecteplase was found to be equivalent with alteplase in terms of mortality reduction, and also appeared to be associated with a lower risk of major bleeding. Following a number of case reports and small series proving the efficacy and safety of the molecule in PE patients, this study of Becattini and Agnelly was the first randomized, double-blind placebo-controlled study aimed at assessing the effect of TNK-t-PA on right ventricular dysfunction in clinically stable PE patients [16].

Methodology

TIPES study was a phase II, multicenter, double-blind, placebo-controlled study performed in 15 centers in Italy. Inclusion criteria: consecutive patients, aged between 18 and 85 years, with an objective diagnosis of PE, and (1) onset of symptoms <10 days, (2) normal blood pressure (systolic blood pressure ≥100 mmHg), and (3) right ventricular dysfunction at echocardiography performed within 24 h from PE diagnosis.

Diagnosis was performed by multidetector CT-scan, pulmonary angiography, or lung scan (either high probability or intermediate probability associated to confirmed deep venous thrombosis). Exclusion: chronic pulmonary hypertension, severe COPD, or systemic hypertension (systolic blood pressure >180 mmHg and/or diastolic blood pressure >110 mmHg). Clinically relevant bleeding within the last 6 months or hemorrhagic diathesis, active peptic ulcer, arterial aneurysm, or arterial/venous malformation, cancer at increased risk for bleeding, history of stroke, and intracranial or spinal surgery [15].

Additional exclusion criteria: Major surgery, biopsy or trauma in the 2 months preceding the admission, if they had received therapeutic doses of heparin (unfractionated or low-molecular-weight heparin) >72 h prior to randomization, or thrombolytic treatment within the previous 4 days or glycoprotein IIb/IIIa antagonists within the preceding 7 days; if they were on oral anticoagulation or had prolonged cardiopulmonary resuscitation (>10 min) in the last 2 weeks. Also severe hepatic or renal failure and subacute bacterial endocarditis. Women were excluded in case of pregnancy, lactation, or delivery in the 30 days before randomization [15].

Eligible patients with objectively confirmed acute PE were randomized in a 1:1 ratio to receive TNK-t-PA or placebo as an intravenous single-bolus injection. Tenecteplase was given as an intravenous weight adjusted bolus (given over 5 s) at a dose ranging from 30 to 50 mg, with a 5 mg step every 10 kg from <60 to ≥90 kg. This regimen was currently recommended for the treatment of acute myocardial infarction. Bolus of TNK-t-PA or placebo were scheduled to be given within 6 h from baseline echocardiography [15].

All patients received unfractionated heparin (80 IU/kg intravenous bolus, followed by an infusion of 18 IU/kg/h), with a maximum bolus dose of 5000 IU (4000 IU for patients with body weight <67 kg). Heparin dose was adjusted to achieve and maintain the activated partial thromboplastin time at 2.0–2.5 times control. Vitamin K antagonists were started preferably on the same day of study treatment administration or as soon as possible. Heparin was continued until the INR was in therapeutic range (2.0–3.0) in 2 consecutive days. For patients already on heparin treatment at the time of inclusion in the study, bolus administration was omitted [15].

Right ventricular dysfunction was defined as right/left ventricle end-diastolic dimension ratio >1 in apical four-chamber view and/or >0.7 in parasternal long axis, in the absence of right ventricle hypertrophy. Echocardiography was scheduled to be repeated 24 h and 7 days after study treatment administration. Echocardiograms should be electrocardiogram-gated to allow end-diastolic diameter measurement on the R wave. Baseline, 24-h and 7-day echocardiography had to be recorded for central blinded adjudication [15].

Primary efficacy endpoint was right ventricular dysfunction reduction on at echocardiography performed 24 h after randomization. The secondary study endpoints were: reduction of right ventricular dysfunction at 7 days from randomization or at hospital discharge (whichever came first); clinical deterioration requiring escalation of treatment within 7 days or before discharge (whichever came first); PE recurrence or death at 30 days from randomization. Clinical deterioration was defined as one or more among the following: catecholamine infusion for sustained hypotension or shock, endotracheal intubation, thrombolytic treatment, cardiopulmonary resuscitation, emergency surgical embolectomy or catheter fragmentation [15].

Clinical suspicion of PE recurrence had to be objectively confirmed by the presence of at least one of the following: (a) a new filling defect revealed by pulmonary angiography or spiral computed tomography; (b) a new V/Q lung scan high probability perfusion defect; (c) sudden otherwise unexplained death. Major bleedings occurring within 7 days from randomization or before discharge (if this occurred earlier) and serious adverse events were considered as safety study endpoints. Major bleeding definition: if it was fatal, intracranial, required transfusions or intervention for hemodynamic deterioration. All bleeding episodes not fulfilling criteria for major bleeding were considered as minor [15].

Results

Overall, 58 patients were included in the study, 28 in tenecteplase plus heparin group and 30 in placebo plus heparin group. Patients assigned to TNK-t-PA plus heparin group were older than those assigned to placebo plus heparin group (72.1 ± 1.2 and 64.5 ± 2.5, respectively $p=0.01$). Heart rate at randomization was lower in patients assigned to TNK-t-PA plus heparin than in placebo plus heparin group ($p=0.04$). The two groups were well matched with regard to other major clinical features at randomization. Clinical presentation was similar in the two groups [15].

All patients had baseline and 24 h echocardiography. Median time between baseline echocardiography and study treatment administration was 70 min (range 10–300 min), with no significant difference between both treatment groups. Baseline and 24 h echocardiograms were available for central reading in 53 patients (recording not available for central reading in 4 patients and not evaluable in 1), and 7-day echocardiograms in 46 patients. Both baseline and 24-h apical four-chamber views were evaluable in 51 patients (23 randomized to tenecteplase plus heparin and 28 randomized to placebo plus heparin) [15].

Both baseline and 24-h parasternal long axis or subcostal four-chamber views were available for central adjudication in 43 patients (19 randomized to TNK-t-PA plus heparin and 24 randomized to placebo plus heparin). Patients with apical four-chamber views were included in the analysis of the primary endpoint. The mean right ventricle end-diastolic dimension was similar in the two treatment groups at baseline echocardiography (49 ± 1.60 and 47 ± 1.71 mm in TNK-t-PA plus heparin and placebo plus heparin patients, respectively), as it was the right/left ventricle end-diastolic dimension ratio (1.36 ± 0.05 and 1.32 ± 0.03 in TNK-t-PA plus heparin and placebo plus heparin groups). Right ventricle end-diastolic dimension and right/left end-diastolic dimension ratio at 24 h were significantly reduced in patients receiving thrombolysis compared with heparin alone [15].

The mean absolute reduction of the right/left ventricle end-diastolic dimension ratio at 24 h after study drug administration was 0.31 ± 0.08 in patients randomized to TNK-t-PA plus heparin compared to 0.10 ± 0.07 in placebo plus heparin group ($p = 0.04$). The analysis of the time course of right/left end-diastolic dimension ratio during the 7 day study period showed a significant reduction in TNK-t-PA plus heparin group in comparison with placebo plus heparin patients ($p = 0.043$). The mean absolute reduction of the right/left ventricle end-diastolic dimension ratio evaluated at 7 days after randomization was 0.47 ± 0.07 in thrombolysis group and 0.34 ± 0.05 in control group (p = ns) [15].

One patient who received placebo plus heparin had clinical deterioration leading to cardiopulmonary resuscitation on day 3 after treatment. Although PE recurrence was suspected, it was not confirmed. Two patients had symptomatic recurrent PE: one TNK-t-PA plus heparin patient at day 3 and 1 placebo plus heparin patient at day 9. Recurrent PE was confirmed by CT angiography or by perfusion lung scan. One patient died within 30 days from randomization. This event occurred in a 64 year-old woman randomized to placebo plus heparin and she died at day 5. Death was attributed to acute myocardial infarction; necropsy was not performed. There were the only clinical events related with recurrence or death occurred within 30 days [15].

Overall, 3 patients had a major nonfatal bleeding. A 73-year-old man in TNK-t-PA plus heparin group had neurological symptoms starting at day 5 after treatment due to intracerebral bleeding confirmed by cerebral CT. Patient fully recovered after 6 months. A 69-year-old man had major gastrointestinal bleeding at 12 h after TNK-t-PA bolus plus heparin administration which required hemodynamic support, transfusions and vena cava filter insertion. Patient had a metastatic prostatic cancer. In placebo plus heparin group, a 67 year-old woman suffered a large intra-abdominal hematoma with compression of the urinary bladder at day 6 after treatment as shown by abdominal CT and required multiple transfusions. Both patients who bled after day 1 had supra therapeutic prolongation of the aPTT (>100 s in repeated evaluations) related to heparin overdosing. At the time of bleeding, both had started warfarin and their INR had reached therapeutic levels. In TNK-t-PA plus heparin group, 13 patients had minor bleedings as compared to one patient in placebo plus heparin group. Minor bleedings were mainly cutaneous hematoma (8 patients). Minor epistaxis occurred in 2 patients, gum bleeding, hematuria and positive stool blood in one patient each [15].

Lessons Learned from This Study

Previously to TIPES study, in the setting of PE, TNK-t-PA was limited to case reports and cohort series. Overall, these paper reports on 22 patients, 12 of them had clinical instability. So, this was the first randomized study in acute PE patients showing the feasibility and safety of this third-generation thrombolytic agent. Additionally, the findings suggest that TNK-t-PA could be used in acute PE patients. Considering the lack of specific data, the dose schedule for tenecteplase was retained from ST-elevation myocardial infarction patients [15].

The results of TIPES study suggesting that TNK-t-PA plus heparin is more effective than heparin alone in obtaining an early reduction of right ventricular dysfunction in clinically stable acute PE patients. These results are consistent with those seen with other thrombolytic agents that were more effective than heparin in achieving a rapid improvement of pulmonary perfusion and regression of right ventricular dysfunction. As with other thrombolytic agents, the advantage is shown by TNK-t-PA at 24 h decreases after 7 days.

As right ventricular dysfunction at echocardiography have been shown to be a predictor of adverse outcome regardless of blood pressure at presentation, authors assessed the efficacy of tenecteplase by measuring its effect on right ventricular dysfunction. A limitation of this study was the need for recording echocardiograms, which required dedicated operators around the clock and contributed to make study enrolment slower than expected and was a main limit for study enrolment and one of the main points when deciding to early terminate the study [15].

Given the benefit from TNK-t-PA observed in patients without clinical instability but with moderately-severe right ventricular dysfunction, Becattini and Agnelli considered that according previous evidence and current guidelines, it was possible that the combination of right ventricular dysfunction by echocardiogram plus troponin expression would allow the identification of a subgroup of clinical stable acute PE patients at particularly high risk of mortality and clinical deterioration. Considering this a correct hypothesis, patients with right ventricle dysfunction (hypokinesis) and acute cellular injury (troponin) could achieve a clearer net clinical benefit from TNK-t-PA than the population included in TIPES study [15].

This hypothesis has been evaluated in a randomized clinical trial (PEITHO) [15]. However, an important limitation was that troponin expression is observed in only 30 % of cases in right ventricular dysfunction (with or without hypokinesis) PE patients with severe pulmonary hypertension (systolic pulmonary pressure >50 mmHg by echocardiography). So, an important number of PE patients with right ventricular dysfunction and severe pulmonary hypertension with or without hypokinesis, will not have troponin expression. Possibly, a biomarker of ventricular dysfunction, brain natriuretic peptide type-B, has to be considered as well [15].

Another important evidence coming from TIPES study was the intravenous anticoagulant strategy. Unfractionated heparin was given without discontinuation close to the TNK-t-PA bolus and continued for at least 48 h after bolus. The absence of discontinuation of unfractionated heparin treatment during the infusion of thrombolytic agents established a difference among TIPES and previous trials in patients with PE. Some regulatory agencies recommend to discontinue intravenous heparin infusion during 2-h alteplase infusion, whereas the infusion is continued during the alteplase infusion in many other countries. Considering that this two therapeutic approaches have never been compared, both are recommended in guidelines [15].

Thus, in the absence of specific data, Becattini and Agnelly decided to use heparin concurrently with TNK-t-PA. The regimen of unfractionated heparin was derived from that used in ST-elevation myocardial infarction patients treated with TNK-t-PA. However, in these studies, a major benefit with a low-molecular-weight heparin, enoxaparin was obtained. Authors, did not explain, why enoxaparin was not used in TIPES trial. In another hand, the incidence of major bleedings was low; 2 patients in TNK-t-PA plus heparin group and 1 in placebo plus heparin group. In 2 out of 3 patients, major bleeding complication was related with over anticoagulation during 2 or 3 days immediately before bleeding event [15]. In spite of these results, authors suggested the need for carefully assessing the net clinical benefit of thrombolysis in clinically stable PE patients [15]. Finally, the results of TIPES study showed that a single bolus of TNK-t-PA plus unfractionated heparin as adjunctive treatment was associated with an early right ventricular dysfunction reduction in clinically stable PE patients. Whether this benefit could be associated with clinical improvement without excessive bleeding is still to be defined [15].

Six-Month Echocardiographic Study in Patients with Submassive Pulmonary Embolism and Right Ventricle Dysfunction: Comparison of Thrombolysis with Heparin

Background

Since the original description from Goldhaber in 1993 [12], the prognosis of acute PE was bounded to the right ventricle dysfunction. Right ventricular failure, as the most common cause of death in acute PE, has been confirmed by echocardiography and by autopsy, which shows right ventricular damage secondary to severe pulmonary hypertension and right ventricular strain and even right ventricular myocardial infarction [16]. In fact, right ventricular dysfunction assessed by echocardiography has been associated with adverse in-hospital outcome. When present, in-hospital mortality ranges from 5 to 17 % in stable PE patients [17].

In spite of previous evidences, thrombolytic treatment was recommended in shocked or severely hypotensive PE patients. However, the clinical benefit of thrombolytic agents in clinically stable PE patients and right ventricular dysfunction remains to be defined. Under this hypothesis, authors conducted a randomized, double-blind, placebo-controlled study aimed to assess the effect of thrombolysis on right ventricular dysfunction in clinically stable patients, namely, submassive PE; additionally, to identify if thrombolysis could be more effective than heparin in first episode of submassive PE patients. The main endpoints were: (a) feasibility and safety, (b) effects on echocardiographic parameters and finally, (c) clinical outcome during hospitalization and in the first 180 days after admission [17].

Methodology

Inclusion criteria: first episode of acute submassive PE, onset symptoms <6 h, normal blood pressure (systolic blood pressure >100 mmHg), echocardiogram with right ventricular dysfunction, positive lung spiral computed tomography (CT). Additionally, dyspnea, chest pain, tachypnea, hypoxemia PO_2 <75 mmHg, PCO_2 <40 mmHg, oxygen saturation <90 % in room air, D-dimer elevation, electrocardiogram with S1-Q3-T3 pattern, inversion of T waves in V1 to V4, a right bundle-branch block or right axis deviation were considered.

Exclusion criteria: active internal or recent intracranial bleeding, intracranial tumor or seizure history, ischemic stroke within 2 months, neurosurgery within 1 month, recent surgery <10 days, punction of uncompressible vessel within 10 days, trauma within 15 days. Also, uncontrolled hypertension (SBP >180 mmHg and diastolic BP >110 mmHg), hemorrhagic disorder of thrombocytopenia (<100,000/mm^3), severe impaired hepatic or renal function, gastrointestinal bleeding within 10 days, pregnancy, age >75 years [17].

Other exclusion criteria were: arterial aneurysm or arterial/venous malformation and cancer at increased risk for bleeding, chronic pulmonary hypertension, severe COPD and therapeutic doses of heparin (unfractionated or low-molecular-weight heparin) for more than 72 h before randomization. Thrombolytic treatment within the previous 4 days, or glycoprotein IIb/IIIa antagonists within the preceding 7 days were also excluded, and also patients who were under oral anticoagulation [17].

The study was designed as a prospective, randomized, double-blind, placebo-controlled trial. Study population was screened from all patients admitted to emergency department within 6 h from onset of sudden acute dyspnea. Patients immediately underwent clinical and ECG evaluation, arterial blood gases, oxygen saturation, D-dimer were determined and chest X-ray was requested. Patients with high probability PE and blood pressure <90 mmHg (massive PE) were excluded [17].

High clinical suspicion submassive PE patients (blood pressure >100 mmHg, dyspnea, chest pain, tachypnea, oxygen saturation <90 % in room air, hypoxemia PO_2 <75 mmHg, PCO_2 <40 mmHg, suggestive history of thrombosis risk and/or predisposing factors for venous thromboembolism and electrocardiogram alterations) were included in the study. All patients received an intravenous bolus of 5000 U of unfractionated heparin and then randomized in two groups before undergoing further diagnostic workup. After randomization, patients underwent echocardiographic examination and spiral CT. In addition, plasma samples were also obtained for troponin I and brain natriuretic peptide type-B plasma levels determination [17].

When final diagnosis of submassive PE was established, patients were assigned to 100 mg of rtPA, alteplase 10 mg bolus, followed by a 90 mg intravenous infusion over a 2 h period, or placebo. In addition to alteplase or placebo, both groups received unfractionated heparin treatment (1000 U/h and/or accordingly activated partial thromboplastin time (aPTT)), in combination with warfarin (started on day 1 after randomization), until the international normalized ratio was within the therapeutic range for 2 consecutive days; after this point, heparin was stopped. Measurements of aPTT were performed at 6-h intervals on day 1 after randomization and at 12-h intervals thereafter for at least 4 days [17].

Patients were under careful follow-up including: Blood pressure and heart rate every 6 h for the first 24 h, then every 12 h until clinical stabilization and subsequently daily up to discharge. In spite of anticoagulation and thrombolysis, arterial blood gas were measured every 30 min from treatment, and then every 6 h up to stabilization; electrocardiogram and echocardiogram were also performed 6 and 12 h after treatment and daily up to discharge and during follow-up to control right ventricular function and electrocardiogram evolution. In the subsequent days after treatment (2–3 days), inferior limbs Doppler echography was also performed. Lung spiral CT, lower abdominal CT and Doppler echography of the inferior limbs were repeated before discharge [17].

After discharge, the patients were followed as outpatients every week for the first month and every 2 weeks for the subsequent 3 months and every month successively for the next 6 months (total follow-up 6 months) to evaluate PE recurrences; and at every follow-up evaluation clinical, electrocardiogram, echocardiographic and laboratory assessments were performed. In addition, spiral CT, and lower abdominal CT and Doppler echography of the inferior limbs were repeated 3 and 6 months after. Two blinded physicians evaluated the clinical status and if recurrence of PE was present and side effects of warfarin treatment (bleedings) were recorded [17].

Submassive diagnostic PE criteria: at least one of the following: stable hemodynamic status (SBP >100 mmHg, hypoxemia PO_2 <75 mmHg, PCO_2 <40 mmHg, D-dimer elevation, electrocardiogram alterations, echocardiographic signs of right ventricular dysfunction and positive lung spiral CT). Echocardiographic right ventricular dysfunction: qualitative hypokinesis of the right ventricular wall—McConnell sign—in apical or subcostal view; tricuspid annular plane systolic excursion. Paradoxical systolic septal motion or a newly developed tricuspid regurgitation (tricuspid regurgitation with jet velocity <2.8 m/s and tricuspid regurgitation with jet velocity <2.5 m/s in the absence of inferior vena cava collapse on inspiration). Dilatation of the right ventricle [end-diastolic diameter >30 mm (precordial and subcostal views)] and right/left ventricle end-diastolic diameter ratio >1 in the apical four-chamber view and/or >0.7 in parasternal long axis, both in the absence of right ventricle hypertrophy [17].

The primary efficacy endpoint was the reduction of right ventricular dysfunction at echocardiogram performed at admission, in subsequent days up to discharge, and at 180 days. Secondary endpoints were PE recurrence or death and clinical events during hospitalization and at 180 days from randomization. Recurrent PE was confirmed by at least one of the following criteria: a new filling defect revealed by spiral CT and sudden otherwise unexplained death. Clinical deterioration was defined as the need for 1 or more among the following: catecholamine infusion for sustained hypotension or shock, endotracheal intubation, cardiopulmonary resuscitation, emergency surgical embolectomy or catheter fragmentation [17].

Major bleedings occurring before discharge and serious adverse events were considered as safety study endpoints. Major bleeding: when it was fatal, intracranial, required transfusions or intervention for hemodynamic deterioration. All bleeding episodes not fulfilling criteria for major bleeding were considered as minor bleedings.

Results

From January 2005 to June 2009, 72 consecutive patients aged between 18 and 75 years, with a first episode of submassive PE were included. Of the 2318 patients admitted to hospital within 6 h from onset of sudden acute dyspnea, 1025 were patients with acute coronary syndrome (ST-elevation myocardial infarction or non-ST elevation myocardial infarction). Another 368 with severe chronic obstructive pulmonary disease, 761 with acute heart failure, 7 with recent intracranial bleeding, 5 had recent ischemic stroke (<2 months), 4 had recent surgery (<10 days). Six had hemorrhagic disorder with thrombocytopenia (<100,000), 9 with important impaired renal function (clearance <35 mL), 22 older than 75 years, 2 had aortic aneurysm, 7 cancer; 12 were on oral anticoagulation, 7 had massive PE with hypotension and 4 were not confirmed as submassive PE. Considering the extensive and strict exclusion criteria, only 72 patients were included, 37 assigned to thrombolysis and 35 to placebo [17].

All patients underwent echocardiogram and spiral CT just after randomization, and the same controls were repeated as stated in the protocol. Time between baseline echocardiography and study treatment administration was <30 min (range, 15–30 min), with no significant difference between the two treatment groups. Baseline and serial echocardiograms (24, 48 and 72 h, 6 days, discharge and 3 and 6 months) were available in all patients except for those dead during hospitalization or follow-up and those with recurrent PE who were excluded from final analysis.

Apical four-chamber and parasternal long axis or subcostal four-chamber views were available in all patients. Mean right ventricular end-diastolic dimension was similar in the two treatment groups at baseline echocardiography (48 ± 2.3 and 49 ± 2.4 mm, respectively), as it was for the right/left ventricle end-diastolic dimension ratio (1.42 ± 0.04 and 1.41 ± 0.05, respectively). Both groups also showed similar results regarding pulmonary hypertension, inferior vein cava, Doppler acceleration time, paradoxical systolic septal motion, and tricuspid annular plane systolic excursion and brain natriuretic peptides type-B values [17].

All echocardiographic parameters of right ventricular function significantly improved in both groups, with earlier improvement in thrombolysis group compared with heparin group, being this benefit evident after 24 h and during the hospitalization period. In addition, parameters of right ventricular function were also significantly reduced during follow-up in the thrombolysis group compared to heparin one. Brain natriuretic peptide type-B showed a faster reduction in thrombolysis group compared to placebo during hospitalization; however both groups showed normal values of this biomarker at 6 days after admission [17].

In-hospital mortality was lower in thrombolysis group, but this difference was not significant (0 vs. 5 patients in heparin group, 3 for recurrent fatal PE and 2 for irreversible right ventricular dysfunction). Besides, heparin group showed additional clinical events during follow-up, in particular one PE (nonfatal) and one death occurred on day 90 (fatal PE). During follow-up, 3 patients in placebo group had clinical deterioration due to right ventricular dysfunction and were rehospitalized for right heart failure treatment and 5 patients showed deep venous thrombosis persistence. Recurrent PE and deep venous thrombosis were confirmed by CT angiography, lower abdominal CT and Doppler echography of the inferior limbs [17].

Chest and lower extremities Doppler and CT venograms performed at 3 and 6 months did not show any recurrence of PE and deep venous thrombosis in all remaining patients. Mortality during hospitalization and follow-up occurred in 6 cases in the heparin group vs. 0 cases in thrombolysis group ($p<0.02$). Analysis of combined events including death, PE recurrence, right ventricular dysfunction, major bleedings, and deep venous thrombosis, showed highly significant difference in favor for thrombolysis group (16 vs. 2 cases, $p<0.005$) [17].

Overall, 3 patients had major nonfatal bleeding. A 64-year-old man randomized to thrombolysis had important hematuria starting at day 2 after treatment, which required blood transfusion in two occasions and was finally proven to be caused by bladder papilloma. A 49-year-old man suffered a gastrointestinal bleeding at 72 h after thrombolysis administration; two transfusions and no hemodynamic support were required. And a 55-year-old woman randomized to heparin group had abdominal bleeding at day 2 after treatment as shown by abdominal CT and required one blood transfusion. All these patients had abnormal aPTT (>100 s) related to heparin overdosing.

Additionally, at the time of bleeding, all patients had been started with warfarin with INR reaching therapeutic levels. No major bleeding was observed in the subsequent follow-up; 11 patients in thrombolysis group had minor bleeding compared with 4 patients in placebo group. Minor bleedings mainly accounted were by cutaneous hematoma (9 patients), epistaxis (3 patients) and hematuria (3 patients). In the follow-up, 9 cases of minor bleedings occurred because of warfarin overdosing (epistaxis or hematuria). Reducing warfarin dose was effective to achieve stop bleeding [17].

Lessons Learned from This Study

This randomized control trial and thrombolysis was the first to use high clinical suspicion concept and biomarkers (D-dimer and brain natriuretic peptide type-B) in the screening of PE and right ventricular dysfunction patients. Although brain natriuretic peptide type-B returned to normal levels during hospitalization in those patients with a favorable outcome, this biomarker was not considered in the risk stratification. Additionally, the study showed the feasibility of thrombolysis treatment in patients with acute submassive PE and did not raise safety concerns. The results also, suggests that thrombolysis is more effective than heparin in obtaining an early reduction of right ventricular dysfunction in clinically stable patients with subsequent beneficial effects in the 180-day follow-up [17].

An interesting observation was the nonsignificant favorable trend in incidence of deep venous thrombosis and PE during follow-up. The necessity for larger sample of patients could be an explanation.

Authors considered that according preceding results and guidelines recommendations it is possible that right ventricular dysfunction on echocardiogram allows the identification of a subgroup of clinically stable PE patients at particularly high-risk mortality and clinical deterioration. Previous studies showed that pulmonary artery systolic pressure >50 mmHg and right ventricular dysfunction in PE patients were three times more likely to develop persistent pulmonary hypertension and right ventricular dysfunction, major mortality at 5 years and more likely to require pulmonary thromboendarterectomy. Given this hypothesis, it is right to consider that patients with these characteristics could achieve a clearer net clinical benefit from thrombolysis [17].

The results reiterate the need for carefully assessing the net clinical benefit of thrombolysis in clinically stable PE patients. The presence or absence of right ventricular dysfunction plays a pivotal role for therapeutically decision making and determining the prognosis during the setting of acute PE. As an echocardiography limitation, cannot establishes when troponin expression occurs and when troponin increases. However, troponin expression could be evident approximately 4–6 h from onset symptoms; in addition, in severe right ventricular dysfunction PE patients, troponin expression increases in only 30 % of cases. This study complements similar previous studies, which compared thrombolysis with heparin in clinically stable PE patients. Unfortunately, in an emergency, high-quality echocardiography is not always available nor is it achievable in every patient. The increasing use of bedside ultrasonography in the acute care setting could help in diagnosis and therapeutic decision in PE patients.

The most difference with other reports was the longer follow-up, the immediate echocardiography before randomization, the early treatment (within 6 h from symptoms onset), the use multiple echocardiographic parameters either during hospitalization or during follow-up and the inclusion of the research of deep venous thromboembolism. Unfortunately, the positivity of troponin test or brain natriuretic peptide type-B evaluation was not considered for randomization. Furthermore, patients received the treatments according to randomization, and escalation treatment or thrombolysis was not added. In this way, the comparison was not affected by subsequent treatment, which might change outcome [17].

Finally, authors considered the necessity that these results have to be reproduced and their possible therapeutic implications have to be tested in prospective management trials.

Moderate Pulmonary Embolism Treated with Thrombolysis (MOPETT) Trial

Background

Thrombolysis is an effective tool in the treatment of massive PE, and has also have been recommended in clinically stable PE patients with right ventricular dysfunction (enlargement or hypokinesia) or with abnormal expression of right ventricular biomarker injury. In another hand, intracranial hemorrhage has been noted in 0.7–6 % of PE patients submitted to intravenous thrombolysis. This frequency had caused a reluctance in the systematic thrombolysis use in acute PE with clinical stability [18].

Previous experience from professor Sharifi using percutaneous endovenous intervention for deep venous thrombosis with low-dose thrombolysis showed a favorable pulmonary response. It is therefore intriguing to postulate that a lower dose of the thrombolytic drug might be effective in PE, with the additional benefit of enhancing its safety profile [18]. No data are available on peripheral intravenous administration of low-dose thrombolysis for moderate PE in the reduction of pulmonary artery pressures after 2 years [18].

Methodology

The MOPETT trial was a prospective, controlled, randomized, single-center open study in patients with symptomatic moderate PE. Patients presenting with signs and symptoms suggestive of PE plus imaging documentation on computed tomographic angiography or V/Q scanning were eligible: Moderate PE definition: signs and symptoms of PE plus computed tomographic pulmonary angiographic involvement of >70 % of thrombus in >2 lobar or left or right main pulmonary arteries or high probability V/Q scan showing ventilation/ perfusion mismatch in >2 lobes [18].

To be eligible, patients were required to have a minimum of >2 new signs and symptoms consisting of chest pain, tachypnea (respiratory rate at rest >22 breaths/min), tachycardia (heart rate at rest >90 beats/min), dyspnea, cough, oxygen desaturation (oxygen partial pressure <95 %) or elevated jugular venous pressure >12 cm H_2O; right ventricular enlargement or hypokinesia and elevation of biomarkers of right ventricular injury (troponin I and brain natriuretic peptide type-B), although measured, were not a requirement for enrollment [18].

Primary end points: development of pulmonary hypertension as assessed by echocardiography and the composite end point of pulmonary hypertension and recurrent PE at intermediate-term follow-up. Secondary end points were total mortality, duration of hospital stay and bleeding at index hospitalization, recurrent PE, and the composite end points of mortality and recurrent PE [18].

Exclusion criteria: onset symptoms >10 days; >8 h since the start of parenteral anticoagulation; systemic arterial systolic blood pressure <95 or >200/100 mmHg; contraindication to unfractionated or low-molecular-weight heparin; severe thrombocytopenia (platelet count <50,000/mm^3); major bleeding within <2 months requiring transfusion; surgery or major trauma within <2 weeks; brain mass; neurologic surgery, intracerebral hemorrhage, or subdural hematoma within <1 year; end-stage illness with no plan for PE treatment; and an inability to perform echocardiography (chest deformities, bandages, or catheters) [18].

Echocardiography was performed within 2 h after randomization and before administration of alteplase and then, 24–48 h after and at 6-month intervals. Pulmonary artery systolic pressure was estimated from the tricuspid valve regurgitant jet velocity using the modified Bernoulli equation. The right atrial pressure was estimated at 10, 15, and 18 mmHg for mild, moderate, and severe right atrial enlargement, respectively. In the standard four-chamber view if the maximum dimension of the right atrium/left atrium was 1–1.2, right atrial enlargement was arbitrarily considered as mild, 1.3–1.5 as moderate, and >1.5 as severe. In the latter case, the diameter of the inferior vena cava had to be >2.5 cm as an additional requirement to assign a value of 18 mmHg for the right atrial pressure, otherwise it was still considered moderate right atrial enlargement. If the right atrial size was less than that of the left atrium, the right atrial pressure was assumed to be 5 mmHg [18].

Echocardiography definitions: Pulmonary hypertension, pulmonary artery systolic pressure of >40 mmHg. Right ventricular enlargement: right ventricular/left ventricular ratio >0.9. Right ventricular hypokinesia: reduction in the anticipated normal wall motion of right ventricular myocardium [18].

All patients received either unfractionated heparin or subcutaneous enoxaparin, with initial preference given to the latter drug. Administration of unfractionated heparin was determined by the presence of renal insufficiency or patient preference. In rt-PA group, enoxaparin was given as 1 mg/kg subcutaneously twice daily, with the initial dose not to exceed 80 mg. For unfractionated heparin in the same group, it was given at 70 U/kg as a bolus but not to exceed 6000 U, with subsequent dose adjustment to keep the activated partial thromboplastin time at 1.5–2 times the baseline value. Although alteplase was infused, the maintenance dose of unfractionated heparin was kept at 10 U/kg/h and not to exceed 1000 U/h. At 3 h after termination of thrombolysis, the dose of unfractionated heparin was increased to 18 U/kg/h [18].

In heparin group, enoxaparin was given at 1 mg/kg subcutaneously twice daily and unfractionated heparin at 80 U/kg as a bolus followed by 18 U/kg/h, with the same partial thromboplastin time target. Alteplase dose was <50 % of the standard PE dose (100 mg) and was termed: safe dose thrombolysis. For patients weighing >50 kg, the total dose was 50 mg, given as a 10 mg bolus by an intravenous push within 1 min followed by infusion of the remaining 40 mg within 2 h. For those weighing <50 kg, the total dose was calculated as 0.5 mg/kg, which was given as a 10-mg initial bolus followed by the remaining within 2 h. Warfarin was started in all patients. A significant paucity of data is available on the changes of pulmonary artery systolic pressure from before treatment to intermediate follow-up in patients with moderate PE, who have received thrombolysis vs. anticoagulation alone [18].

Results

During a 22-month period from May 2008, 178 patients with PE were considered for enrollment, but ultimately, 121 patients were randomized, 61 patients to alteplase group and 60 to heparin group. Baseline clinical characteristics were similar in both. Follow-up was obtained for 58 patients in the alteplase group and for 56 in heparin group. The mean follow-up period was 28 ± 5 months. RV enlargement on the initial echocardiogram was noted in 12 of 61 (20 %) of the alteplase group and 14 of 60 (23 %) of heparin group. Right ventricular hypokinesia, in 3 of 61 (5 %) of alteplase group and 4 of 60 (7 %) of heparin group. An elevation in brain natriuretic peptide type-B or troponin I was seen in 40 of 61 (66 %) of alteplase group and 42 of 60 (70 %) of heparin group. All differences were nonsignificant. Enoxaparin was given to 48 of 61 (79 %) of alteplase group and 49 of 60 (81 %) in heparin group [18].

Pulmonary hypertension and the composite end point developed in 9 of 58 patients (16 %) in alteplase group and 32 of 56 patients (57 %) in heparin group ($p<0.001$) and 9 of 58 patients (16 %) in alteplase group and 35 of 56 patients (63 %) in heparin group ($p<0.001$), respectively. The secondary end points were total mortality, in-hospital stay duration, bleeding at the index hospitalization, recurrent PE, and mortality and recurrent PE combined. Duration of hospitalization was 2.2 ± 0.5 days in alteplase group and 4.9 ± 0.8 days in heparin group ($p<0.001$). The combination of death plus recurrent PE was 1 (2 %) in alteplase group and 6 (10 %) in heparin group ($p<0.04$). No bleeding occurred in any group, and despite a positive trend in favor of a safe dose thrombolysis, no significant difference was noted in the rate of individual outcomes of death and recurrent PE when assessed independently [18].

Lessons Learned from This Study

The results have demonstrated that a reduced alteplase dose was safe and effective in the treatment of moderate PE, leading to a significant early reduction in the pulmonary artery systolic pressure that was maintained through the intermediate term. An important question in this study, it is why authors decided to use pulmonary artery systolic pressure as main target? Authors analyze four previous reports addressing effects of pulmonary artery pressure changes after thrombolysis from a total of 257 PE patients. The largest of these was a prospective, nonrandomized study that consisted of 200 normotensive patients with PE, with 21 of them receiving 100 mg of alteplase. In this group, right ventricular systolic pressure was 45 mmHg, which decreased to 20 mmHg at 6 months (55 % decrease). Patients who did not receive thrombolysis had only a 15 % decrease in right ventricular systolic pressure [18].

One half of the patients treated with anticoagulation alone manifested an increased or persistently elevated right ventricular systolic pressure, 46 % of whom had either dyspnea at rest or exercise intolerance. This was in contrast with the absence of worsening of right ventricular systolic pressure in any patient of the thrombolysis group. In a small series of 7 patients who underwent catheter-directed thrombolysis with urokinase and heparin for massive PE, the pulmonary artery systolic pressure decreased from a pretreatment value of 61 mmHg to 25 and 24 mmHg at 6 days and 15 months, respectively. The dreaded complication of thrombolysis is intracerebral hemorrhage, which has dissuaded physicians from embracing this form of therapy, even when there is clear indication for its use [18].

The results from a multicenter registry reported a major bleeding rate of 21.9 % in patients receiving thrombolysis compared to 8 % with standard therapy. All these patients had major PE. However, in a randomized trial by the same lead investigator, major bleeding in the thrombolysis group was only 0.8 %, with no intracerebral hemorrhage or fatal bleeding. Levine cited an 8 % incidence of major bleeding and a fatal hemorrhage rate of 2 % in patients receiving thrombolysis for PE. The ICOPER registry reported a 3 % incidence of intracerebral hemorrhage. In another report, the frequency of intracerebral hemorrhage was 2.1 %.16 The very high incidence of major bleeding reported in older studies is not consistent with the contemporary data or our experience and the authors considered all of these evidence as historic interest.

The absence of major or minor bleeding had several explanations. The modification of parenteral anticoagulation dose administered concomitantly with alteplase and the validity of the concept of "safe dose" thrombolysis. It is important to modify the existing "standard parenteral anticoagulation protocols" in many hospitals if thrombolytic therapy is to be administered. By doing so, the intense fluctuations in the partial thromboplastin time, which is usually noted during the first 1–2 days, is eliminated. Targeting a lower partial thromboplastin time of 1.5–2 times baseline was another contributing factor in reducing the bleeding risk. In the present study, no recurrent PE was found in patients in alteplase group but it occurred in 3 patients (5 %) in heparin group. Previously professor Konstantinides reported no significant difference in the 4 % (4 of 118) rate of recurrent PE in their thrombolysis group compared to the 3 % (4 of 138) rate noted in the heparin group.

Professor Sharifi proposed the administration of "safe dose" thrombolysis by expanding its use for moderate PE in which the risk of bleeding is reduced and its benefits are retained. In addition, even lower doses of alteplase used in MOPPET trial proved effectiveness. Very low doses of 0.5–4 mg of alteplase given as bolus have been successfully used in the treatment of intracardiac thrombus and PE during liver transplantation. There are some common sense concepts that deserve attention. One has to consider the uniqueness of the lungs and their exquisite sensitivity to thrombolysis. In contrast to any other organ, which receives a fraction of the cardiac output, the lungs receive it entirely (in the absence of shunting). From the existing guidelines, the "standard practice" uses the same or similar alteplase dose for PE that is used for thrombolysis in the systemic arterial circulation.

For example, in ST-elevation myocardial infarction, 100 mg of tPA is given within 90 min for a coronary thrombis, which receives only 5 % of the cardiac output. Similarly, 0.9 mg/kg of alteplase has been used in acute ischemic stroke in which the cerebral circulation receives 15 % of the cardiac output. These doses have the potency to withstand "route attrition": alteplase is given into the venous circulation, it traverses the lung capillaries, enters the arterial circulation, reaches a steady state, and is still capable of dissolving arterial clots. The 100 mg of alteplase is poised to effectively meet these "challenges." However, the key question is whether it is necessary to use the same dose that has been designed for thrombolysis in the systemic circulation for the lungs? It is clear that all alteplase molecules, no matter through which venous access site they are given, converge in the lungs. It stands to reason that a "first-pass" effect might exist, especially with a bolus dose, that would have a favorable effect in the lungs, thereby achieving thrombolysis with a much lower dose.

The corollary of this perspective might be applied to catheter-directed thrombolysis. In contrast to almost every other vascular bed with thrombosis, which would benefit from catheter-directed thrombolysis, in the lungs it would probably not be necessary, because the lungs are the center of convergence of all venous flow, and, ultimately, all administered molecules of alteplase would reach the lungs. In conclusion, the results from the present prospective randomized trial suggests that "safe dose" thrombolysis is safe and effective in the treatment of moderate PE, with a significant immediate reduction in the pulmonary artery pressure that was maintained at 28 months.

Fibrinolysis for Patients with Intermediate-Risk Pulmonary Embolism: PEITHO Trial

Background

The PEITHO study has been the most anticipated trial in the history of thrombolysis and PE. All available evidence showed that acute right ventricular pressure overload at diagnosis was an important determinant of the severity and early clinical outcome of PE [19].

Patients having acute right ventricular dysfunction and myocardial injury, even without overt hemodynamic compromise, may be at intermediate risk for an adverse early outcome. Randomized controlled studies, testing thrombolytic agents vs. heparin alone in acute PE patients have enrolled less than 1000 patients over the past 40 years [5–18]. Previous evidence proved that thrombolytic agents rapidly improve hemodynamic variables; however, effects on the clinical outcome, particularly in PE patients without clinical instability at presentation, have not been determined [19].

The PEITHO trial was designed to investigate the clinical efficacy and safety of thrombolytic therapy with a single-bolus injection of TNK-t-PA, in addition to standard anticoagulation therapy with heparin, in normotensive acute PE with an intermediate risk of an adverse outcome [19].

Methodology

This was a multicenter, double-blind, placebo-controlled randomized, initiated by the investigators and sponsored by Direction de la Recherche Clinique at Assistance Publique–Hôpitaux de Paris, a consortium of university hospitals in Paris. Trial funding was provided by Programme Hospitalier de Recherche Clinique in France, by the Federal Ministry of Education and Research in Germany, and by a grant from Boehringer Ingelheim [19]. The protocol was written by three academic principal investigators and reviewed, modified, and approved by the trial steering committee [19].

Inclusion criteria: age >18 years, objectively confirmed acute PE with an onset of symptoms 15 days or less, right ventricular dysfunction confirmed by echocardiography or chest spiral computed tomography, and myocardial cell injury confirmed by a positive test for troponin I or troponin T [19].

Eligible patients underwent central randomization with an internet based system. Randomization was performed within 2 h after documenting both right ventricular dysfunction (by echocardiography or spiral computed tomography) and myocardial injury (positive cardiac troponin test). Patients assigned to thrombolysis received a single weight-based intravenous bolus of the fibrinolytic agent TNK-t-PA. Weight adjusted dose ranged from 30 to 50 mg, and were administered over a period of 5–10 s [19]. Unfractionated heparin was started as an intravenous bolus immediately after randomization in both groups. The initial bolus of unfractionated heparin was omitted in patients who had already received an intravenous bolus or infusion of unfractionated heparin, and also in patients receiving a therapeutic dose of low-molecular-weight heparin or fondaparinux, cases in which infusion was delayed until 12 h after the last injection of low-molecular-weight heparin or until 24 h after the last injection of fondaparinux [19].

The heparin infusion rate was adjusted to achieve and maintain an activated partial thromboplastin time 2.0–2.5 times the upper limit of normal range, corresponding to therapeutic heparin levels (equivalent to factor Xa inhibition of 0.3–0.7 IU/mL). The use of anticoagulant agents other than unfractionated heparin was not allowed until 48 h after randomization [19].

Patients had 30 days follow-up and were evaluated for death, hemodynamic decompensation (or collapse), bleeding, stroke, recurrent PE, and serious adverse events. An independent clinical-events committee, unaware of the treatment group assignments [19] adjudicated all efficacy and safety outcomes.

Primary efficacy outcome: clinical composite of death from any cause or hemodynamic decompensation (or collapse) within 7 days after randomization. Secondary outcomes: death within 7 days after randomization, hemodynamic decompensation within 7 days, confirmed symptomatic recurrence of PE within 7 days, death within 30 days, and major adverse events within 30 days. Safety outcomes were defined as ischemic or hemorrhagic stroke (including hemorrhagic conversion of ischemic stroke) within 7 days after randomization, extracranial major (moderate or severe) bleeding within 7 days, and serious adverse events within 30 days. Major bleeding, was defined according to the criteria of the International Society on Thrombosis and Hemostasis [19].

Results

From November 2007 through July 2012, a total of 1006 patients were enrolled at 76 sites in 13 European countries. Of these, 506 were randomly assigned to treatment with TNK-t-PA plus unfractionated heparin, and 500 were randomly assigned to placebo plus unfractionated heparin. One patient was excluded, so the intention-to-treat population consisted of 1005 patients [19].

Demographic data, clinical status, and medical history were well matched between the two treatment groups. The median age was 70 years. All patients were normotensive at randomization. In the vast majority of cases, the diagnosis of PE was confirmed by CT pulmonary angiography in both thrombolysis and placebo group (95 and 95 %). Right ventricular dysfunction was diagnosed by echocardiography (54 and 51 %) or CT (14 and 14 %) or both studies (30 and 35 %) in all cases. Myocardial injury was confirmed with a test for cardiac troponin I (72 and 72 %) or troponin T (32 and 33 %) in all but 9 patients. Low-molecular-weight heparin or fondaparinux was administered before randomization in 34 and 27 %, and the remaining patients received unfractionated heparin before randomization or at the time of randomization [19].

The primary efficacy outcome occurred in 13 patients (2.6 %) between randomization and day 7 in TNK-t-PA group, as compared with 28 patients (5.6 %) in heparin group (odds ratio, 0.44; 95 % confidence interval [CI], 0.23–0.87; $p=0.02$). Six patients (1.2 %) in TNK-t-PA group and 9 patients (2 %) in heparin group died between randomization and day 7 ($p=0.42$), and hemodynamic decompensation or collapse occurred in 8 patients (2 %) in TNK-t-PA group and in 25 patients (5.0 %) in heparin group ($p=0.002$). Persistent hypotension or a drop in blood pressure was recorded in 8 patients in tenecteplase group and in 18 patients in placebo group; catecholamines were administered to 3 patients in TNK-t-PA group and 14 patients in heparin group, and one patient in TNK-t-PA group and 5 patients in heparin group required cardiopulmonary resuscitation [19].

Eight patients in TNK-t-PA group required mechanical ventilation, as compared with 15 patients in the heparin group. More patients in the heparin group than in the TNK-t-PA group underwent open-label rescue fibrinolysis; in accordance with the protocol, this treatment was administered only after the primary outcome had occurred, with the exception of 9 patients. By day 30 after randomization, 12 patients (2 %) in the TNK-t-PA group had died, as compared with 16 patients (3 %) in the placebo group ($p=0.42$) [19].

Major bleeding occurred between randomization and day 7 in 58 patients (12 %) in TNK-t-PA group and in 12 patients (2 %) in heparin group. Major extracranial bleeding occurred in 32 patients (6 %) in TNK-t-PA group and in 6 patients (1 %) in heparin group ($p<0.001$). Twelve patients (2 %) in TNK-t-PA group had a stroke within 7 days after randomization; in 10 of these patients, the stroke was hemorrhagic. By comparison, only one patient in heparin group had a stroke ($p=0.003$), and it was a hemorrhagic stroke. Six of the 10 patients in TNK-t-PA group who had a hemorrhagic stroke were alive 30 days after randomization, corresponding to a fatality rate of 40 %; mild or moderate disability persisted in most of the survivors [19].

Prespecified subgroups were defined by age (≤75 vs. >75 years) and male and female patients. In terms of death and hemodynamic decompensation all prespecified groups had better outcome in TNK-t-PA group compared with heparin group. The rate of extracranial major bleeding in the prespecified subgroups of age and sex was better in heparin group. Among 75 years or younger patients, the primary efficacy outcome occurred in 2 % of those assigned to TNK-t-PA and 5 % of those assigned to heparin, corresponding to an odds ratio of 0.33 (95 % CI, 0.13–0.85) in favor of TNK-t-PA; by comparison, the odds ratio was 0.63 (95 % CI, 0.24–1.66) among patients older than 75 years. However, on the basis of interaction testing, this difference was not significant ($p=0.36$) [19]. Among patients treated with TNK-t-PA, older patients had a higher rate of major extracranial bleeding compared to younger patients; the difference was not significant ($p=0.09$). The rates of these efficacy and safety outcomes also did not differ significantly between men and women [19].

Lessons Learned from This Study

In PEITHO trial, intermediate-risk PE patients treated with standard anticoagulation had a 6 % incidence of death or hemodynamic decompensation (the primary efficacy outcome) within the first 7 days after randomization. A single-bolus injection of TNK-t-PA, in a weight-based dose, resulted in a significantly lower risk of the primary outcome (3 %). Thrombolysis was associated with a 2 % rate of hemorrhagic stroke and a 6 % rate of major extracranial hemorrhage [19].

Authors established that normotensive PE patients could have an elevated risk of early death or major complications when right ventricular dysfunction and/or myocardium injury are identified. Thrombolytic agents promptly reduce pulmonary artery resistance, pressure improving right ventricular dysfunction and myocardial injury. In spite, all guidelines supporting its use in massive or high-risk PE patients, the efficacy of thrombolytic agents in improving the outcome in intermediate-risk PE patients remains controversial. The main gray zone in this issue was the lack of trials with statistical power in terms of sample and focus in specific population [19].

PEITHO trial results indicate that prompt fibrinolysis can reduce the risk of hemodynamic decompensation or death in normotensive acute PE patients with right ventricular dysfunction, by echocardiography or CT, and myocardial injury, as indicated by a positive cardiac troponin test. Considering that the efficacy of thrombolysis was mainly driven by the prevention of hemodynamic decompensation; the study was not powered to detect differences in rates of death, which occurred relatively infrequently in the two treatment groups [19].

Additionally, definition of hemodynamic decompensation or collapse included a persistent, isolated drop in systolic blood pressure, which could be of questionable clinical significance. Nevertheless, 14 patients with hemodynamic decompensation in heparin group needed inotropic support and 5 underwent cardiopulmonary resuscitation. It is possible that the prognosis for some of these patients would have been worse if they had not been closely monitored and promptly treated when decompensation occurred [19].

Fibrinolytic treatment is known to carry a risk of major bleeding, including intracranial hemorrhage. The results involving single bolus TNK-t-PA, confirm previous observations. The risk of hemorrhagic stroke was 2 % among hemodynamically stable acute PE patients. In previous studies, increasing age and the presence of coexisting conditions have been associated with a higher risk of bleeding complications. However, in PEITHO trial thrombolysis was associated with a lower risk of bleeding in younger patients than in patients >75 years of age, although this difference was not significant [19].

In a recently published trial of TNK-t-PA treatment in ST-elevation myocardial infarction patients the incidence of intracranial hemorrhage had significant reduction when TNK-t-PA dose was decreased by 50 % in patients 75 years of age or older. In this study primary ischemic strokes were more frequent in thrombolysis group than in the primary percutaneous coronary intervention group. After the dose reduction of TNK-t-PA in patients 75 years of age or older, there were no cases of intracranial hemorrhage (0 of 97 patients), as compared with 3 of 37 patients (8.1 %) in this age group before the amendment. The rate of major nonintracranial bleeding was 7 % in thrombolysis group, and 5 % in the primary percutaneous coronary intervention primary group, a not significant difference ($p=0.11$). The rates of blood transfusions were also similar in the two study groups (2.9 % and 2.3 %, respectively; $p=0.47$) [20]. Considering this evidence, if a reduced-dose strategy TNK-t-PA might also be beneficial in intermediate-risk PE patients remains as an open question.

Despite some trial limitations PEITHO data strengthen the case for risk stratification and for careful monitoring of patients who have an intermediate risk of death. The findings suggest that careful monitoring and rescue fibrinolysis can minimize deaths from PE. In this trial, only 17 of 500 patients (3 %) who were assigned to initial treatment with an anticoagulant and placebo received rescue thrombolysis. This approach averts the increased risk of major bleeding, especially hemorrhagic stroke, for the majority of patients. Although patients who were at increased risk for major bleeding were excluded, the rate of hemorrhagic stroke in thrombolysis group (2 %) was ten times as high as that in the heparin group (0.2 %) [21].

Finally, in normotensive intermediate-risk PE patients, the composite primary outcome of early death or hemodynamic decompensation was reduced after treatment with a single intravenous bolus of TNK-t-PA. However, TNK-t-PA was also associated with a significant increase in the risk of intracranial and other major bleeding. Therefore, great caution is warranted when considering thrombolysis for clinically stable PE patients, right ventricular dysfunction, and a acute myocardial cell damage by cardiac troponin expression. What course should physicians chart when confronted with a normotensive acute PE patients with acute pulmonary embolism? Data from the PEITHO trial provide valuable insight but no definitive answer [21].

Treatment of Submassive Pulmonary Embolism with Tenecteplase or Placebo: Cardiopulmonary Outcomes at 3 Months: Multicenter Double-Blind, Placebo-Controlled Randomized Trial—TOPCOAT Trial

Background

From the viewpoint of Professor Kline, thrombolysis use in acute submassive PE remains controversial. For patients without contraindications, all clinical guidelines consistently recommend thrombolysis for massive PE, defined as clinical instability identified as systolic arterial hypotension. However, the same guidelines have conflict in their recommendations for submassive PE, defined as PE with acute pulmonary arterial hypertension and right ventricular dysfunction that does not cause systolic arterial hypotension [22].

Mortality as a primary outcome hampers clinical trials of submassive PE because the short-term mortality rate directly attributable to PE is below 2 %. This implies the need for an impractically large sample size, compelling the need for a composite endpoint, which is more likely to have larger differences between treatment groups. In addition to risk of death, submassive PE patients may suffer persistent right ventricular dysfunction that can impair their quality of life by causing dyspnea and exercise intolerance. If associated with deep vein thrombosis, their quality of life can be further degraded by the post-thrombotic syndrome [22].

Professor Kleine and colleagues [22] designed a primary composite outcome from the perspective of patients: to survive PE without need for life supporting interventions in-hospital and on follow-up, and to have good functional capacity at 90 days. This was defined as normal right ventricular function on echocardiography, New York Heart Association functional class >3, and adequate exercise tolerance on 6-min walk test, and perception of wellness on the physical component portion of the SF-36 no worse than two standard deviations below normal.

In TOPOAC trial all patients received standard therapy with low-molecular-weight heparin followed by random assignment to either a weight-based, single bolus of placebo or TNK-t-PA. Authors hypothesized that a larger proportion of patients who received TNK-t-PA would have a favorable composite outcome.

Methodology

TOPCOAT was a multicenter, double-blinded, intention-to-treat, placebo-controlled, randomized controlled efficacy trial. Inclusion criteria: age >17 years, PE proved on computed tomographic pulmonary angiography performed within 24 h, normal arterial systolic blood pressure with evidence of right ventricular strain characterized by hypokinesis on echocardiography, elevated troponin I or T (values exceeding the 99 percentile with coefficient of variability <10 %) or brain natriuretic peptide type-B measurement >90 pg/mL or NT proBNP >900 pg/mL. The initial echocardiography had to be ordered as part of standard care. Severity criteria initially included a pulse oximetry reading <95 % within the previous 2 h. As usually, the study had 24 exclusion criteria. Exclusions: systolic hypotension (<90 mmHg), inability to walk, contraindications to fibrinolysis, and end-stage conditions [22].

All patients were treated with full dose of a low-molecular-weight heparin, enoxaparin 1 mg/kg or weight-based dalteparin, 200 U/kg, administered subcutaneously prior to injection of study drug or placebo. If patient was receiving unfractionated heparin, this was discontinued and low-molecular-weight heparin was started. Patients received titrated dose TNK-t-PA in accordance with the TNKase insert. Decisions about long-term anticoagulant therapy were at the discretion of the clinical care team [22].

Five-day adverse outcomes were considered as PE-related or treatment-related. Adverse outcomes from PE were death, circulatory shock (hypotension requiring vasopressor infusion), or need for intubation. Adverse outcomes from treatment were death from hemorrhage, any intracranial or intraspinal hemorrhage, active bleeding with >2 g/dL drop in hemoglobin within 24 h requiring transfusion, and any bleeding that required surgery, endoscopic or intravascular treatment [22].

All patients had a complete blood count and fibrinogen concentration measured at enrollment and on days 1 and 2. After discharge, all patients without active cancer were treated with warfarin sodium with a target international normalized ratio (INR) for the prothrombin time between 2 and 3. Patients with active cancer were treated with low-molecular-weight heparin injections. The quality of anticoagulation was assessed by the time in therapeutic range (TTR), defined as the percentage of INR found between 2 and 3 in the timeframe of 1 week after discharge and 90-day follow-up [22].

At 90 days, all survivors returned for measurements to assess for adverse outcomes defined as venous thromboembolism recurrence, poor functional capacity or poor physical health-related quality of life. All patients had transthoracic echocardiography, with a specific protocol to assess for right ventricular size, pressure and systolic function. Adverse outcomes within 90 days were assessed: Venous thromboembolism recurrence (proven by new pulmonary arterial filling defect observed on repeat CT pulmonary angiography), or a new deep venous thrombosis observed on compression ultrasound [22].

Poor functional capacity outcome required two components: (a) Right ventricular hypokinesis or dilation (right ventricle > left ventricle in apical four-chamber view), or an estimated right ventricular systolic pressure >45 mmHg, assessed on transthoracic echocardiography. (b) Dyspnea at rest or exercise intolerance defined as inability to walk 330 m using the 6-min walk test. Severe dyspnea was defined by a New York Heart Association functional class 3 or 4; poor physical health-related quality of life outcome required a normalized Physical Component Summary score from the Standard Form 36 (SF 36™) below 30 (i.e., <2 standard deviations below the normative score of 50) [10, 22]. Impact of post-thrombotic syndrome was assessed with the VEINES QOL survey [22].

Secondary outcomes measured within 5 days included dependence upon intensive care services, rate of unblinding, rate of hospital discharge, hemoglobin and fibrinogen concentrations, total number of days of minor bleeding, and frequency of all-cause Good Clinical Practice-defined adverse events. Secondary outcomes measured at 90 days included the proportion with a New York Heart Association functional class ≥3, and the mean 6-min walk distance, change in pulse oximetry with walking, the mental health component score from the SF-36, the VEINES-QOL score, and the patients' self-assessment of their overall health status on a 1–10 scale, with 1 indicating the worst possible and 10 the best possible health [22].

Summary of the composite criterion standard for an adverse outcome (1) Any PE-related or treatment-related serious adverse outcomes within 5 days of enrollment. (2) Image-confirmed recurrent PE or deep venous thrombosis within 3 months. (3) Poor functional capacity at 3 months. (4) [22]. A normalized Physical Component Summary score <30 from the SF-36. (5) A VEINES QOL score <40 in patients with known deep venous thrombosis. Patients with an adverse outcome within 5 days were invited to follow-up at 90 days, but each patient was only counted once in the summation of patients with an adverse outcome [22].

Results

From August 2008 until October 2012, 643 patients were screened, and 83 were randomized, 40 to TNK-t-PA, and 40 to placebo and low-molecular-weight heparin. Clinical characteristics of study population, including the demographic data, frequency of comorbid conditions indicating the severity of the PE were stratified by treatment group. None of the variables were significantly different between groups, although the data suggest a trend ($p<0.20$) with gender, Hispanic ethnicity, malignancy and COPD [22].

Biomarkers for severity were performed as follows: echocardiography in 54 (65 %), brain natriuretic peptide 69 (83 %) and troponin in 83 (100 %). There were no significant differences in the frequency or location of deep venous thrombosis between the two groups. Regarding quality of anticoagulation during the 3 months after discharge, patients randomized to TNK-t-PA had a mean TTR of 48 % (SD 24 %) and a median TTR of 50 % (first to third quartiles, 33–67 %). Patients randomized to low-molecular-weight heparin had a mean TTR of 49 % (SD 20 %) and a median TTR of 50 % (first–third quartiles, 33–60 %) [22].

Three patients treated with placebo had an adverse outcome within 5 days, including one who died from cardiac arrest that was directly attributed to PE, and 2 who required endotracheal intubation, vasopressor support and catheter thrombectomy. One patient treated with TNK-t-PA died from intracranial hemorrhage that occurred 5 h after drug administration, representing the only patient with a major bleed that occurred during the 5-day period of surveillance. No patient died in the period between hospital discharge and 90 days. Complete follow-up data was obtained on 39/43 survivors from the placebo group (90 %) and 37/39 (94 %) of TNK-t-PA group [22].

At follow-up, 13 (30 %; 95 % CI, 17–46) patients treated with placebo developed a study-defined adverse outcome, compared with 5 (12.5 %; 95 % CI, 4–27) patients treated with TNK-t-PA. None of these 18 patients had a prior serious adverse outcome. Thus, including the patients with adverse outcomes that occurred within 5 days, 16/43 patients (37 %; 95 % CI, 23–53) treated with placebo and 6/40 patients (15 %; 95 % CI, 6–30) treated with TNK-t-PA, had an adverse outcome (95 % confidence interval for the difference of 22 %, 3.2–40; $p=0.017$; Fisher's exact $p=0.027$) [22].

No patient had a VEINES QOL score <40, but 4 patients in the placebo group had a score worse than two standard deviations below the mean compared with no patients in the tenecteplase-treated group. Secondary outcomes measured in-hospital included level of care, hospital dependency, laboratory values and bleeding events. Regarding hospital dependency, the proportion of patients who remained in the intensive care unit on day 2 was significantly higher with placebo (20.5 %) compared with tenecteplase (5 %, $p=0.03$). On days 1 and 2, the mean fibrinogen concentration was 417 ± 146 and 451 ± 189 mg dL, respectively, in low-molecular-weight heparin group and 370 ± 162 and 391 ± 185 mg dL±respectively in TNK-t-PA group ($p=0.2$) [22].

Hemoglobin values were not different on day 2: 12.7 ± 1.8 g dL for placebo vs. 12.3 ± 1.8 g dL for TNK-t-PA group ($p = 0.4$). Members of the clinical care team opened the sealed envelope to reveal the randomization assignment in 3 patients treated with placebo and two treated with tenecteplase. All but one of these patients had a serious adverse outcome that prompted unblinding. The one patient without a serious adverse event was a low-molecular-weight heparin-treated patient. The total number of hospital days on which patients experienced any clinically observable bleeding in the first 5 days after enrollment was 11 days in the placebo group and 19 days in TNK-t-PA group [22].

Of note, one patient treated with TNK-t-PA who had undergone hysterectomy 31 days prior developed vaginal bleeding that produced transient hypotension, requiring fluid resuscitation, but the bleeding event did not meet the predefined criteria as a treatment-related adverse outcome. During the entire hospitalization, the total number of Good Clinical Practice-reportable adverse events of any type that were not part of the main composite outcome were similar between groups, with 23 (53 %) in the placebo treated group and 24 (55 %) in the tenecteplase-treated group [22].

Authors found no clinically important difference between groups in the mean 6-min walk distance or any of the scales used in the Mental Component Summary score from the SF-36. The only significant difference was a higher patient self-assessment of overall health using a 1–10 scale in the tenecteplase group [22].

Regarding the 2 patients in the placebo group with low perception of wellness based on the SF-36 as their only adverse outcome, one patient had a prior history of COPD and the other had none of the comorbid conditions. If the SF-36 results were removed as a criterion for an adverse outcome, the significance level would decrease: 14/43 placebo patients vs. 6/40 patients (two-sided $p = 0.048$; Fisher's exact $p = 0.075$). If one more patient met an endpoint in the tenecteplase group, the p values would be 0.03 from the exact binomial and 0.053 by Fisher's exact [22].

Lessons Learned from This Study

TOPCOAT reports a clinical trial of fibrinolysis to treat acute submassive PE that employed a patient-oriented, composite outcome that included measurements that assess quality of life. This composite outcome was motivated by data from interviews and surveys of patients with submassive PE, administered hours, months and years after diagnosis [22].

Immediately after diagnosis, acutely symptomatic submassive PE patients consistently indicate their desire to survive without the need for life supporting measures at any time, avoid PE recurrence, and to achieve resolution from dyspnea and exercise intolerance. In TOPCOAT authors therefore compiled an endpoint that included death, circulatory shock requiring vasopressor support, respiratory distress requiring intubation, and the 90-day endpoint of poor functional capacity or low self-perception of physical health. TOPCOAT differs from previous TNK-t-PA PE studies in the outcome, and the use of low-molecular-weight heparin instead of unfractionated heparin as the anticoagulant. Authors considered that low-molecular-weight heparin simplifies the treatment protocol and provides more reliable anticoagulation [22].

Patients with PE randomized to low-molecular-weight heparin were more likely to have an undesirable outcome than patients randomized to TNK-t-PA. The main drivers of this effect were the composite endpoint of impaired functional capacity and a low self-assessment of physical wellness from the SF-36 measured 3 months after PE diagnosis. Patients treated with TNK-t-PA spent less time in the intensive care unit and less overall time in the hospital and had no increase in adverse events or total days of any bleeding. The extensive exclusion criteria were designed to lower the risk of bleeding with fibrinolysis, but this sample included patients with higher risk criteria, including 13 with active malignancy, eight over age 75 years, and five with surgery within 6 weeks [22].

These outcomes provide clinicians and patients with the first data that enable an evidence-based discussion that can include the short-term risks together with potential longer term health benefits of fibrinolysis for acute submassive PE. However, the data also suggest that clinicians should discuss an increased risk of bleeding, including the worst-case scenario of a disabling or fatal intracranial hemorrhage [22].

The study limitations included: The study had to be terminated early, as a direct result of the principal investigator relocating to a new institution that led to insurmountable legal and administrative barriers. The study was closed prior to unblinding. Secondary analyses of prematurely closed randomized trials have suggested that *p* values fluctuate randomly early during enrollment, and early termination may have caused unrecognized bias if it were coincident with a chance nadir in *p* value.

Quality of life improvements would be associated with improved right ventricular function, but we found no difference in the frequency of right ventricular dilation or hypokinesis between groups at 90 day follow-up. It remains possible that observed differences in right ventricular pressures if measured during exercise were acquired. When TOPCOAT was planned in 2008, no instrument had been specifically derived to assess quality of life after PE, the SF-36 was used because of its long history as a standard tool to assess quality of life in clinical trials of many cardiopulmonary diseases, including pulmonary embolism.

Finally, TOPCOAT, a small trial found that submassive PE patients treated with a single bolus of TNK-t-PA had a modestly increased probability of a good functional outcome, but the sample size was too small to assess whether TNK-t-PA increases the risk of intracranial hemorrhage compared with low-molecular-weight heparin.

References

1. Konstantinides S, Torbicki A. Management of venous thromboembolism: an update. Eur Heart J. 2014;35:2855–63.
2. Tapson VF. Thrombolytic therapy for acute pulmonary embolism. Semin Thromb Hemost. 2013;39:452–8.
3. Konstantinides S, Goldhaber SZ. Pulmonary embolism: risk assessment and management. Eur Heart J. 2012;33:3014–22.

4. Chatterjee S, Chakraborty A, Weinberg I, Kadakia M, Wilensky RL, Sardar P, Kumbhani DJ, Mukherjee D, Jaff MR, Giri J. Thrombolysis for pulmonary embolism and risk of all-cause mortality, major bleeding, and intracranial hemorrhage: a meta-analysis. JAMA. 2014;311:2414–21.
5. The Urokinase Pulmonary Embolism Trial. Urokinase pulmonary embolism trial: phase 1 results: a cooperative study. JAMA. 1970;214:2163–72.
6. Tibbutt DA, Davies JA, Anderson JA, Fletcher EWL, Hamill J, Holt JM, Thomas ML, Lee G, Miller GAH, Sharp AA, Sutton GC. Comparison by controlled clinical trial of streptokinase and heparin in treatment of life-threatening pulmonary embolism. Br Med J. 1974;1:343–7.
7. Ly B, Arnesen H, Eie H, Hol R. A controlled clinical trial of streptokinase and heparin in the treatment of major pulmonary embolism. Acta Med Scand. 1978;203:465–70.
8. Marini C, Di Ricco G, Rossi G, Rindi M, Palla R, Giuntini C. Fibrinolytic effects of urokinase and heparin in acute pulmonary embolism: a randomized clinical trial. Respiration. 1988;54:162–73.
9. Levine M, Hirsh J, Weitz J, Cruickshank M, Neemeh J, Turpie AG, Gent M. A randomized trial of a single bolus dosage regimen of recombinant tissue plasminogen activator in patients with acute pulmonary embolism. Chest. 1990;98:1473–9.
10. PIOPED Investigators. Tissue plasminogen activator for the treatment of acute pulmonary embolism: a collaborative study by the PIOPED Investigators. Chest. 1990;97:528–33.
11. Dalla-Volta S, Palla A, Santolicandro A, Giuntini C, Pengo V, Visioli O, Zonzin P, Zanuttini D, Barbaresi F, Agnelli G, Morpurgo M, Marini MG, Visani L. PAIMS 2: alteplase combined with heparin versus heparin in the treatment of acute pulmonary embolism: Plasminogen Activator Italian Multicenter Study 2. J Am Coll Cardiol. 1992;20:520–6.
12. Goldhaber SZ, Come PC, Lee RT, Braunwald E, Parker JA, Haire WD, Feldstein ML, Miller M, Toltzis R, Smith JL, da Silva AM T, Mogtader A, McDonough TJ. Alteplase versus heparin in acute pulmonary embolism: randomised trial assessing right-ventricular function and pulmonary perfusion. Lancet. 1993;341:507–11.
13. Jerjes-Sanchez C, Ramirez-Rivera A, Garcia ML, Arriaga-Nava R, Valencia S, Rosado-Buzzo A, Rosas E. Streptokinase and heparin vs heparin alone in massive pulmonary embolism: a randomized controlled trial. J Thromb Thrombolysis. 1995;2:227–9.
14. Konstantinides S, Geibel A, Heusel G, Heinrich F, Kasper W. Management strategies and prognosis of pulmonary embolism-3 trial investigators. Heparin plus alteplase compared with heparin alone in patients with submassive pulmonary embolism. N Engl J Med. 2002;347:1143–50.
15. Becattini C, Agnelli G, Salvi A, Grifoni S, Pancladi LG, Enea I, Blasemin F, Campanini M, Ghirarduzzi A, Casazza F, TIPES Study Group. Bolus tenecteplase for right ventricle dysfunction in hemodynamically stable patients with pulmonary embolism. Thromb Res. 2010;125:e82–6.
16. Lankeit M, Konstantinides S. Tenecteplase can be given to patients with intermediate-risk pulmonary embolism—but should it? Thromb Res. 2010;126:e407–8.
17. Fasullo S, Scalzo S, Maringhini G, Ganci F, Canizzaro S, Basile I, Cangemi D, Terrazzino G, Parrinello G, Sarullo FM, Baglini R, Paterna S, Di Pascuale P. Six-month echocardiographic study in patients with submassive pulmonary embolism and right ventricle dysfunction: comparison of thrombolysis with heparin. Am J Med Sci. 2011;341:33–9.
18. Sharifi M, Bay C, Skrocki L, Rahimi F, Mehdipour M, for the "MOPETT" Investigators. Moderate pulmonary embolism treated with thrombolysis (from the "MOPETT" Trial). Am J Cardiol. 2013;111:273–7.
19. Meyer G, Vicaut E, Danays T, Agnelli G, Becattini C, Beyer-Westendorf J, Bluhmki E, Bouvaist H, Brenner B, Couturaud F, Dellas C, Empen K, Granca A, Galiè N, Geibel A, Goldhaber SZ, Jimenez D, Kozak M, Kupatt C, Kucher N, Lang IM, Lankeit M, Meneveau N, Pacouret G, Palazzini M, Petris A, Pruszczyk P, Rugolotto M, Salvi A, Schellong S, Sebbane M, Sobkowicz B, Stefanovic BS, Thiele H, Torbicki A, Verschuren F, Konstantinides SV, PEITHO Investigators. Fibrinolysis for patients with intermediate-risk pulmonary embolism. N Engl J Med. 2014;370:1402–11.

20. Paul W, Armstrong PW, Gershlick AH, Goldstein P, Wilcox R, Danays T, Lambert Y, Sulimov V, Rosell Ortiz F, Ostojic M, Welsh RC, Carvalho AC, Nanas J, Arntz HR, Halvorsen S, Huber K, Grajek S, Fresco C, Bluhmki E, Regelin A, Vandenberghe K, Bogaerts K, Van de Werf F, for the STREAM Investigative Team. Fibrinolysis or primary PCI in ST-segment elevation myocardial infarction. N Engl J Med. 2014;368:1379–87.
21. Elliot CG. Fibrinolysis of pulmonary emboli–steer closer to Scylla. N Engl J Med. 2014;370: 1457–8.
22. Kline JA, Nordenholz KE, Courtney DM, Kabrhel C, Jones AE, Rondina MT, Diercks DB, Klinger JR, Hernandez J. Treatment of submassive pulmonary embolism with tenecteplase or placebo: cardiopulmonary outcomes at 3 months: multicenter double-blind, placebo-controlled randomized trial. J Thromb Haemost. 2014;12:459–68.

Chapter 4
Patients for Thrombolysis

Carlos Jerjes-Sánchez and Pedro Gutierrez Fajardo

Acute pulmonary embolism (PE) is a cardiovascular emergency. It is a condition related with high morbidity and mortality. In spite of the advances on thrombosis prophylaxis, cardiac imaging studies and pharmacological treatment, it is still the third most frequent cardiovascular disease after acute coronary syndrome and stroke. It could be under diagnosed often, mainly due to its wide spectrum of presentation as it goes from mild symptomatic patient to cardiogenic shock and risk of death. It affects both genders and it is present in all age groups, though is more prevalent between fifth and sixth decade of life, occurring 23–69/100,000 people per year in the United States and 100–200/100,000 in Europe [1–3]. Both medical and surgical conditions are related with PE and a most objective focused stratification protocol in order to determine how the treatment should be selected is mandatory.

Several aspects must be taken into account for a primary treatment. Clinical suspicions and level of risk are common terms used in the scenarios of PE approach. In brief, patients must be categorized in either high or low risk, depending on hemodynamic derangement or the degree of right ventricle dysfunction. Triggering a stratification protocol should be based on clinical presentation, level of biomarkers, and noninvasive imaging studies to determine right ventricular status and pulmonary vascular obstruction [4–8]. Patients who survived the acute phase can evolve to chronic and deteriorating disease if vascular obstruction was not resolved.

C. Jerjes-Sánchez, M.D., F.C.C.P., F.A.C.C. (✉)
Sistema Nacional de Investigadores, Nivel II – Clinical Research Director,
Instituto de Cardiologia y Medicina Vascular, TEC Salud

Escuela de Medicina, Tecnológico de Monterrey San Pedro Garza Garcia, Nuevo León, Mexico

Unidad de Investigacion Clinica en Medicina SC Monterrey, Nuevo León, Mexico
e-mail: jerjes@prodigy.net.mx

P. G. Fajardo, M.D., F.A.S.E., M.E.A.C.I.
Echocardiography Laboratory, Hospital Bernardette, Instituto Cardiovascular
de Guadalajara, Jalisco, Mexico
e-mail: drpedrogutierrez@yahoo.com

C. Jerjes-Sánchez, *Thrombolysis in Pulmonary Embolism*,
DOI 10.1007/978-3-319-19707-4_4

Identifying Patients for Thrombolysis

High-Clinical Suspicion

The relevance of categorizing a patient in a high-clinical suspicion level attempt to an accurate testing and is based on clinical bases focus on risk factors as well as, cardiovascular and respiratory symptoms and signs; patients with submassive or massive PE could present with cardiopulmonary arrest or sudden dyspnea (rest or on exertion) associated to ischemic-like chest pain, and/or near-syncope and/or syncope; as well as tachypnea, tachycardia, and diaphoresis. Jugular venous distension and cyanosis are infrequent specifically in patients with early onset of symptoms that come early to the emergency room department. Cyanosis has to be related with severe right ventricular dysfunction and cardiogenic shock or other clinical situation (COPD, pulmonary hypertension).

On cardiac examination right ventricular lift, increased P_2, third and fourth heart sound suggesting pulmonary hypertension and right ventricular dysfunction; listening an attenuate and low P_2 it is a confounder and has been related with severe right ventricular dysfunction. Also, hypotension can be present as cardiogenic shock expression; however normal blood pressure cannot exclude impending clinical instability. In minor, submassive or massive PE it is possible identified leg pain, warmth, swelling, and Homans' sign suggesting deep venous thrombosis; however, these symptoms and signs could not be observed in some high-risk PE patients.

In the setting of venous thromboembolism, risk factors and clinical presentation are of utmost importance to establish a high-clinical suspicion. PE can occur in patients with temporary predisposing factors and are usually identified as secondary or provoked PE. When the acute event occurs in the absence of any identifiable risk factors it is considered as idiopathic or unprovoked PE. Patients with minor PE without right ventricular dysfunction may present with an extensive variety of cardiorespiratory symptoms, such as shortness of breath, exertion or rest dyspnea, pleuritic chest pain, cough, palpitations, either new onset or evolving for several days, hemoptysis. Physicians have to be in warning, because symptoms and signs suggesting a critical condition are not specific to PE [8] (Table 4.1). In high-clinical suspicion of submassive or massive PE several differential diagnosis as acute myocardial infarction, aortic dissection, pericardial tamponade, acute valve prosthesis dysfunction, extensive pneumonia, hypertensive pneumothorax, as well as pulmonary arterial hypertension have to be considered.

Current data coming from EMPEROR registry suggests an "atypical" PE presentation related with emerging risk factors. This was a prospective contemporary registry in Emergency Department patients to identify data specific of race or ethnicity, to compare the availability and contemporaneous use of risk stratification methods, including serum biomarkers and, the frequency of use of empiric anticoagulation, an intervention that may affect outcome [8].

In this study, 1880 acute PE patients were confirmed by computerized tomographic pulmonary angiogram in 88 % of cases. Patients represented both sexes equally, and racial and ethnic composition paralleled the overall US Emergency

Table 4.1 Clinical characteristics of patients with suspected pulmonary embolism

	PE confirmed ($n=1880$) (%)	PE not confirmed ($n=528$) (%)
Symptoms		
Dyspnea	50	51
Pleuritic chest pain	39	28
Substernal chest pain	15	17
Syncope	6	6
Unilateral leg pain	6	5
Signs		
Cough	23	23
Fever	10	10
Hemoptysis	8	4
Signs of deep venous thrombosis	24	18
Diaphoresis	7	5
Respiratory distress	16	13

Modified from Pollack et al. J Am Coll Cardiol 2011; 57:700, with permission

Department population. An unexpected clinical profile included young male, Caucasian or African American, employed, living independently, with a high incidence of atherosclerosis risk factors, and, with dyspnea on exertion [8]. Additionally, this "atypical" clinical profile had two confounding factors: an increase in the incidence of male gender and dyspnea with exertion. Because effort dyspnea has been related with COPD, heart failure with preserved or not ejection fraction, asthma, ischemic heart disease, and pulmonary arterial hypertension, physicians have to be in warning with this clinical presentation.

Although white-collar employment is usually equivalent with a sedentary lifestyle and long periods of sitting behind a computer (eThrombosis), such a relationship was not explored. Emergency physicians have to be in warning and should not limit their thinking suspicion to the "typical" presentations of PE (chronic or incurable disease, hospitalization, cancer, major surgery, bed-bound, etc.), and avoid misdiagnosis of acute coronary syndromes.

Risk Factors

Current approach to classify risk factors is considering that venous thromboembolism results from both interaction between patient-related risk factor and setting-related risk factors [9–11] (Table 4.2). The first, are considered to be permanent, whereas the second, temporary. Risk factor evidence including age, past history of deep venous thrombosis, major trauma, lower limb fractures, spinal cord injury, left ventricular dysfunction, cancer, chronic obstructive pulmonary disease, and infection can interact predisposing hospitalization and deep venous thrombosis.

Table 4.2 Risk factors for venous thromboembolism

	Temporary	Permanent
Patient-related risk factors—hereditary		
Activated protein C resistance without factor V Leiden		+
Antithrombin deficiency		+
Dysfibrinogenemia		+
Factor V Leiden		+
Protein C deficiency		+
Protein S deficiency		+
Prothrombin gene mutation		+
Plasminogen deficiency		+
Patient-related risk factors—setting		
Acute medical illness	+	
Advanced age		+
Cancer	+	+
Central venous catheter	+	
Chemotherapy	+	
Chronic obstructive pulmonary disease		+
Hormonereplacement therapy	+	+
Immobilizer or plaster cast	+	
Infection	+	
Major surgery	+	
Left ventricular dysfunction	+	+
Obesity	+	+
Oral contraceptives	+	
Pregnancy and post partum period	+	
Prolonged travel (air or ground)	+	
Reduced mobility (prolonged)	+	+
Spinal cord injury	+	+
Trauma	+	

Interestingly, the predictive weighs for these factors are unequal and venous thromboembolism could occur in patients without any identifiable predisposing factor [10] in up to 30 % of PE patients. In women, oral contraception use, even in reduced dose of estrogen, represent still an increased risk [12]. Pregnancy and postpartum period are related with venous thromboembolism and is an important cause of maternal morbidity and mortality. The risk is highest by the last trimester of pregnancy and 6 weeks after delivery [12–14]. Due to nonspecific presentation, PE could be a challenging ruling-out disorder. However, a prompt stratification and expedite diagnosis are fundamental to offer an early directed treatment. Being aware of patient's particular profile together with risk factors could help physician choosing a most appropriate stratification and diagnostic approach.

Current European Cardiology Society guidelines on PE classified the risk factors regarding the odds ratios are as follows: Strong risk factors (odds ratio >10): Fracture of lower limb previous 3 months, hip or knee replacement, major trauma, myocardial infarction (within previous 3 months), previous venous thromboembolism, and spinal cord injury. Moderate risk factors (odds ratio 2–9): arthroscopic knee surgery, auto–immune diseases, blood transfusion, central venous lines, chemotherapy, congestive heart or respiratory failure, erythropoiesis-stimulating agents, hormone replacement therapy (depends on formulation), in vitro fertilization, cancer (highest risk in metastatic disease), oral contraceptive therapy, paralytic stroke, postpartum period, and thrombophilia. Weak risk factors (odds ratio <2): Bed rest >3 days, diabetes mellitus, hypertension, immobility due to sitting (e.g., prolonged car or air travel), increasing age, laparoscopic surgery (e.g., cholecystectomy), obesity, pregnancy, and varicose veins [7]. An interesting observation is that stronger risk factors with odds ratio ranging from <2 to >10 were all involved with inflammation, coagulation cascade, and platelet activation.

From our point of view, risk factors could be classified on molecular bases [15]. A reorganization of the risk factors, taking into account the molecular evidence, is shown in Table 4.3. Inflammation involves several conditions in health and disease related historically with deep venous thrombosis and PE. Secondary thrombophilia includes factors associated with the coagulation cascade and platelet activation to a greater or lesser degree; as well as other mechanisms observed in different clinical situations. Molecular thrombophilia was separated in acquired and hereditary. Finally, independent of the risk factors, stasis or infections are the triggers for acute thromboembolic event.

Different calculation rules have been validated in predicting probability (low, moderate, or high-clinical probability, PE likely or unlikely) (Table 4.4), and adverse outcome [16, 17] (Table 4.5). These scores account both for the clinical severity of an acute event and the patient's comorbidity. The Pulmonary Embolism Severity Index (PESI) has been widely validated. One of its major strength is ruling out an adverse outcome as evidenced by the high negative predictive value of the classes II and I. On the other hand, a weak of the original PESI score is the many unequally weighed variables that can become a quite multipart calculate, reducing eventually its workability in an emergency setting. A simplified version (sPESI) assesses only six equally weighed variables and accurately identifies patients with PE who are at low risk of death and other complications [18]. Those patients with moderate or high pretest probability should continue their assessment with an imaging modality.

Considering that dyspnea plus near-syncope or syncope or dyspnea associated to ischemic-like chest pain in PE patients has been associated with >50 % of pulmonary arterial obstruction in pulmonary angiography and with severe right ventricular dysfunction, respectively, we considered that both conditions could be added to proposed PSI score, maintaining pulse, systolic blood pressure, respiratory rate, and oxygen saturation. This simple tool could be used in emergency department by physicians with or without experience. Our proposal required clinical validation.

Table 4.3 Risk factors on molecular bases

Risk factor	Clinical expression
Inflammation	Smoking, obesity, dysglycemia, diabetes mellitus, metabolic syndrome, dyslipidemia, ischemic heart disease, acute coronary syndromes, stroke, peripheral artery disease, hypertension, COPD, acute or chronic heart failure, respiratory failure, atrial fibrillation, connective tissue diseases (systemic lupus erythematosus, rheumatoid arthritis, etc.), renal chronic failure, nephrotic syndrome, Behcet's disease
Secondary thrombophilia	
Coagulation cascade and platelet activation	Fracture, hip or knee replacement, major or minor surgery, major trauma, spinal cord injury, arthroscopic knee surgery, secondary polycythemia, vaginal delivery and cesarean section
Miscellaneous mechanisms	• *Physiologic hypercoagulable state*: age >40 years, aging, pregnancy, postpartum
	• *Procoagulant effects*: malignancy
	• *Therapeutic action*: chemotherapy, hormone replacement and oral contraceptive therapy, pacemaker or implantable cardiac defibrillator leads and indwelling venous catheters, heparin-induced thrombocytopenia
Molecular thrombophilia	
Acquired	Lupus anticoagulant, antiphospholipid antibody syndrome, hyperhomocystinemia (less commonly inherited secondary to a mutation in methylenetetrahydrofolate reductase), deficiency of dysfibrinogenemia, myeloproliferative disorders such as polycythemia rubra vera, elevated levels of lipoprotein (a)
Hereditary	Deficiency of antithrombin III, protein C or protein S, factor V Leiden mutation, prothrombin gene mutation, primary thrombocytopenia, hypercoagulability syndromes, deficit or abnormalities of plasminogen, dysplasminogenemia, hyperprothrombinemia, deficiency of factor XII, factor VIII increase, deficiency or abnormalities of plasminogen, increase plasminogen activator inhibitor type-1, paroxysmal nocturnal hemoglobinuria
Triggers	• *Stasis*: prolonged car or air travel, bed-bound, computer works, or immobilities related to the home: convalescence secondary to chronic heart failure, pulmonary or neurological diseases, cancer, degenerative osteoarthropathy, and obesity
	• *Chronic or acute infections*: periodontitis, upper or lower respiratory tract, gastrointestinal, urinary, prostate, etc.

Modified from [15]

Suggestive Electrocardiogram

In the stratification approach, this accessible tool provides important findings to identify severe right ventricular pressure overload and ventricular ischemia. An electrocardiogram never will be normal in submassive or massive PE. The traditional right axis deviation is not always present, specifically during the early state of the acute event. In Fig. 4.1 a normal preoperative ECG, then in-hospital patient had a massive PE complicated with patent foramen ovale and paradoxical embolism to right coronary artery. In Fig. 4.2, there is not a right axis deviation expected in

Table 4.4 Clinical prediction rules for pulmonary embolism

Variable	Clinical decision rule points	
	Original version	Simplified version
Wells rule		
Previous pulmonary or deep venous thrombosis	1.5	1
Heart rate ≥100 beats per minute	1.5	1
Surgery or immobilization within past 4 weeks	1.5	1
Hemoptysis	1	1
Active cancer	1	1
Clinical signs of deep venous thrombosis	3	1
Clinical probability		
Three-level score		
Low	0–1	N/A
Intermediate	2–6	N/A
High	≥7	N/A
Two-level score		
Pulmonary embolism unlikely	0–4	0–1
Pulmonary embolism likely	≥5	≥2
Revised Geneve score		
Previous pulmonary embolism or DVT	3	1
Heart rate		
75–94 beat per minute	3	1
≥95	5	2
Surgery or fracture within the past month	2	1
Hemoptysis	2	1
Active cancer	2	1
Unilateral lower limb pain	3	1
Pain on lower limb deep venous and unilateral edema	4	1
Age >65 years	1	1
Clinical probability		
Three-level score		
Low	0–3	0–1
Intermediate	4–10	2–4
High	≥11	≥5
Two-level score		
Pulmonary embolism unlikely	0–5	0–2
Pulmonary embolism likely	≥6	≥3

DVT deep venous thrombosis. Eur Heart J 2014; 35:3033–3080, with permission

massive PE; however there is almost 60° axis deviation compared with the first electrocardiogram; also other electrocardiogram findings described in massive PE are observed; lead standard DI, aVL, chest leads V2, V3, and V4 ST depression, aVR-ST elevation [19] and chest lead V1 with qR and ST elevation: ST elevation in standard inferior leads are secondary to right coronary paradoxical embolism.

Table 4.5 Original, simplified and proposed pulmonary embolism severity index (PESI)

Variable	Original PESI[a] Score	Simplified PESI[b] Score	Proposed PESI Score
Dyspnea plus near-syncope or syncope			1
Dyspnea plus ischemic-like chest pain			1
Age >80 years	Age in years	1	–
Male sex	+10	–	–
History of cancer	+30	1	–
History of heart failure	+10	1[c]	–
History of chronic lung disease	+10		–
Pulse ≥110 beats per minute	+20	1	1
Systolic blood pressure <100 mmHg	+30	1	1
Respiratory rate ≥30 breaths per minute	+20	–	1
Temperature <36 °C	+20	–	–
Altered mental status[d]	+60	–	–
Arterial oxygen saturation <90 %[e]	+20	1	1

Modified from Thromb Haemost 2011; 106:423–28
[a]A total point score for a given patient is obtained by summing the patient's age in years and the points for each applicable prognostic variable. The five following risk classes are defined on patient's total point score: class I (≤65 points), class II (66–85 points), class III (86–105 points), class IV (106–125 points), and class V (>125 points). Patients in risk classes I/II are considered low risk
[b]A total point score for a given patient is obtained by summing the patient's age in years and the points for each applicable prognostic variable. Patients with 0 points are considered low risk
[c]The variables were combined into a single category of chronic cardiopulmonary disease
[d]Altered mental status was defined as disorientation, lethargy, stupor, or coma
[e]Arterial oxygen saturation was defined with and without the administration of supplemental oxygen

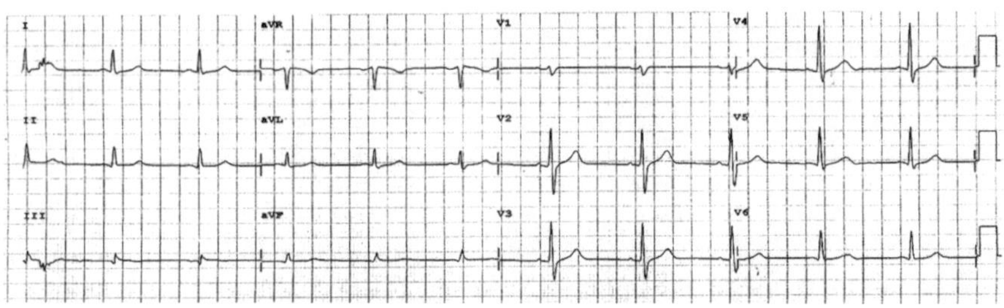

Fig. 4.1 Before surgery normal electrocardiogram

In the setting of PE patients, on admission aVR-ST elevation was present in 34.3 % ($n=136$). Presence of aVR-ST elevation was associated with more severe clinical presentation (dyspnea at rest 44.9 % vs. 29.2 %; $p=0.002$, hypotension 17.0 % vs. 6.5 %; $p=0.001$, syncope 16.2 % vs. 6.5 %; $p=0.002$), higher median troponin T levels (0.035 [0.01–0.2] vs. 0.01 [0.01–0.02]; p 0.001), more frequent right ventricular dysfunction (74.5 % vs. 46.6 %; p 0.001), and central located thrombi (50.8 vs. 29.2; p 0.001). Thrombolysis was used more frequently (29.1 % vs. 7.5 %; p 0.001) and in-hospital-mortality was increased (10.3 % vs. 5.4 %; $p=0.07$) when compared to patients without that sign. Mortality in intermediate-risk

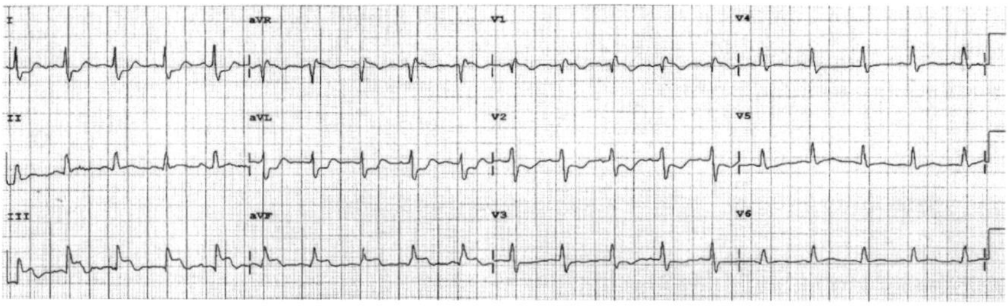

Fig. 4.2 Compared with electrocardiogram in Fig. 4.1, there is right axis deviation and ST depression in DI, aVL, V2 to V3 related with massive pulmonary embolism. Also ST elevation in inferior leads was secondary right coronary artery paroximal embolism. qR in V1 is related with right atrial dilatation. ST elevation in aVR and V1 could be explained for right ventricular ischemia and infarction respectively

PE patients with aVR-ST elevation was 8.9 % compared to 0 % in those without ($p=0.04$). In contrast, the presence of other classical electrocardiogram pattern of PE did not further increase mortality in intermediate-risk patients. Finally, ST elevation in lead aVR is associated with a more severe course of PE, especially in patients with intermediate-risk. Therefore, aVR-ST elevation might be useful in risk stratification of PE [20].

aVR-ST elevation identified right ventricular ischemia because lead aVR has a frontal plane vector of −150 directly facing the thinner wall of the right ventricular outflow area and through it the basal aspect of the interventricular septum below the aortic and pulmonary valves. Lead aVR faces through the left ventricular cavity the inner side of the apex and lateral wall and is directionally opposite to standard leads I and II and chest leads V5 and V6. The basal septum receives blood supply usually from very proximal septal branches of the left anterior descending artery [21].

Findings indicating RV overload such as qR pattern and ST elevation in lead V_1 has been associated with major in-hospital mortality; qR expressed right atrium intracavitary lead suggesting acute right atrium dilatation; ST elevation has been related with right ventricular myocardial infarction [22, 23]. Additionally, left axis deviation has been attributed to right anterior fascicular block [24].

Other electrocardiogram findings are inversion of T waves in leads V_1–V_4, D_{III} and aVF, $S_1S_2S_3$, $S_1Q_3T_3$ patterns, incomplete or advanced right bundle-branch block, especially in severe cases of PE. Also nonspecific T wave, ST segment depression, and ST segment elevation can be found. In spite that electrocardiogram changes could be considered unspecific, they likely represent right ventricular dilatation and/or right ventricular ischemia [25, 26].

Another classical electrocardiogram finding is tachycardia, however, in special group of PE patients, bradycardia (heart rate <60 beats/min) could be identified at the beginning of the acute event. Among 400 consecutive cases of PE, 13 patients with proved PE by high probability VQ scan or pulmonary angiography had bradycardia. Three groups were identified, AV block and malfunctioning pacemaker generator, COPD, and ischemic heart disease. The main clinical manifestations were sudden dyspnea and congestive heart failure. Among these patients, PE diagnosis was not considered until 3 or 7 days. In 13 patients with heterogeneous cardiopulmonary disease and proved non massive PE, bradycardia in the acute phase was attributed to primary or secondary conduction system disease (anti-dysrhythmic and anti-ischemic medication) [27].

It is important to note that electrocardiogram is not a method to rule out PE, however, it is helpful in predicting adverse clinical outcomes in confirmed PE. Also it is useful when acute coronary syndrome is considered as a differential diagnosis. Rhythm disturbances are not frequent but atrial fibrillation or flutter may be present.

Chest Radiograph

This study is obtained in all patients with PE high-clinical suspicion. Chest radiograph in minor PE could be normal. In massive or submassive PE is possible identified classic radiographic findings as Westermark sign characterized by a clarified area with diminished vascularity corresponding to the extent of the embolized artery; Hampton sign classical is a triangle with base to the pleura and the vertex directed to a branch of the pulmonary artery; frequently is associated with elevated diaphragm and small pleural effusion and has been associated with pulmonary infarction; when pulmonary obstruction is >35 % acute pulmonary arterial hypertension occurs inducing pulmonary artery and right ventricular remodeling, its radiographic expression are right and/or left pulmonary artery dilatation, main pulmonary artery dilatation, as well as, right ventricular dilatation. Also elevated diaphragm could be observed. In Fig. 4.3, it is possible to identify bilateral and extensive Westermark sign in both lungs, also right artery dilatation and left artery amputation is observed. In Fig. 4.4, it is possible to identify Westermark sign with more precision. The chest radiograph of female with submassive PE is shown in Fig. 4.5; where Westermark signs in right upper and left inferior lobe, also left artery amputation and right artery dilatation is observed; left low lobe had normal circulation. In a lateral view, retrosternal space is obliterated by right ventricular dilatation (Fig. 4.6).

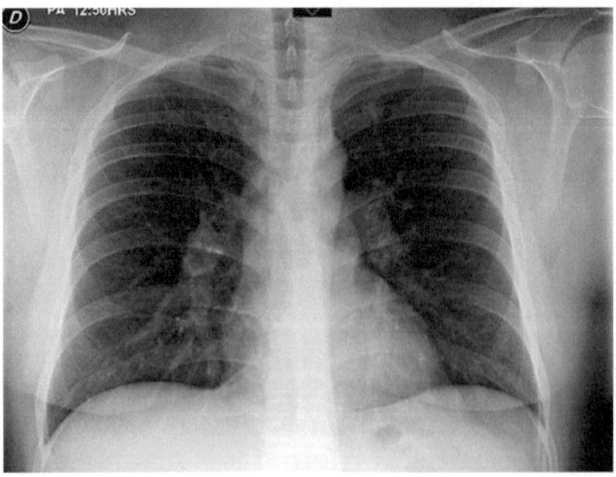

Fig. 4.3 Chest radiograph in a young man with effort dyspnea as clinical manifestation to acute pulmonary embolism. Bilateral Westermark sign, also right artery dilatation and left artery amputation

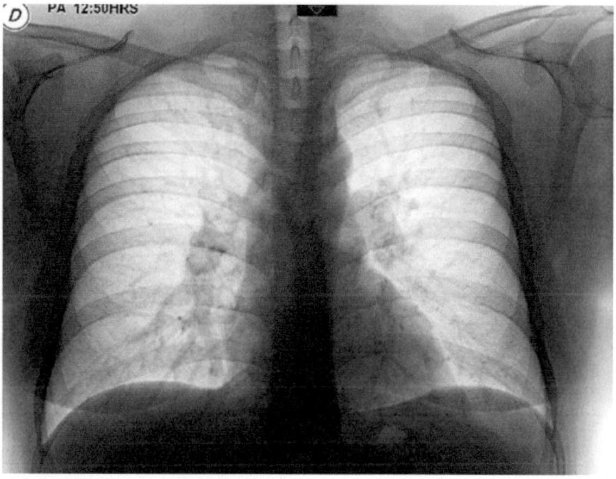

Fig. 4.4 A negative view of radiograph of Fig. 4.3, there it is possible to identify acute radiographic signs of acute pulmonary embolism

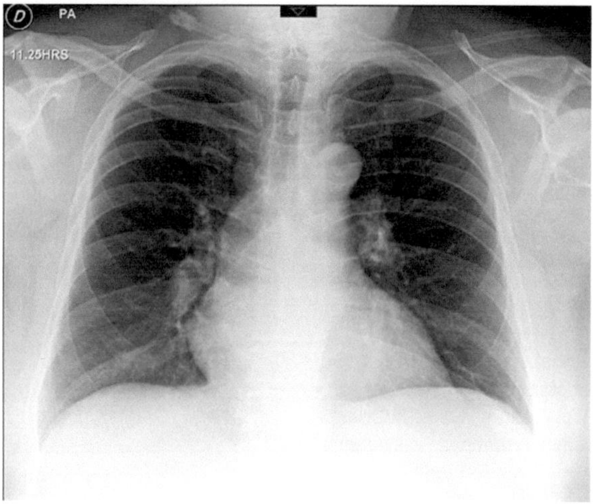

Fig. 4.5 Female patient with submassive pulmonary embolism. Westermark signs in right upper and left inferior lobe, left artery amputation, and right artery dilatation is observed

In patients with submassive or massive PE, the majority of chest radiographs are obtained bedside. In this situation, it is no easy to identify classic signs; however in this condition chest radiograph allows to exclude another clinical situation mimicking PE (acute pulmonary edema, COPD exacerbation, cardiac tamponade, extensive pneumothorax, etc.) In Fig. 4.7, a portable chest radiograph of a massive PE patient with extensive Westermark sign in both lungs with pulmonary vasculature preserved in left upper lobe only is shown. Another chest radiograph of a male patient with massive PE showed bilateral Westermark sign, elevated diaphragm, as well as both pulmonary arteries dilated (Fig. 4.8). In all of these cases an important observation is that main artery and right ventricular dilatation are absent.

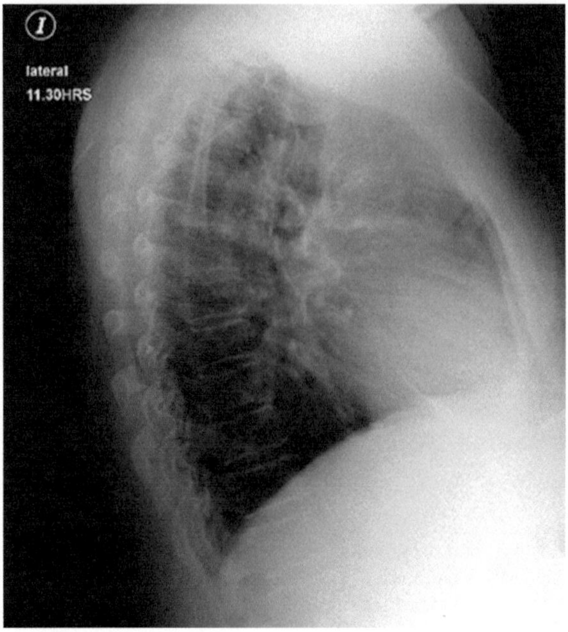

Fig. 4.6 Right lateral view showing retrosternal space obliteration as expression of right ventricular dilatation

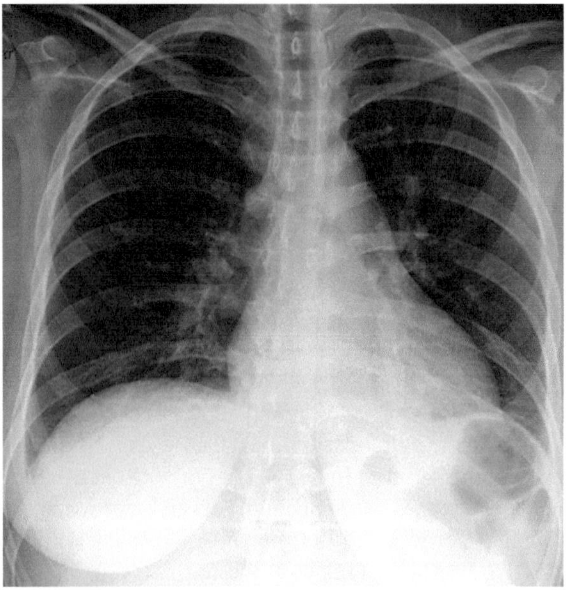

Fig. 4.7 A portable chest radiograph of a patient with massive pulmonary embolism. It is possible to observe extensive Westermark sign in both lungs, pulmonary vasculature remains in left upper lobe only

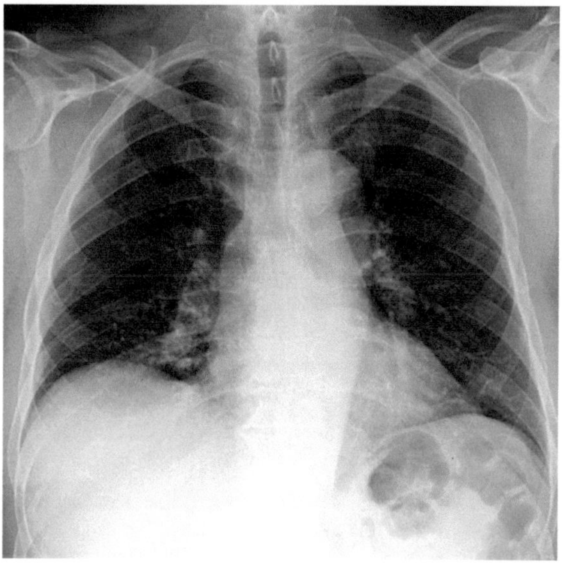

Fig. 4.8 Chest radiograph of a male patient with massive pulmonary embolism showing bilateral Westermark sign, elevated diaphragm, and pulmonary arteries dilatation

High-Risk Stratification

Different medical groups and societies [28–31] have emphasized the importance of identifying high-risk patients, considering as the most important predictors (a) clinical markers (especially systemic arterial hypotension), (b) biomarkers, and (c) noninvasive imaging studies, with evidence of right ventricular dilatation at the time of screening. The rationale for categorizing patients at high-risk is predicting a subsequent worsening condition and death. Contrasting to other diseases, treatment in PE is defined by the assessment of the patient's early death risk, closely related to the level of right ventricular dysfunction. Accordingly, while some patients will be stable with anticoagulation only, others will require systemic thrombolysis, catheter-directed thrombectomy, thrombolysis, or surgical thrombectomy (Fig. 4.9) to guarantee a prompt revascularization to revert right ventricular dysfunction, in an attempt of improving survival and avoiding recurrence.

Clinically defining an acute PE will depend on the classification used in this setting. Whereas some groups classify PE in acute massive, acute submassive, acute small, and subacute massive, with or without previous cardiopulmonary disease [29], with cardiogenic shock or normotensive, others use different systems of classification according to the individual risk of early mortality taking into account risk markers [32]. Any classification will emphasize right ventricular function/dysfunction and the hemodynamic impact on systemic blood pressure (shock or persistent low pressure) as the critical elements affecting survival and prognosis [33].

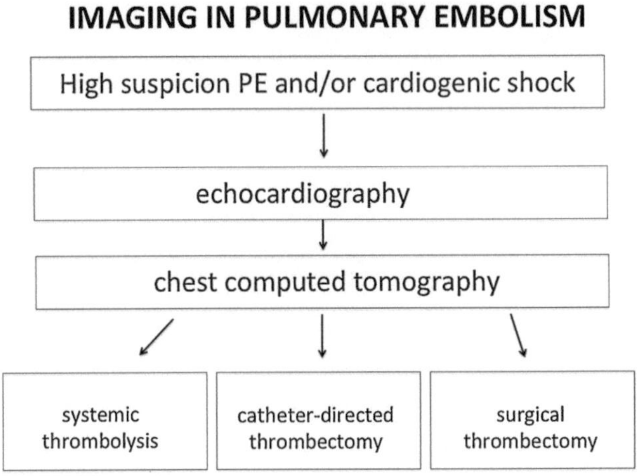

Fig. 4.9 Flow chart for pulmonary reperfusion. Pathway based on high-clinical suspicion, echocardiogram and chest computed tomography. For echocardiogram accessibility, low cost and no radiation could be preferred to chest computed tomography

Clinical Markers

Serious conditions including cardiorespiratory arrest, cardiogenic sock and hypotension, reflect the possibility that significant obstruction of pulmonary vasculature secondary to a huge clot or several small clots have lodged into the pulmonary artery lumen producing an increase in pulmonary vascular resistance that exceeds the ability of right ventricular to cope with an acute increase in afterload. Normally, right ventricular pumps blood into a low resistance circuit; as a conductance chamber, it does not have conditioning to overcome an acute increase in afterload. In PE, initially, the rise in pulmonary artery pressure and afterload leads to an increase in right ventricular wall tension, and a higher myocardial oxygen demand, generating an imbalance in the supply–demand relationship. Simultaneously, as compensatory mechanism, right ventricle dilates and prolongs its contraction time, overlapping into left ventricle early diastole causing leftward bowing in the interventricular septum.

Also, neurohumoral response leads to inotropic–chronotropic stimulation. If obstruction is not resolved, compensatory mechanisms fail, leading to right ventricular ischemia and reducing myocite contractile forces with detrimental effects on circulation worsening right ventricular ischemia, and even in the absence of significant artery coronary plaques, although rarely, right ventricular infarction can occur. An ischemic RV continues dilating even to a greater size than left ventricle, affecting the normal right ventricular/left ventricular (RV/LV) ratio. The hypotension response and the state of shock could be the result of spiraling cycle of RV/LV deterioration function where low cardiac output, neurohormonal and inflammatory response culminate in global cardiac failure and death [34–37]. Thirty to fifty percent of patients with APE are "hemodynamically" stable but with some degree or RV strain. These patients are at higher risk of collapsing and dying later on [31].

Biomarkers

Echocardiography and other imaging modalities are important tools in assessing PE; however, they all reveal right ventricular mechanical changes due to acute afterload [35]. In massive or major PE, an enlarged right ventricle and other right ventricular dysfunction surrogates are expected. When right ventricular dysfunction findings are found in normotensive patients or in submassive PE, they may represent a worse prognosis [32]. It is not difficult to consider that abnormal right ventricular size, free-wall motion abnormalities, changes in RV/LV ratio, could in fact be a kind of accompaniment to thrombosis initiation, myocardial damage, and neurohormonal activation, developing simultaneously, permitting some serum markers be detected. Usefulness of biomarkers is based on their ability for elucidating that myocardial damage is occurring and that neurohormonal response has switched on [7].

A major role for cardiac biomarkers is differentiating risk patients in a diagnosed PE that is related also with severity of right ventricular dysfunction. It is well known the sensitivity of troponin I and T for detecting myocardial injury. In contrast with patients with acute coronary syndrome, elevations of troponin levels in patients with PE are brief and subtle but they have a good correlation with the extent of right ventricular dysfunction especially in massive PE [38, 39]. It seems that elevations in troponin level are secondary to myocardial ischemia or elevated post load, due to imbalance in oxygen demand and supply, even in the absence of angiographic coronary obstruction [40]. Elevation in natriuretic peptides are associated with right ventricular dysfunction, consequently, they are useful in diagnostic stratification approach. Mechanism for synthesis and secretion of brain natriuretic peptide type-B responds to myocyte stretching from acute pressure overload. It has been reported that biomarkers elevation to be related to increased risk of adverse outcomes, including death, requiring close monitoring and prompt treatment [41, 42].

Those patients with low troponin and low brain natriuretic peptide type-B levels would be considered in the low-risk group as reflected by their high negative predictive value for adverse events. On the other hand, the hemodynamically stable patient but with increased biomarker levels, right ventricle dysfunction should be assessed by echocardiography [43]. Likewise, D-dimer is in the stratification scenario, reflecting that coagulation and fibrinolysis are activated. D-dimer fibrin is the result of the activation of coagulation system, whose product is a fibrin clot that is subsequently lysed by the activation of fibrinolytic system, which breaks the fibrin clot to fibrin degradation products. Consequently, D-dimer is a fibrin-derived fragment that is released into the circulation when cross-linked fibrin is broken down by the fibrinolytic system [44]. Although, a positive D-dimer test may be useful as indicated that venous thrombosis has not preditive value. In general, D-dimer is preferred for those patients with low probability of PE. Although is a sensitive test (91–97 % for enzyme-linked immunofluorescence), it has a low to moderate specificity (43–50 %) since positive results may be found in elderly patients, in pregnant women and in patients with cancer, trauma, infection and inflammatory diseases [45–47], thus decisions on treatment cannot be taken. D-dimer test should be considered in the context of clinical probability, especially in patients with clinical stability, but due to its limited value, not in patients with moderate to high probability as well as in-hospital patients [48].

Noninvasive Imaging Studies

Although transthoracic echocardiography could be considered an imaging technique with low sensitivity in PE, it is a most useful noninvasive study as the initial approach for stratification of patients suspecting PE, due to its availability, portability, low cost, nonradiation, non-contrast use, and immediate results, as provides strong information. Bedside transthoracic echocardiography can rapidly differentiate conditions mimicking PE but whose treatment is tremendously dissimilar, such as acute myocardial infarction, aortic dissection, pericardial tamponade, also allowing a rapid life-saving treatment (Table 4.6). On the other hand, transthoracic echocardiography can be done several times when close monitoring of right ventricular function or treatment result is required, as is harmless for patient and does not have any accumulative effect.

Table 4.6 Role of echocardiography in acute pulmonary embolism

Assess
Right ventricle size and thickness
Right ventricle shape
Right ventricle/left ventricle ratio
Right ventricle free-wall and apex motion
Inferior cava vein diameter and inspiratory collapse
Pulmonary pressure
Detect (eventually)
Thrombus
Inferior vena cava
Right chambers
Pulmonary trunk
Proximal pulmonary branches
Rule out
Acute diseases simulating acute pulmonary embolism
Acute myocardial infarction
Aortic dissection
Cardiac tamponade
Acute valve prosthesis dysfunction
Helps in determining cause
State of shock
Cardiac arrest

In patients with poor acoustic window, transesophageal echocardiography allows a better right ventricular examination and eventually thrombus in main pulmonary artery and proximal branches can be found. In some centers, transthoracic echocardiography/transesophageal echocardiography findings together with clinical and biomarkers changes, are enough to start thrombolysis in high-risk patients considering that the severity of right ventricular dysfunction is directly proportional to the degree of vascular obstruction. The more abnormal ventricular function, the more embolus loads in pulmonary vessels. It has been shown that right ventricular dysfunction on echocardiography is a powerful and independent predictor of mortality, even in patients with normal systemic blood pressure [49].

Up to 40 % of patients with PE can present with echocardiographic abnormalities due to acute pulmonary hypertension reflecting right ventricular dysfunction, these include: (a) Right ventricle dilatation, qualitatively, in a four-apical chamber view RV/LV change ratio, 1:1 ratio 2:1 ratio or more than 2:1 ratio [50]; and quantitatively, RV/LV end-diastolic dimension ratio >0.6 in parasternal long axis view or more than 0.9 in four-chamber view [16], (b) right ventricular free-wall abnormalities-hypokinesis, akinesis [51], right ventricular apex hyperkinesis (McConnell's sign) [52] (c) signs of right ventricular pressure overload, such as paradoxical interventricular systolic septum motion, flattened interventricular septum, right atrium dilatation, inferior vena cava dilatation with reduced or absence of inspiratory collapse, interatrial septum shift to the left, tricuspid regurgitation (more than mild grade), pulmonary regurgitation (more than mild grade), pulmonary artery trunk enlargement, and

Table 4.7 Echocardiography findings in PE with hemodynamic compromise

Right chambers dilatation (right ventricle—right atrium)
Right ventricle/left ventricle inversion ratio
1:1
2:1
>2:1
Wall motion abnormalities
Right ventricle free-wall basal and midsegments hypokinesis
McConell sign (right ventricular apex hyperkinesis)
Reduced TAPSE
Interventricular septum paradoxical motion
Decreased left ventricle diastolic diameter
Interatrial septum bowing to left
Tricuspid valve regurgitation (greater than mild)
Pulmonary valve regurgitation (greater than mild)
Dilated inferior venous cava and lack of inspiratory collapse
Dilated hepatic veins
Elevated pulmonary pressure
Dilated artery pulmonary trunk
Patent foramen ovale (rarely a thrombus straddling)
Right ventricular hypertrophy absence (a must for considering acute pulmonary embolism)

Table 4.8 Right atrium pressure estimation with IVC response to inhaling

Right atrium pressure (mmHg)	Inferior vena cava
5	Full collapse
10	Collapse ≥50 % of initial diameter
15	Collapse ≤50 % of initial diameter
20	No collapse

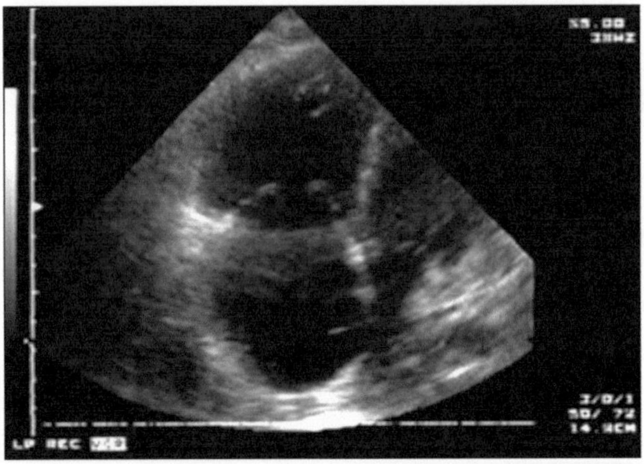

Fig. 4.10 Four-chamber view transthoracic echocardiogram showing severe right ventricular and atrium dilatation

elevated pulmonary artery pressure (Tables 4.7 and 4.8). In Fig. 4.10 a four-chamber view transthoracic echocardiogram has shown severe right ventricular and atrium dilatation. Accordingly, it is not expected that a subsegmental pulmonary thrombus provoke any significant echocardiographic abnormality. Thus, a normal or near normal echocardiogram should not be used to rule out PE when clinical suspicion exists.

Diagnosis

Hemodynamic impact is the main demanding rapid diagnosis component in massive PE. In the past, pulmonary angiography was considered the gold standard to demonstrate emboli in arterial tree; now its use has decreased due to chest CT advancement and other imaging modalities showing right ventricular dysfunction. In the setting of suspecting PE, where available, in high-risk patient a CT angiography should be done. Chest CT has shown to be as accurate as invasive pulmonary angiography with good negative predictive value in the assessment of PE,

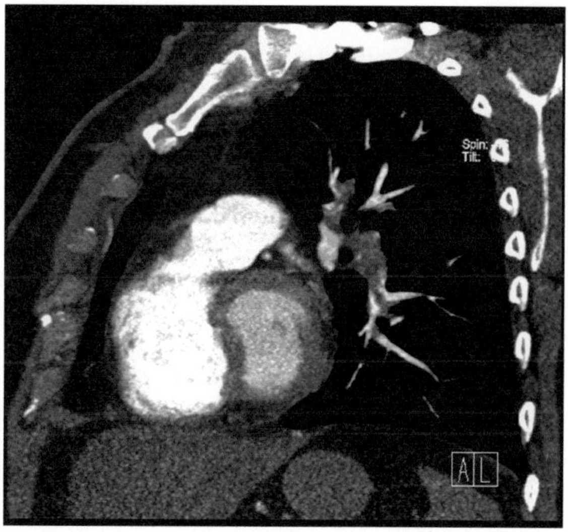

Fig. 4.11 Chest computed tomography with a thrombus occluding left main pulmonary artery, also severe right ventricular and atrial dilatation are observed

especially with multidetector row pulmonary angiography [53–55] (CTPA) that used in combination with clinical risk prediction scores can exclude PE; in fact, CTPA has increased detection of PE and subsegmental embolisms [56, 57].

Similarly to echocardiography, CT has demonstrated the prognostic utility of including signs of right ventricular dysfunction, such as RV/LV dimension ratios, interventricular septal motion abnormality and inferior vena cava diameter. CT angiography sagittal view with severe right ventricular dilatation, septal deviation and a thrombus occluding left main pulmonary artery, also several segmentary intraluminal defects are observed (Fig. 4.11). In spite of the diagnostic images obtained with CT, technical limitations such as poor contrast enhancement of pulmonary vessels, patient respiratory motion, irregular rhythm, and increased image noise due to obesity could produce a nondiagnostic study. Also, intravenous use of contrast can precipitate renal failure mainly in patients with poor kidney function reserve. Irradiation amount is a point of concern, especially in younger people.

Currently new techniques as dual-energy CT ventilation/perfusion imaging can provide high-spatial-resolution morphological and functional ventilation/perfusion information of the lung in patients with suspected PE, with CT as a single investigation. Despite its limitations dual-energy CT ventilation/perfusion imaging can visualize PE-related ventilation/perfusion mismatch even in peripheral lung regions and may thus have a role in improving the detection of peripheral PE in selected patients with suspected PE [58].

Magnetic resonance angiography is considered a good imaging modality for detecting PE when thrombus is proximal. Compared to CT it has similar specificity [59]. MR has several advantages over CT, essentially for the lack of contrast requirement of ionizing or iodinated products. Magnetic resonance allows assessment of both right and left ventricles; using techniques as three-dimensional gadolinium-enhanced MR angiography, direct thrombus imaging magnetic resonance, as well as, perfusion imaging. This study looks like an attractive option in PE patients.

Additionally magnetic resonance is rapidly evolving and the inherent advantages of noninvasiveness, nonionizing radiation requirement, the use of safer (or completes absence of) contrast agents, and the versatile sequences employed to assess various tissues in the chest render it of potential value for the future. In addition to technical considerations, the availability and the cost remain problematic in the majority of the hospitals [60]. Currently, the accuracy of this method is similar to 16-slice CT. Magnetic resonance angiography emerge as interest option for PE diagnosis, specially in patients with allergic reactions to iodated contrast media and in pediatric patients because it does not involve ionizing radiation [61].

Ventilation/perfusion lung scanning (V/Q) used to be the pivotal noninvasive diagnostic test for suspected PE for many years but due to nondiagnostic scanning and complex terminology now is almost replaced by chest CT. Recently complex terminology was modified for diagnosis or not diagnosis [29]. Current European Cardiology Society guidelines establish that is an established diagnostic test for suspected PE. It is safe and few allergic reactions have been described. The test is based on the intravenous injection of technetium (Tc)-99m-labelled macroaggregated albumin particles, which block a small fraction of the pulmonary capillaries and thereby enable scintigraphic assessment of lung perfusion [7].

Perfusion scans are combined with ventilation studies, for which multiple tracers such as xenon-133 gas, Tc-99m-labelled aerosols, or Tc-99m-labelled carbon microparticles (Technegas) can be used. The purpose of the ventilation scan is to increase specificity: in acute PE, ventilation is expected to be normal in hypoperfused segments (mismatch). According to the International Commission on Radiological Protection, the radiation exposure from a lung scan with 100 MBq of Tc-99m macroaggregated albumin particles is 1.1 mSv for an average sized adult, and thus is significantly lower than that of CT angiography (2–6 mSv).

Being a radiation- and contrast medium-sparing procedure, the V/Q scan may preferentially be applied in outpatients with low clinical probability and a normal chest X-ray, in young (particularly female) patients, in pregnancy, in patients with history of contrast medium-induced anaphylaxis and strong allergic history, in severe renal failure, and in patients with myeloma and paraproteinemia. The high frequency of nondiagnostic intermediate probability scans has been a cause for criticism, because they indicate the necessity for further diagnostic testing.

Considering current evidence, identifying a high-risk PE patient for thrombolysis is a process that included high-clinical suspicion based on experience and expertise. At present time, a careful risk factor, clinical symptoms and signs analysis at presentation is mandatory; the simplified or proposed PESI is an excellent toll to identify in an easy way not technology dependent high-risk PE patients. The second step consists in identifying bleeding complication risk through relative or absolute contraindications for thrombolysis [7, 29]. In addition, it is important to avoid puncture in arterial or venous major vessels; as well as high-risk variables to bleeding complications including elderly fragile patients have to be considered. The third step required to establish objectively the presence or not of right ventricular dysfunction by echocardiogram, CT angiogram, and right ventricular and acute cellular damage biomarkers. In patients with clinical instability, all evidences that we have recommend thrombolysis. In patients with right ventricular dysfunction and clinical stability, we have over 30 years of controversy. Since our experience, we are using thrombolysis in PE patients with clinical stability and right ventricular dysfunction with success and practically without bleeding complications. Finally the best stratification approach will be depending on experience, expertise, and available technology in each center.

References

1. Wood KE. Major pulmonary embolism. Chest. 2002;121:877–905.
2. Horlander KT, Mannino DM, Leeper Schcreiber KV. Pulmonary embolism in the United States, 1979-1998: an analysis using multiple cause-mortality data. Arch Intern Med. 2003;163: 1711–17.
3. Cohen AT, Agnelli G, Anderson FA, Arcelus JI, Bergqvist D, Brecht JG, Greer IA, Heit JA, Hutchinson JL, Kakkar AK, Mottier D, Oger E, Samama MM, Spangl M. Venous thromboembolism (VTE) in Europe. The number of VTE events and associated morbidity and mortality. Thromb Haemost. 2007;98:756–64.
4. Anderson Jr FA, Spencer FA. Risk factors for venous thromboembolism. Circulation. 2003;107:19S–16.
5. Stein PD, Henry JW. Prevalence of acute pulmonary embolism among patients in a general hospital and at autopsy. Chest. 1995;108:978–81.
6. Kyrle PA, Rosendaal FR, Eichinger S. Risk assessment for recurrent venous thrombosis. Lancet. 2010;376:2032–39.
7. Konstantinides SV, Torbicki A, Agnelli G, Danchin N, Fitzmaurice D, Galie N, Gibss JSR, Huisman MV, Humbert M, Kucher N, Lang I, Lankeit M, Lekakis J, Maack C, Mayer E, Meneveau N, Perrier A, Pruszczyk P, Rasmussen LH, Schindler TH, Svitil P, Vonk Noodergraff A, Zamorano JL, Zampotari M. 2014 ESC Guidelines on the diagnosis and management of acute pulmonary embolism. The Task Force for the diagnosis and management of acute pulmonary embolism of the European Society of Cardiology. Eur Heart J. 2014;35: 3033–80.
8. Pollack CV, Schcreiber D, Goldhaber SZ, Slattery D, Fanikos J, O'Neil BJ, Thompson JR, Hiestand B, Briese BA, Pendleton RC, Miller CD, Kline JA. Clinical characteristics, management and outcomes of patients diagnosed with acute pulmonary embolism in the emergency department: initial report of EMPEROR (Multicenter Emergency Medicine Pulmonary Embolism in the real world registry). J Am Coll Cardiol. 2011;57:700–6.
9. Squizzato A, Kuciani D, Rubboli A, Di Gennaro L, Landolfi R, De Luca C, Porro F, Moia M, Testa S, Imberti D, Bertolini G. Differential diagnosis of pulmonary embolism in outpatients with non-specific cardiopulmonary symptoms. Intern Emerg Med. 2013;8:695–702.
10. Anderson Jr FA, Spencer FA. Risk factors for venous thromboembolism. Circulation. 2003;107:I9–15.
11. Rogers MA, Levine DA, Blumberg N, Flanders SA, Chopra V, Langa KM. Triggers of hospitalization for venous thromboembolism. Circulation. 2012;125:2092–99.
12. Vanderbroucke JP, Rosing J, Bloemenkamp KWM, Middeldorp S, Helmerhorst FM, Bouma BN, Rosendaal F. Oral contraceptives and the risk of venous thrombosis. N Engl J Med. 2001;344:1527–35.
13. Blanco-Molina A, Rotta LL, DiMicco P, Brenner B, Trujillo-Santos J, Ruiz-Gamietea A, Monreal M. Venous thromboembolism during pregnancy, postpartum or during contraceptive use. Thromb Haemost. 2010;103:306–11.

14. Pomp ER, Leselnik AM, Rosendaal FR, Doggen JM. Pregnancy, the postpartum period and prothrombotic defects: risk of venous thrombosis in the MEGA study. J Thromb Haemost. 2008;6:632–37.
15. Jerjes-Sánchez C. Pulmonary embolism. From molecular basis to clinical practice. In: Wright NJ, Smith A, editors. Pulmonary embolism: causes, symptoms and treatment, Pulmonary and respiratory diseases and disorders. Hauppauge: Nova; 2012. p. 1–20.
16. Wicki J, Perrier A, Perneger TV, Bounameaux H, Junod AF. Predicting adverse outcome in patients with acute pulmonary embolism: a risk score. Thromb Haemost. 2000;84:548–52.
17. Zhou XY, Ben SQ, Chen HL, Ni SS. The prognostic value of pulmonary embolism severity index in acute pulmonary embolism: a meta-analysis. Respir Res. 2012;4:111–122.
18. Venet C, Jimenez D, Mean M, Aujesky D. A comparison of the original and simplified Pulmonary Embolism Severity Index. Thromb Haemost. 2011;106:423–28.
19. Zhong-Qun Z, Chong-Quan W, Nikus KC, Sclarovsky S. A new electrocardiogram finding for massive pulmonary embolism: ST elevation in lead aVR with ST depression in leads I and V4 to V6. AJEM. 2013;31:456.e5–8.
20. Janata K, Höchtl T, Wenzel C, Jarai R, Fellner B, Geppert A, Smetana P, Havranek V, Huber K. The role of ST-segment elevation in lead aVR in the risk assessment of patients with acute pulmonary embolism. Clin Res Cardiol. 2012;101:329–37.
21. Wong C-K, Gao W, Stewart RAH, Benatar J, French JK, Aylward PEG, White HD, for the HERO-2 Investigators. aVR ST elevation: an important but neglected sign in ST elevation acute myocardial infarction. Eur Heart J. 2010;31:1845–53.
22. Kucher N, Walpoth N, Wustmann K, Novenu M, Gertsch M. QR in V1—and ECG sign associated with right ventricular strain and adverse clinical outcome in pulmonary embolism. Eur Heart J. 2003;24:107–19.
23. Reyes E, Jerjes-Sanchez C, Ramirez-Rivera A, Gutierrez-Fajardo P, Garza A, Decanini H, Cantú F. Valor predictivo de qR asociado a desnivel positivo del segmento ST-T en V1 para el diagnóstico de infarto del ventrículo derecho secundario a TEP. Arch Inst Cardiol Mex. 1997;6:148.
24. Jerjes-Sanchez C, Ramirez-Rivera A, Gonzalez CVM, Garcia CA. Tromboembolia pulmonar masiva con desviación del eje eléctrico a la derecha y bajo voltaje. Arch Cardiol Mex. 1987;57:301–5.
25. Adelasis J, Morge J, Alberca D, Grenho MF, Arroja I, Aleixo AM. Electrocardiographic presentation of massive and submassive pulmonary embolism. Rev Port Cardiol. 2008;27:591–610.
26. Stein PD, Dalen JE, McIntyre KM, Sasahara MM, Wnger NK, Willis PW. The electrocardiogram in acute pulmonary embolism. Prog Cardiovasc Dis. 1975;17:247–57.
27. Jerjes-Sanchez C, Ramirez-Rivera A, Ibarra-Perez C. Pulmonary embolism and bradycardia. Interconti Cardiol. 1996;5:27–9.
28. Campbell IA, Fennerty A, Miller AC, Baglin T, Gibss S, Hansel D, Reid J, Bonameux H, Remy-Jardin M, Wells P. British Thoracic Society Guidelines for the management of suspected acute pulmonary embolism. Thorax. 2003;58:470–84.
29. Jerjes-Sanchez DC, Elizalde-Gonzalez JJ, Sandoval-Zarate J, Gutierrez-Fajardo P, Seoane M, Ramirez-Rivera A, Pulido T, Beltran M, Santos E, Bautista E, Ibarra-Perez C, Arriaga-Nava R. Diagnostico, estratificación y tratamiento de la tromboembolia pulmonar aguda. Guias y Recomendaciones del Capitulo de Circulacion Pulmonar de la Sociedad Mexicana de Cardiologia. Arch Cardiol Mex. 2004;74:S547–85.
30. Laporte S, Mismetti P, DecousUS H, Uresandi F, Otero R, Lobo JL, Monreal M. Clinical predictors for fatal pulmonary embolism in 15520 patients with venous thromboembolism: findings from the Registro Informatizado de la Enfermedad TromboEmbolica Venosa (RIETE) Registry. Circulation. 2008;117:1711–16.
31. Jaff MR, McCurtry MS, Archer SL, Cushman M, Goldbenger N, Golhaber SZ, Jenkins JS, Kline JA, Michaelis AD, Thistlewaite P, Vedantham S, White RJ, Zierler BK. Management of massive and submassive pulmonary embolism, iliofemoral deep venous thrombosis and

chronic thrombotic pulmonary hypertension: a scientific statement from American Heart Association. Circulation. 2012;125:1788–830.
32. Lualdi JC, Goldhaber SZ. Right ventricular dysfunction after acute pulmonary embolism: pathophysiologic factors, detection, and therapeutic implications. Am Heart J. 1995;130: 1276–82.
33. Konstantinides S. Pulmonary embolism: impact of right ventricular dysfunction. Curr Opin Cardiol. 2005;20:496–501.
34. Grignola JC, Gines F. Mecanica del ventriculo derecho. Actas Fisiologia. 2000;6:131–63.
35. Bleeker GB, Steendijk P, Holman ER, Yu CM, Breithardt OA, Kaandorp TAM, Shalij MJ, van der Wall EE, Bax JJ, Nihonyannopoulos P. Acquired right ventricular dysfunction. Heart. 2006;92:i14–8.
36. Chung T, Emmet L, Mansber R, Peters M, Kritharides L. Natural history of right ventricular dysfunction after acute pulmonary embolism. J Am Soc Echocardiogr. 2007;20:885–94.
37. Dell'Italia LJ. Anatomy and physiology of the right ventricle. Cardiol Clin. 2012;30:167–87.
38. Gianitis E, Muller-Bardoff M, Kurowski V, Weidtmann B, Wiegand U, Kampan M, Katus HA. Independent prognostic value of cardiac troponin T in patients with confirmed pulmonary embolism. Circulation. 2000;102:211–7.
39. Konstantinides S, Geibel A, Olschewski M, Kasper W, Hruska N, Jacle S, Binder L. Importance of cardiac troponin T I and T in risk stratification of patients with acute pulmonary embolism. Circulation. 2002;106:1263–8.
40. ten Wolde M, Tulevski II, Mulder JWM, Shone M, Boosma F, Mulder BJM, Buller HR. Brain natriuretic peptide as a predictor of adverse outcome in patients with pulmonary embolism. Circulation. 2003;86:2082–4.
41. Kucher N, Goldhaber SZ. Cardiac biomarkers for risk stratification of patients with acute pulmonary embolism. Circulation. 2003;108:2191–94.
42. Kucher N, Printzen G, Goldhaber SZ. Prognostic role of brain natriuretic peptide in acute pulmonary embolism. Circulation. 2003;107:2545–47.
43. Pruszczyk P, Bochowicz A, Torbicki A, Szulc M, Kurzyna M, Fijalkowska A, Kuch-Wocial A. Cardiac troponin T monitoring identifies high-risk group of normotensive patients with acute pulmonary embolism. Chest. 2003;123:1947–52.
44. Wells PS, Anderson DR, Rodger M, Stiell I, Dreyer JF, Barnes D, Forgie M, Kovacs G, Ward J, Kovacs MJ. Excluding pulmonary embolism at the bedside without diagnostic imaging: management of patients with suspected pulmonary embolism presenting to the emergency room department by using a simple clinical model and d-dimer. Ann Intern Med. 2001;135:98–107.
45. Righini M, Van EJ, den Exter PL, Roy PM, Verschuren F, Ghuysen A, Rutschman OT, Sanchez O, Jaffrelot M, Trinh-Duc A, Le Gall C, Mustafa PM, van Kralingen KW, Grootenboers MJ, Durian MF, Cheung YW, Meyer G, Bounameux H, Huisman MV, Kamphuisen PE, Le Gal G. Age-adjusted D-dimer cutoff levels to rule out pulmonary embolism: the ADJUST PE study. JAMA. 2014;311:1117–24.
46. Chabloz P, Reber G, Boehlen F, Hohlfeld P, de Moerloose P. TAFI antigen and D-dimer levels during normal pregnancy and at delivery. Br J Haematol. 2001;115:150–52.
47. Righini M, Le Gall G, De Lucia S, Roy PM, Meyer G, Aujesky D, Bounameaux H, Perrier A. Clinical usefulness of D-dimer testing in cancer patients suspected pulmonary embolism. Thromb Haemost. 2006;95:715–19.
48. Di Nisio M, Squizzato A, Rutjes AWS, Buller HR, Zwinderman AH, Bossuyt PMM. Diagnostic accuracy of D-dimer test for exclusion of venous thromboembolism. A systematic review. J Thromb Haemost. 2007;5:296–304.
49. Kucher N, Rossi E, de la Rosa M, Goldhaber SZ. Prognostic role of echocardiography in patients with acute PE and a systemic arterial pressure of 90 mmHg or higher. Arch Intern Med. 2005;165:1777–81.
50. Jerjes Sanchez C, Gutierrez-Fajardo P, Ramírez-Rivera A. Qualitative echocardiographic stratification in pulmonary embolism: significance of inversion of diastolic right/left ventricles ratio. Chest. 1998;114:392S.

51. Jerjes Sanchez C, Gutierrez-Fajardo P, Ramírez-Rivera A, Hernandez-Chavez G. Infarto agudo del miocardio del ventriculo derecho secundario a tromboembolia pulmonary masiva. Arch Inst Cardiol Mex. 1995;65:65–73.
52. McConell MV, Solomon SD, Rayan ME. Regional right ventricular dysfunction detected by echocardiography in acute pulmonary embolism. Am J Cardiol. 1996;78:469–73.
53. van Belle A, Buller HR, Huisman MV, Huisman PM, Kaasjager K, Kamphuisen PW, Kramer MH, Kruip MJ, Kwakkel-van Erp JM, Leebeek FW, Nijkeuter M, Prins MH, Sohne M, Tick LW. Effectiveness of managing suspected pulmonary embolism using an algorithm combining clinical probability, D-dimer testing and computed tomography. JAMA. 2006;295:172–79.
54. Shoepf UJ, Costello P. CT angiography for diagnosis of pulmonary embolism: state of the art. Radiology. 2004;230:329–37.
55. Perrier A, Roy PM, Sanchez O, Le Gal G, Meyer G, Gourdier AL, Furber A, Revel MP, Howarth N, Davido A, Bounameaux H. Multidetector-row computed tomography in suspected pulmonary embolism. N Engl J Med. 2005;352:1760–68.
56. Wiener RS, Schartz LM, Woloshin S. Time trends in pulmonary embolism in the United States: evidence of overdiagnosis. Arch Intern Med. 2001;171:831–37.
57. Carrier M, Righini M, Wells PS, Perrier A, Anderson DR, Rodger A, Pleasance S, Le Gal G. Subsegmental pulmonary diagnosed by computed tomography: incidence and clinical implications. A systematic review and meta-analysis of the management outcome studies. J Thromb Haemost. 2010;8:1716–22.
58. Zhang LJ, Zhou CS, Schoepf UJ, Sheng HX, Wu CY, Krazinski AW, Silverman JR, Meinel FG, Zhao YE, Zhang ZJ, Lu GM. Dual-energy CT lung ventilation/perfusion imaging for diagnosing pulmonary embolism. Eur Radiol. 2013;23:2666–75.
59. Sostman HD, Layish DT, Tapson VF, Spritzer CE, Delong DM, Trotter RTP, Macfall JR, Patz EF, Goodman PC, Wodard PK, Foo TKF, Farber JL. Prospective comparison of helical CT and MR imaging in clinically suspected acute pulmonary embolism. J Magn Reson Imaging. 1996;6:275–81.
60. van Beek EJR, Wild JM, Fink C, Moody AR, Kauczor H-U, Oudkerk M. MRI for the diagnosis of pulmonary embolism. J Magn Reson Imaging. 2003;18:627–40.
61. Hochhegger B, Ley-zaporozhan J, Marchiori E, Irion K, Soares Souza Jr A, Moreira J, Kaucsor HU, Ley S. Magnetic resonance imaging findings in acute pulmonary embolism. Br J Radiol. 2011;84:282–7.

Chapter 5
Anticoagulation as Adjunctive Treatment and One-Hour Alteplase Infusion

Carlos Jerjes-Sánchez

In the setting of acute pulmonary embolism (PE) parenteral or subcutaneous anticoagulation is the cornerstone of the initial treatment. The main target of initial pharmacologic anticoagulation is: to reduce thrombus size, avoid thrombin expression, and prevent extension reducing recurrence and mortality; additionally, to establish a bridge to start oral anticoagulation with vitamin-K antagonists or activated factors anticoagulants. Both approaches are improving the outcome of PE patients in any clinical stage.

Current guidelines recommendation suggest that in high or intermediate clinical probability PE patients, parenteral anticoagulation have to be initiated using intravenous unfractionated heparin or subcutaneous low-molecular-weight heparin or fondaparinux whilst awaiting diagnostic tests. In high-risk PE patients characterized by severe right ventricular dysfunction with or without troponin expression considered to thrombolysis, unfractionated heparin is recommended. This recommendation is based on its short half-life, the ease monitoring of anticoagulant effects (activated partial thromboplastin time), as well as its rapid reversal anticoagulant effect through a specific antidote, protamine [1].

Unfractionated heparin infusion should be stopped during administration of streptokinase but it can be continued during recombinant human tissue-type plasminogen activator (rt-PA) infusion. In patients receiving low-molecular-weight heparin or fondaparinux at the time of starting thrombolysis, infusion of unfractionated heparin should be delayed until 12 h after the last low-molecular-weight heparin injection (given twice daily), or until 24 h after the last low-molecular-weight heparin or

C. Jerjes-Sánchez, M.D., F.C.C.P., F.A.C.C. (✉)
Sistema Nacional de Investigadores, Nivel II – Clinical Research Director, Instituto de Cardiologia y Medicina Vascular, TEC Salud

Escuela de Medicina, Tecnológico de Monterrey San Pedro Garza Garcia, Nuevo León, Mexico

Unidad de Investigacion Clinica en Medicina SC Monterrey, Nuevo León, Mexico
e-mail: jerjes@prodigy.net.mx

C. Jerjes-Sánchez, *Thrombolysis in Pulmonary Embolism*,
DOI 10.1007/978-3-319-19707-4_5

fondaparinux injection (given once daily). Given the bleeding risks associated with thrombolysis and the possibility of needing immediate discontinuation or reversal of the anticoagulant effect of heparin, it appears reasonable to continue anticoagulation with unfractionated heparin for several hours after the end of thrombolytic treatment before switching to low-molecular-weight heparin or fondaparinux [1].

Previously, guidelines recommendations coming from American Heart Association suggest that therapeutic anticoagulation with subcutaneous low-molecular-weight heparin, intravenous or subcutaneous unfractionated heparin with monitoring, unmonitored weight-based subcutaneous unfractionated heparin, or subcutaneous fondaparinux should be given to patients with objectively confirmed PE and no contraindications to anticoagulation. Therapeutic anticoagulation during the diagnostic workup should be given to patients with intermediate or high clinical probability of PE and no contraindications to anticoagulation. In the suggested treatment algorithm for thrombolysis used to treat acute PE, heparin anticoagulation is considered as initial treatment in low-risk, submassive and massive PE [2].

The American College of Chest Physicians guidelines and recommendations [3], identified in randomized and nonrandomized trials of PE patients submitted to thrombolysis. Intravenous unfractionated heparin should be given in full therapeutic doses before thrombolysis administration. It is acceptable to continue or stop intravenous infusion during thrombolysis. However, both practices have never been compared. FDA recommends intravenous unfractionated heparin suspension during rt-PA 2-h infusion, while in other countries infusion is continued. US authorities recommend checking the activated partial thromboplastin time immediately after completion of the rt-PA infusion and, if the activated antithrombin time is not >80 s, it is possible to restart intravenous unfractionated heparin without a bolus at the same infusion rate used before the rt-PA administration.

Recommendations coming from current guidelines agree on the use of unfractionated heparin as adjunctive treatment in acute PE patients submitted to thrombolysis. However, several answers remain open. Do we need to start with unfractionated heparin bolus or not? And which is the best bolus (5000 or 10,000 U or less) to start previous thrombolysis? Could another subcutaneous or intravenous anticoagulant with more anticoagulation activity be used in this group of patients?

Fondaparinux as Adjunctive Treatment

In 2009 year, Janin et al. [4] used fondaparinux as adjunctive treatment in high- and intermediate PE submitted to thrombolysis. At that time, no data were available on the efficacy and safety of a combination of fondaparinux and thrombolysis in the setting of acute PE.

Fondaparinux is a synthetic and selective inhibitor of factor Xa that has proven its efficacy and safety at different dose regimens as a primary prevention and as initial treatment of venous thromboembolism compared with a low-molecular-weight heparin, enoxaparin [5–7]. The main advantages over low-molecular-weight heparin are: pharmacokinetic properties allow a simple, fixed dose, once-daily regimen of subcutaneous injection without monitoring. The pharmacokinetic and pharmacodynamics curves, in spite of subcutaneous administration, allow a fast anticoagulation action, similar than observed by intravenous route. When used as pharmacological prophylaxis in patients undergoing major orthopedic surgery a trend of and increased risk of major bleeding was observed. However, it was not confirmed when higher therapeutic dosing regimens were used in deep venous thrombosis and low-risk PE patients [4–7].

Unfractionated heparin was the only recommended molecule as adjunctive treatment in PE patients submitted to thrombolysis. Considering the safety and efficacy of 2.5 mg of fondaparinux given once daily compared with unfractionated heparin observed in ST-elevation myocardial infarction patients [8], an important consideration emerges: Whether similar results could be extrapolated to high and intermediate-risk PE patients is unknown, since higher fondaparinux doses as adjunctive treatment to thrombolysis could be associated with an increase of bleeding complications.

Patient Selection

Based on these observations Janin and colleagues [4] conducted a prospective one center trial to evaluate safety and efficacy of a combination of fondaparinux and thrombolysis in the setting of acute high- and intermediate-risk PE. Patients were selected if they had a at least one of the following criteria: Cardiogenic shock, systolic blood pressure ≤90 mmHg, or a pressure drop of ≥40 mmHg, associated with clinical signs of organ hypoperfusion and hypoxia; syncope; one or more proximal thrombo-embolus at CT scan; positive troponin. Also, at least an echocardiogram finding suggesting right ventricular dysfunction: as right/left ventricular end diastolic diameter ratio ≥1 in four-chamber view, paradoxical septal systolic motion or pulmonary hypertension by right ventricular/atrial gradient ≥30 mmHg. Patients were not included by: contraindication to thrombolytic therapy; or renal failure on admission, creatinine clearance <30 mL/min [4].

Study Treatment

Streptokinase or rt-PA was considered as thrombolytic regimens. Streptokinase was administered as a continuous intravenous infusion of 1.5 million IU over 2 h (started after an infusion of 40 mg of methylprednisolone). rt-PA was infused at a dose of 70 or 100 mg over 2 h, according to body weight (if body weight >70 kg, bolus of 10 mg followed by 90 mg over 2 h; if body weight <70 kg, bolus of 7 mg followed by 63 mg over 2 h). Streptokinase or rt-PA were only administered once fibrinogen level rose above 1 g/L. Fondaparinux was given immediately at the beginning of thrombolytic infusion or before starting thrombolysis while waiting for the confirmation of the diagnosis [4].

In patients who previously received heparin and were transferred for thrombolysis, fondaparinux was administered 12 h after the last injection of low-molecular-weight heparin. All patients received a single daily subcutaneous injection of 5.0 mg fondaparinux when the body weight was <50 kg, 7.5 mg if their body weight was 50–100 kg, or 10.0 mg in those with body weight was >100 kg [4].

Vitamin-K antagonists (fluindione) were initiated when the patients were hemodynamically stable (48–72 h after thrombolytic infusion). Doses were adjusted to obtain an INR target of 2.5 (range 2.0–3.0), for at least 6 months. Fondaparinux was stopped when the INR was between 2.0 and 3.0 for at least 2 consecutive days [4].

Efficacy End Point

Combined end point in-hospital course included persistent clinical instability and residual echocardiographic right ventricular dysfunction within the first 36 h. Persistent clinical instability was considered as the presence of at least two of: refractory cardiogenic shock; systemic arterial hypotension (defined as systolic blood pressure of ≤90 mmHg or a pressure drop of ≥40 mmHg for >15 min if not caused by new-onset arrhythmia, hypovolemia, or sepsis); severe hypoxemia (i.e., room-air pulse oximetry of ≤90 % or PaO_2 ≥55 mmHg without oxygen therapy); or tachycardia (heart rate, ≥110 beats/min). Residual echocardiographic right ventricular dysfunction was defined as the persistence of at least two initial right ventricular dysfunction criteria [4].

Adverse events such as death, recurrent PE, repeated thrombolysis, surgical embolectomy, and bleeding complications were noted throughout the hospital stay. Perfusion lung scans were performed within 6–8 days after onset of treatment. Perfusion impairment was graded as to the proportion of lung not perfused. Patients with symptoms suggesting PE and with new perfusion defects on the lung scan or pulmonary angiogram were interpreted as having recurrent PE [4].

Safety End Point

They included major and important bleeding complications. Major bleeding complications were defined as: Any bleeding event that required blood transfusion, surgical control, discontinuation of thrombolytic or anticoagulant treatment; hemorrhagic stroke confirmed by computed tomography or autopsy; or any bleeding causing death or defined as a fall of 15 % in hematocrit. Important bleedings, defined as: fall of 10 % in hematocrit. Other bleeding events were considered as minor bleedings, and were not included in the safety end point [4].

Clinical Presentation

Twenty seven patients with proven recent high and intermediate-risk PE (symptom onset <15 days) were included between October 2006 and January 2008. The major proportion was female and in productive social life; the most important demographic characteristics were thromboembolic disease history 33 %; onset symptoms ≤5 days 44 % and hypertension ≥56 %. Considering the proportion of right ventricular overload on electrocardiogram (74 %), brain natriuretic type-B expression (63 %) tachycardia (52 %), troponin expression of myocardial infarction (44 %) cardiogenic shock (37 %), syncope (30 %) is clear that the majority of the patients had high-risk PE [4].

Twenty five proximal pulmonary embolisms were diagnosed with CT scan and one with ventilation-perfusion lung scintigraphy. In only one PE patient with cardiogenic shock thrombolysis was driven by echocardiographic findings of severe RV overload before spiral CT scan examination. The remaining 9 patients (33 %) without cardiogenic shock and considered with clinical stability had initially with high troponin I (TnI >0.15 ng/mL) and brain natriuretic peptide type-B >200 pg/mL levels [4]. All patients had echocardiographic criteria of right ventricular dysfunction. Mean systolic pulmonary artery pressure was 56 ± 15 mmHg and all patients had a RV/atrial gradient >30 mmHg [4].

Treatment and In-Hospital Course

Twenty two patients (81.5 %) received rt-PA and 5 (18.5 %) streptokinase. Mean duration of fondaparinux administration was 8.6 ± 4.0 days. In terms of safety there was one major bleeding, and on important bleeding (two events, 7.4 %). The major bleeding and important bleedings occurred in a 71-year-old man who had undergone elective hip replacement 2 weeks previously. The bleeding was in the surgical site. This patient required blood transfusion. Fondaparinux was replaced by unfractionated heparin. Infusion of recombinant coagulation factor VIIa and surgery were not required. A 57-year-old man with cirrhosis experienced an important bleeding complication without any identifiable bleeding site. Fondaparinux was not stopped. Clinical evolution of these 2 patients was favorable [4].

Fondaparinux is a synthetic and selective inhibitor of factor Xa that has been used with efficacy and safety in the treatment of thromboembolic disease. An important advantage is the predictable and sustained anticoagulant effect for 24 h allowing once-daily injection, additionally, it does not cross-react with heparin-induced antibodies, and platelet count monitoring is no longer needed. Until our knowledge this is the only evidence in which fondaparinux was used in the setting of high-risk PE patients submitted to thrombolysis [4].

In this study 3 patients (11.1 %) met the clinical efficacy endpoint criteria, one of them died from refractory shock and 2 patients required successful surgical embolectomy for persistent clinical instability. This result confirms previous observations of this group with 8 % of failed thrombolysis in unfractionated heparin-treated patients [9]. Fondaparinux had similar in-hospital efficacy compared to unfractionated heparin in stable PE patients, as occurs in ST-elevation myocardial infarction patients [8].

Considering bleeding complications during in-hospital stay, previous evidence on fondaparinux showed that a 2.5 mg daily dose was associated with a trend towards an increase in the incidence of major bleeding complications in patients undergoing orthopedic surgery [7]. However, in the initial treatment of hemodynamically stable patients with deep venous thrombosis and PE, fondaparinux 5–10 mg was associated with low rates of major bleedings (1.1 % and 1.3 %, respectively) [5, 6]. Although the small sample size does not make possible to draw any definitive conclusions, the combination of fondaparinux and thrombolysis does not seem to be associated with an increase in bleeding events compared with unfractionated heparin alone [4].

This French group has an important experience in the field of PE and thrombolysis, however, considering the lack of control group (unfractionated heparin) and the sample size, as authors wrote, this study has to be considered as pilot trial and the real efficacy and safety of fondaparinux as adjunctive treatment of PE patients submitted to thrombolysis remains waiting for a randomized control trial. This study has not been performed to date.

Improving Adjunctive Treatment

The Role of Enoxaparin and Weight-Adjusted Unfractionated Heparin

Thrombolysis in PE accelerates reversal of right ventricular dysfunction among properly selected patients. Short duration and high concentration regimens plus standard intravenous unfractionated heparin act more rapidly, enhance safety, and reduce recurrence, improving in-hospital course and mortality rate. However, the role of weight-adjusted unfractionated heparin and enoxaparin as adjunct to thrombolysis remains unknown. In the setting of PE and thrombolysis these antithrombotic approaches successfully used in ST-elevation myocardial infarction patients could prolong and simplify traditional heparin treatment improving the outcome and reducing bleeding complications [10].

In 2009, we reported the results of the first prospective multicenter trial in high-risk PE patients in whom a weight-adjusted unfractionated heparin dose followed by enoxaparin as adjunct to one-hour alteplase infusion improved in-hospital and follow-up outcome without increasing bleeding complications compared to unfractionated heparin alone in a prospective, open-label, controlled, multicenter trial, with

2-year follow-up [10]. The main target was efficacy and safety of weight-adjusted unfractionated heparin dose followed by enoxaparin as adjunctive to one-hour alteplase infusion to improve in-hospital and follow-up outcome regarding reduction of major adverse cardiovascular events, treatment escalation, and in-hospital stay without the increase of bleeding complications vs. unfractionated heparin alone [10].

Patients aged >15 years, with high-risk PE, proved PE, referred within 14 days after onset of symptoms entered the study. Patients were excluded in the case of history of severe chronic pulmonary arterial hypertension, absolute contraindication for thrombolysis, any concurrent condition limiting short-term survival [10]. The control group included high-risk PE patients in whom thrombolysis was not used as contraindication, risk of major bleeding superior to benefit, patient reject, and physician in charge decision [10].

Pharmacological Regimen

Patients in thrombolysis group assigned to weight-adjusted intravenous unfractionated heparin received a bolus of 60 U/kg [11] (maximum 4000 U) and then a bolus of 15 mg (>65 years) or 20 mg (<65 years) of recombinant human tissue-type plasminogen activator, alteplase followed by 75 or 80 mg over 1 h infusion [12, 13] by peripheral vein. After thrombolysis a constant heparin infusion (12 U/kg per h, maximum 1000 U/h) adjusted to maintain an activated partial thromboplastin time of 50–70 s for 24–48 h was started. Then, the first subcutaneous dose of 1 mg.kg of enoxaparin was applied [10].

To achieve sustained anticoagulation, this subcutaneous dose was repeated every 12 h until hospital discharge for a maximum of 7 days. In control group UH standard regimen was used: bolus of 5000 or 10,000 U followed by a constant infusion of 1000 U/h of heparin titrated to APTT of 2–2.5 times control by 7 days [14, 15]. In survivors of the acute phase, on the first day to third day, heparin was overlapped with warfarin. The patients were kept on warfarin, aiming for an INR between 2.0 and 3.0 for 6 months or more, depending on the presence of major risk factors [10].

Stratification, Fibrinolytic Therapy and Diagnosis Workup

All patients with high clinical suspicion of PE (major risk factors, clinical manifestations, chest X-ray, electrocardiogram and oximetry) were under a one-hour "fast track" echocardiography evaluation and treatment in the Emergency Department. In patients with high-risk PE with clinical stability, impeding instability or instability an experienced physician administered FT by peripheral vein as soon as possible [14–16] reproducing ST-elevation myocardial infarction strategy to reduce ischemia and right ventricular dysfunction time [10].

Patients with impeding instability or instability were the only in whom V/Q lung scan was performed after starting treatment. When severe right ventricular wall motion abnormalities were excluded, lung scan was performed before starting FT. After fibrinolytic regimen, all patients had clinical, ECG and echocardiographic evaluation. In case of nonsuccessful FT or when in-hospital recurrence, rescue FT, rethrombolysis or percutaneous pulmonary intervention were considered. Twenty-four to 72 h after FT all patients had tests to assess pulmonary circulation and deep venous thrombosis search [10].

Diagnostic and Echocardiogram

V/Q Lung Scans

Baseline, 24 h and at discharge, and 30 and 90 days perfusion scan with intravenously injected 99mTC/DTPA in anterior, posterior, lateral, and oblique views were obtained. Ventilation lung scan was done with 99mTC/MAA aerosol inhalation. Scans were scored through a segmental method that included all views [10].

Echocardiograms

Baseline, 1, 24 h, at discharge and follow-up echocardiograms were done. Echocardiographic examination and interpretation were performed before and after starting thrombolysis. Qualitative: right ventricular end diastolic diameter, regional and global hypokinesis, paradoxical septal motion, loss of inspiratory collapse or the inferior cava vein. Quantitative evaluation: pulmonary artery systolic pressure determined with the modified Bernoulli formula, measurements of right and left ventricular size, ejection fraction, tricuspid and pulmonary regurgitation and right ventricular wall thickness. Echocardiography was standardized using the apical four chambers, parasternal long and short axis. When these positions were not appropriate, a subcostal four-chamber view was used.

Analysis of Efficacy

Baseline and 24 h clinical evaluation included: clinical, electrocardiogram, chest X-ray, oximetry, pulmonary arterial hypertension and right ventricular dysfunction improvement. Pre- and post-treatment lung scans and echocardiograms were analyzed regarding perfusion abnormalities, pulmonary arterial systolic pressure, and right ventricular dysfunction behavior. In-patient mortality, recurrence, treatment escalation, duration of in-hospital stay was evaluated. Follow-up evaluation included functional class, recurrent PE, chronic pulmonary arterial hypertension, post-thrombotic syndrome and mortality.

Follow-Up

Visits at 30, 90, and 180 days and then every 2 months. In the two first subsequent visits electrocardiograms, transthoracic echocardiogram, V/Q lung scan, or any other tests assessing pulmonary circulation were done. At the end visit only ECG and TTE were performed.

Definitions

High-risk PE was defined a priori and three variables of clinical, electrocardiogram and echocardiogram categories were required at least.

Clinical: (a) sudden or persistent dyspnea plus chest pain and or syncope, (b) S3 gallop, (c) hypoxemia, (d) hypotension, (e) shock, (f) cardiac arrest.

Electrocardiogram: (a) new ECG signs of right ventricular strain, (new right bundle branch block or right axis deviation), (b) qR in V1, (c) transitory or persistent ST-elevation >1 mm in leads V1, V2, and V3, (d) transitory or persistent ST depression >1 mm in leads V1, V2, and V3 or over, (e) T wave inversion in leads V1–V4.

Echocardiogram: (a) right ventricular end diastolic diameter/left ventricular end diastolic diameter ratio (RVEDD/LVEDD) ≥2:1, (b) regional or global right ventricular hypokinesis, (c) right ventricular diameter ≥35 mm, c systolic pulmonary arterial pressure ≥50 mmHg [10].

Right ventricular hypokinesis: Moderate or severe systolic hypokinesis of the right ventricular free wall by qualitative assessment. PE proved: by high probability V/Q lung scan, tomography or pulmonary angiography. Mortality secondary to PE: in the first 48 h due to cardiogenic shock or ventricular arrhythmia with echocardiography findings of pulmonary arterial hypertension, right ventricular dysfunction, and PE diagnosis [10].

Major adverse cardiovascular events: mortality secondary to index event or PE recurrence; Global mortality: in-hospital and follow-up mortality secondary to PE. Treatment escalation: use of at least one of the following: infusion of a catecholamine because of persistent clinical instability, hypotension or shock, invasive or noninvasive mechanical ventilation, cardiopulmonary resuscitation and rescue FT, emergency surgical or thrombus fragmentation by catheter [10].

Recurrent PE: proved new PE (new perfusion lung scan defect) in-hospital or in the follow-up event with or without clinical instability. Recurrent deep vein thrombosis: diagnosed by ultrasonography, a new noncompressible venous segment in the proximal veins, an increase of 4 mm or more in thrombus diameter with compression or an increase of 1–4 mm in diameter combined with an extension of at least 4 cm in length. Reperfusion criteria: clinical, ECG, echocardiogram, and V/Q lung scan improvement after FT regimen compared with baseline state [10].

Rethrombolysis: after successful FT (clinical and echocardiographic improvement) another fibrinolysis treatment in the setting of in-hospital PE recurrence. Rescue thrombolysis: a second fibrinolytic regimen immediately performed when nonsuccess FT was identified (persistent or worsening clinical instability with RV dysfunction detected on echocardiogram) [10].

Major hemorrhage: stroke (confirmed by computed tomography), hematoma >5 cm, prolonged external bleeding at puncture site, oral or gastrointestinal bleeding, hematuria or another bleeding with concomitant hypotension that required treatment with intravenous fluids, blood transfusion, surgical control, discontinuation of FT regimen, decrease >15 % points in hematocrit or >5 g/dL in hemoglobin. Minor hemorrhage: decrease among 10–15 % points in hematocrit or 3–5 g/dL in hemoglobin reduction [10].

From October 2002 to December 2004 eighty patients with full inclusion criteria were enrolled. Forty patients were allocated to one-hour alteplase infusion plus unfractionated heparin and enoxaparin and other 40 received unfractionated heparin alone. All patients had proved PE and 2-year follow-up. Demographic characteristics of patients in thrombolysis group compared heparin group were as follows: more often male with previous history of deep venous thrombosis than opposite group. Patients in unfractionated heparin group had higher incidence of surgery. Both groups were well matched among other risk factors including deep venous thrombosis location and high fibrinogen plasmatic levels as an expression of an inflammatory state. On clinical presentation, patients in unfractionated heparin group had more data of respiratory failure and syncope than opposite group. Electrocardiogram findings in thrombolysis group were tachycardia 93 %, inverted T waves 45 %, qR en V1 43 %, transitory ST-elevation 38 %, ST depression 28 % compared with opposite group 98, 45, 55, 30, 33 %. Although, patients under thrombolysis had higher degree of pulmonary arterial hypertension and right ventricular remodeling, there were not differences on PE extension in both groups; segmental perfusion defects were 10.7 ± 1.7 in thrombolysis group compared to 10.5 ± 1.8 in heparin group (p NS). Baseline echocardiogram was performed in all patients and the most important findings were: thrombolysis group patients had pulmonary arterial systolic pressure 62.3 ± 12.4, right ventricular diastolic diameters 43.9 ± 4.4 mm, right ventricular hypokinesis 75 %, McConnell sign 48 % compared with heparin group 58.4 ± 1.8 ($p=0.05$), 41.0 ± 2.9 mm ($p=0.001$), 90 % ($p=0.07$), 43 % ($p=0.41$) [10].

Patients in control group were not considered to receive thrombolysis due to history or recently surgical or medical reasons. Other causes were identified also. Surgical: cesarean section (7 patients), gastrectomy (3 patients), liposuction (2 patients), and retinoplasty, aneurysmectomy, craniotomy and hysterectomy (1 patient each). Medical: acute cerebral vascular disease (2 patients), gastrointestinal bleeding (2 patients), cranioencephalic trauma (2 patients), and traumatic cardiac arrest, hemoptysis, transitory ischemic attack (1 patient each). Other: inexperience on FT use (14 patients), and lack of resources (1 patient) [10].

Analysis of efficacy: Pre- and post-treatment clinical, echocardiographic and lung scan baseline and 24 h assessment in both groups are shown in Table 5.1. Patients under unfractionated heparin had improvement of severe pulmonary arterial hypertension, right ventricular dysfunction, wall motion abnormalities and pulmonary perfusion. Patients with unfractionated heparin alone did not improve and a worsening of right ventricular dysfunction was identified. In this group right ventricular hypokinesis was a persistent echocardiographic finding. The improvement on pulmonary perfusion could be explained by spontaneous fragmentation or endogen lysis [10].

Table 5.1 Treatment evaluation

Fibrinolytic regimen evaluation			
Variable	Pre $n=40$ (%)	Post $n=40$ (%)	p
Right ventricular sound	96	5	<0.0001
Shock	15	0	<0.0001
Respiratory rate	33.5±5.7	25.0±4.4	<0.0001
Cardiac rate	108.9±13.1	94.4±8.9	0.008
Systolic pressure	102.3±19.7	119.5±10	<0.001
Diastolic pressure	61.2 19.6	76.7±8.4	<0.001
Oximetry	84.7±4.3	95.5±3.1	<0.001
Echocardiogram			
PA systolic pressure	62.3±12.4	38.26±12.4	<0.001
RV diastolic diameter	43.9±4.4	32.30±4.8	<0.001
RV hypokinesis	75	18	0.007
McConnell sign	48	8	0.005
V/Q lung scan (32 patients)			
Perfusion defects	10.7±1.7	6.07±3.1	<0.001
Unfractionated heparin evaluation			
Variable	Pre	Post	p
Right ventricular sound	95	95	1
Shock	18	18	1
Respiratory rate	37.5±3.4	38.0±5.6	0.63
Cardiac rate	116.0±10.2	111.0±9.1	0.02
Systolic pressure	103.5±18.5	95±20.4	0.05
Oximetry	83.5±3.6	81.7±5.8	0.06
Echocardiogram			
PA systolic pressure	58.4±1.8	56.2±3.6	0.0009
RV diastolic diameter	41.0±2.9	44.0±4.9	0.001
RV hypokinesis	90	90	1
McConnell sign	43	40	95
V/Q lung scan (32 patients)			
Perfusion defects	10.5±1.8	7.0±2.84	0.001

Modified from: Jerjes-Sanchez C, et al. J Thromb Thrombolysis 2009; 27:154–162
PA pulmonary artery, *RV* right ventricular

In-hospital clinical course and adverse events: Findings regarding major adverse cardiovascular events, escalation treatment, in-hospital stay, and bleeding complications are presented in Table 5.2. Patients under thrombolysis had better outcome than patients under unfractionated heparin alone. Major bleeding complications had a close relationship with venous puncture in both groups [10].

Follow-up and major adverse cardiovascular events: Follow-up was complete in 100 % of the cases (Table 5.2). Within the first 30 and 90 days the most important clinical finding was a pulmonary perfusion improvement in alteplase plus enoxaparin group compared with unfractionated heparin alone. Although a trend to major incidence of major adverse cardiovascular events in unfractionated heparin group was observed, these clinical findings had statistical significance until day 180, including a better right ventricular remodeling. Global mortality was another relevant clinical finding (Table 5.2) [10].

Table 5.2 In-hospital outcome, follow-up, and adverse events

Variable	Alteplase 1 h+ enoxaparin $n=40$ (%)	UH $n=40$ (%)	p
Mortality	3	25	0.009
Recurrence	10	20	0.17
Escalation treatment	3	53	<0.001
In-hospital stay (days)	6.7±1.7	16.4±8.7	<0.001
Rescue thrombolysis	10	0	0.12
Bleeding (total)	13	13	1
Major hemorrhage	8	8	1
Groin hematoma	5	3	0.78
Jugular hematoma	3	5	0.78
Intracranial hematoma	0	0	–
Minor hemorrhage	5	5	1
Cava filter	3	43	<0.001
Pulmonary percutaneous intervention	5	0	0.47
Follow-up and adverse events			
30 days			
Patients	39	30	
Mortality	0	3	0.89
Recurrence PE	0	3	0.06
DVT	0	7	0.36
Bleeding	0	0	–
Perfusion defects	3.4±2.0	5.2±1.6	<0.001
Normal echocardiogram	90	87	0.98
90 days			
Patients	39	29	
Mortality	0	7	0.34
Recurrence PE	3	7	0.79
DVT	0	7	0.34
Bleeding	0	0	–
Perfusion defects	2.8±2.1	4.6±1.5	<0.001
Normal echocardiogram	95	82	0.22
180 days			
Patients	39	27	
Mortality	0	7	0.34
Recurrence PE	0	22	0.007
DVT	0	26	0.003
Bleeding	0	0	–
Normal echocardiogram	97	55	0.01
Patients	40	40	
Global mortality	3	38	0.0002

Modified from: Jerjes-Sanchez C, et al. J Thromb Thrombolysis 2009; 27:154–162
DVT deep venous thrombosis

The Kaplan-Meier survival curve applied to mortality clearly showed the benefit achieved in patients who received thrombolysis compared with unfractionated heparin standard regimen alone ($p=0.0001$). In a 1- and 2-year follow-up patients under thrombolysis had an outcome free of major adverse cardiovascular events as has been previously compared with heparin alone in whose more incidence of PE and deep venous thrombosis was identified [10].

The study has three important findings. First, the efficacy proved by weight-adjusted unfractionated heparin and one-hour alteplase infusion in the acute phase. Second, as compared with the standard regimen of unfractionated heparin, enoxaparin improved pulmonary perfusion, right ventricular remodeling, and reduced recurrence. Third, the low incidence of bleeding complications that accompanies the efficacy of this therapeutic approach improving in-hospital and follow-up outcome [10].

Adjunctive Treatment

In PE patients, weight-adjusted dose of intravenous unfractionated heparin recommended in ST-myocardial infarction was effective and safe. This unfractionated heparin dosing was associated with absence of intracranial hemorrhage. The main advantages of using it as "bridge" before starting enoxaparin are: short half-life, hepatic clearance, effective antidote and available test to know activity. Also, it is possible to stratify renal function to starting low or standard enoxaparin dose reducing bleeding complications [10].

After the high-risk period for bleeding complications enoxaparin improves and simplifies the traditional anticoagulation approach through easier administration, sustained anticoagulation and an enhanced antithrombotic effect (longer half-life, sustained effect, higher action on Xa factor and less important platelet interaction, antigenicity, rebound and sensibility effect) [10].

This antithrombotic profile improves pulmonary perfusion in the follow-up, in contrast with previous evidences in which no differences were observed on pulmonary perfusion rate when unfractionated heparin standard regimen was used. During hospital stay, a recurrence rate reduction was a significant finding with subsequent impact on in-hospital costs. In this study enoxaparin bolus used in myocardial infarction setting was not considered appropriate for safety reasons and lack of evidence in PE [10].

One-Hour Alteplase Infusion

In PE patients with right ventricle hypokinesis, infusions of short duration and high concentration (alteplase 2 h, and streptokinase in 1 or 2 h) act more rapidly, improve outcome and reduce mortality without increasing bleeding complications. The main advantage of current thrombolysis regimens is to achieve a rapid "pharmacological embolectomy" to improve right ventricle dysfunction and consequently the cardiopulmonary and systemic hemodynamic [10].

Considering our previous experiences with one-hour streptokinase regimen [14–16] that has been successfully used in ST-elevation myocardial infarction, we decided to assess the efficacy and safety profile of one-hour alteplase infusion based on the following advantages: (a) the highest TIMI-3 flow in ST-elevation myocardial infarction (81 %) in the history of pharmacological reperfusion [12], (b) it was an effective and safe option in México [13] and (c) low incidence of bleeding complications [13, 17]. Our data suggest that one-hour alteplase infusion plus unfractionated heparin establishes rapid reversal of pulmonary arterial hypertension and right ventricular heart failure without increasing hemorrhagic complications improving the outcome in high-risk PE. The evidence obtained in-hospital and follow-up ascertains that this thrombolytic regimen could reduce major adverse cardiovascular events. These findings support the safety and effectiveness of ST-elevation myocardial infarction thrombolytic regimens on high-risk PE as has been reported previously.

Bleeding Complications

Major bleeding complications are the most threatening adverse effects impairing thrombolysis use. Age of patients, anticoagulation strategy in acute phase and non-invasive design were favorable factors to prevent major hemorrhage complications. The incidence of these complications was low (8 %) compared with evidence coming from pulmonary angiography era (14 % 23 and 36–45 % 24). Higher incidence of cave vein filters used in unfractionated heparin group could overestimate the bleeding rate in this group. Although in this study nonintracranial hemorrhage was observed reproducing our previous results, a careful stratification is mandatory when alteplase in one-hour is considered in elderly patients [10].

Fibrinolytic Therapy Contraindications

Considering our previous results, these patients were used as control group since we consider unethical to use only secondary prevention in PE with right ventricular dysfunction. In fact, pharmacologically thrombolysis plus heparin have major feasibility to induce rapid thrombolysis than heparin alone. On the other hand, in the setting of PE and right ventricular dysfunction, thrombolysis is not considered by the lack of current and strong evidence in terms of mortality, when in the context of a relative contraindication risk bleeding exceeds the benefit, and once an absolute contraindication is identified [10].

Although currently hundreds of patients with PE and right ventricular dysfunction have been under thrombolysis, the outcome of patients with contraindications is unclear. The reason to avoid thrombolysis in surgical and medical patients was the possibility to induce bleeding complications. Nevertheless, thrombolysis was not applied in 35 % (14 patients) of high-risk PE because physicians in charge did not have experience [10].

In addition, percutaneous pulmonary intervention was available in only one tertiary center. These observations coming from a country with middle income provides reliable information on outcome, quality of care, and mortality in this group. In addition, it identifies areas for further improvement of the quality (mechanical and pharmacological strategies) of PE care. Our results broaden our knowledge about how thrombolysis and antithrombotic approaches modify the outcome and what needs to be improved in México [10].

Study advantages: A fast track to starting FT in Emergency Department and a noninvasive strategy reduced the time of right ventricular dysfunction and bleeding complications respectively. High-risk PE stratification used in this study precludes the bias of including low-risk patients [10].

Study limitations: One limitation of this study was the sample size. Another, that it was a not a double-blind, placebo-controlled trial since the ethics review board and our group refused it considering previous results. Another limitation was the relatively early age of our patient population which undoubtedly underestimates the overall risks of major hemorrhagic complications. In the follow-up any test assessing pulmonary circulation was done, so we cannot exclude residual central thrombus which could modify the outcome.

Finally we considered that enoxaparin and weight-adjusted intravenous unfractionated heparin as adjunctive treatment to one-hour alteplase infusion improve in-hospital and follow-up outcome compared to heparin alone in high-risk PE. This therapeutic approach could be another available option. Similar strategy has been used in the most recent and important randomized control trials conducted in PE patients submitted to pharmacological thrombolysis [18–20].

Final Considerations

Considering the evidence that we have, unfractionated heparin has been used in all randomized control trials from 1970 to 2014 [21]. This parenteral anticoagulant has been used with first- and second-generation fibrinolytics, including standard [21] and half-doses [20] with safety and effectivity; recently, considering the unfractionated heparin advantages (short half-life, hepatic clearance, effective antidote and available test to know activity, namely protamine) we use it as a bridge to start low-molecular-weight heparin, in patients submitted to third-generation fibrinolytic [18–20]. So, in spite of other parenteral anticoagulants with more direct action on coagulation cascade, unfractionated heparin remains as cornerstone as adjunctive treatment in PE patients submitted to thrombolysis.

In the last 20-years we had active participation in the decision and the process of thrombolysis in 289 PE patients with severe right ventricular dysfunction [10–15]. One hundred and sixty patients have not been published yet; however all of them can be reviewed in Chap. 7.

In all of these studies we are using different unfractionated heparin bolus. At the beginning 10,000 U of unfractionated heparin was used in 48 patients submitted to one-hour streptokinase infusion [14, 15]. Then, we used half-dose in 131 PE patients submitted to the same thrombolytic regimen. All of these patients were under continuous infusion of 1000 U/h of heparin titrated to a PTT of 2–2.5 times control (Table 5.3); both strategies proved to be safe and effective (Table 5.4)

Table 5.3 Fibrinolytic regimen bolus, adjunctive treatment, and bleeding complications findings in 289 patients with pulmonary embolism

Variable	1992	1992–1994	1996–2002	2002–2004	2009–2011
60 min regimen	SK 1,500,000	SK 1,500,000	SK 1,500,000	rt-PA 100 mg	TNK-t-PA/10 s mg.kg
Number of patients	8	40	131	80	30
Bolus	No	No	No	20 mg <65 years	Yes
				15 mg >65 years	
Unfractionated heparin	Bolus 10,000/1,000/h	Bolus 10,000/1,000/h	Bolus 5000/1000/h	Bolus 60 or 12 U/kg	Bolus 60 or 12 U/kg
Low-molecular-weight heparin	No	No	No	1 mg.kg12 h 24–48 h/7 days	1 mg.kg12 h 24–48 h/7 days
Intracranial hemorrhage (%)	0	0	2	0	0
Major hemorrhage (%)	0	2	8	8	3
Minor hemorrhage (%)	0	0	5	5	10

SK streptokinase; *rt-PA* recombinant human tissue-type plasminogen activator; *TNK-t-PA* tenecteplase-tissue-type plasminogen activator

Table 5.4 Cardiovascular adverse events and therapeutic rescue approaches in 289 patients with pulmonary embolism

Variable	1992	1992–1994	1996–2002	2002–2004	2009–2011
60 min regimen	SK 1,500,000	SK 1,500,000	SK 1,500,000	rt-PA 100 mg	TNK-t-PA/ 10 s, mg.kg
Number of patients	8	40	131	80	30
Mortality	T 0/4 H $p=0.02$	12 (%)	28 (%)/61 (%) RVHK	T 3(%)–25 (%) H	13 (%)
Recurrence	0	18 (%)	11 (%)	T10-H20	3 (%)
Rescue thrombolysis	0	10 (%)	5 (%)	10 (%)	0 (%)
Rethrombolysis	0	–	7 (%)	0 (%)	0 (%)
Residual thrombus	2	18 (%)	26 (%)	10 (%)	7 (%)
Percutaneous pulmonary intervention	0	–	16 (%)	5 (%)	7 (%)
Surgical embolectomy	0	–	2 (%)	0 (%)	0 (%)

SK streptokinase; *rt-PA* recombinant human tissue-type plasminogen activator; *TNK-t-PA* tenecteplase-tissue-type-plasminogen activator; *T* thrombolysis; *H* heparin; *RVHK* right ventricular hypokinesis

Later the same unfractionated heparin dose used in ST-elevation myocardial infarction patients was used [10] as adjunctive treatment to one-hour alteplase infusion. Considering that the window for bleeding complications is around the first 48 h, and that in this period there is not any difference in terms of mortality between unfractionated heparin and low-molecular-weight heparin, starting with unfractionated heparin was an excellent bridge to continue with a low-molecular-weight heparin, enoxaparin, that improves and simplifies the traditional anticoagulation approach through easier administration, sustained anticoagulation and an enhanced antithrombotic effect (longer half-life, sustained effect, higher action on Xa factor and less important platelet interaction, antigenicity, rebound and sensibility effect) [10]. Also, this strategy was safe and effective when used with a second- and third-generation thrombolytic (Tables 5.1 and 5.2). The same unfractionated and low-molecular-weight heparin strategy in tenecteplase-tissue-type plasminogen activator PE patients was safe and effective. We decided to use this therapeutic approach based on results of In-Time 3-trial mortality trial.

Although we do not have any head-to-head study, low unfractionated heparin as bridge to start a low-molecular-weight heparin could be an interesting option in PE patients submitted to one-hour alteplase infusion and tenecteplase-tissue-plasminogen activator.

References

1. Konstantinides SV, Torbicki A, Agnelli G, Danchin N, Fitzmaurice D, Galie N, Gibbs JSR, Huisman MV, Humbert M, Kucher N, Lang I, Lankeit M, Lekakis J, Maack C, Mayer E, Meneveau N, Perrier A, Pruszczyk P, Rasmussen LH, Schindler TH, Svitil P, Noordegraaf AV,

Zamorano JL, Zompatori M. 2014 ESC Guidelines on the diagnosis and management of acute pulmonary embolism. The Task Force for the Diagnosis and Management of Acute Pulmonary Embolism of the European Society of Cardiology (ESC). Eur Heart J. 2014;35:3033–80. doi:10.1093/eurheartj/ehu283.

2. Jaff MR, McMurtry MS, Archer SL, Cushman M, Goldenberg NA, Goldhaber SZ, Jenkins JS, Kline JA, Michaels AD, Thistlethwaite P, Vedantham S, White RJ, Zierler BK, on behalf of the American Heart Association Council on Cardiopulmonary, Critical Care, Perioperative and Resuscitation, Council on Peripheral Vascular Disease, and Council on Arteriosclerosis, Thrombosis and Vascular Biology. Management of massive and submassive pulmonary embolism, iliofemoral deep vein thrombosis, and chronic thromboembolic pulmonary hypertension: a scientific statement from the American Heart Association. Circulation. 2011;123:1788–830. doi:10.1161/CIR.0b013e318214914f.
3. Kearon C, Akl EA, Comerota AJ, Prandoni P, Bounameaux H, Goldhaber SZ, Nelson ME, Wells PS, Gould MK, Dentali F, Crowther M, Kahn SR. Antithrombotic therapy for VTE disease: antithrombotic therapy and prevention of thrombosis, 9th ed: American College of Chest Physicians evidence-based clinical practice guidelines. Chest. 2012;141(2 Suppl):e419S–94.
4. Janin S, Meneveau N, Mahemuti A, Descotes-Genon V, Dutheil J, Chopard R, Seronde MF, Schiele F, Bernard Y, Bassand JP. Safety and efficacy of fondaparinux as an adjunctive treatment to thrombolysis in patients with high and intermediate risk pulmonary embolism. J Thromb Thrombolysis. 2009;28:320–24.
5. Buller HR, Davidson BL, Decousus H. Fondaparinux or enoxaparin for the initial treatment of symptomatic deep venous thrombosis: a randomized trial. Ann Intern Med. 2004;140: 867–73.
6. Buller HR, Davidson BL, Decousus H. Subcutaneous fondaparinux versus intravenous unfractionated heparin in the initial treatment of pulmonary embolism. N Engl J Med. 2003;349: 1695–702.
7. Turpie AG, Bauer KA, Eriksson BI. Fondaparinux vs enoxaparin for the prevention of venous thromboembolism in major orthopedic surgery: a meta-analysis of 4 randomized double-blind studies. Arch Intern Med. 2002;162:1833–40.
8. Yusuf S, Mehta SR, Chrolavicius S. Effects of fondaparinux on mortality and reinfarction in patients with acute ST-segment elevation myocardial infarction: the OASIS-6 randomized trial. JAMA. 2006;295:1519–30.
9. Meneveau N, Seronde MF, Blonde MC. Management of unsuccessful thrombolysis in acute massive pulmonary embolism. Chest. 2006;129:1043–50.
10. Jerjes-Sanchez C, Villarreal-Umaña S, Ramirez-Rivera A, Garcia-Sosa A, Canseco LM, Archondo T, Reyes E, Garza A, Arriaga R, Castillo F, Jasso O, Garcia H, Bermudez M, Hernández JM, Garcia J, Martinez P, Rangel F, Gutierrez J, Comparan A. Improving adjunctive treatment in pulmonary embolism and fibrinolytic therapy. The role of enoxaparin and weight-adjusted unfractionated heparin. J Thromb Thrombolysis. 2009;27:154–62.
11. The Assessment of the Safety and Efficacy of a New Thrombolytic Regimen (ASSENT)-3 Investigators. Efficacy and safety of tenecteplase in combination with enoxaparin, abxicimab, or unfractionated heparin: the ASSENT-3 randomised trial in acute myocardial infarction. Lancet. 2001;358:605–13.
12. Gulba DC, Tanswell P, Dechend R, Sosada M, Weis A, Waigand J, Uhlich F, Hauck S, Jost S, Raffenbeul W, Lichtlen PR, Dietz R. Sixty-minute alteplase protocol: a new accelerated recombinant tissue-type plasminogen activator regimen for thrombolysis in acute myocardial infarction. J Am Coll Cardiol. 1997;30:1611–17.
13. Martinez SC, Dominguez JL, Aguirre SJ, Carrillo J, Chuquiure VE, Franco J. Tratamiento del infarto agudo al miocardio con rt-PA en 60 minutos. Estudio Cooperativo. Arch Inst Cardiol Mex. 1997;67:126–31.
14. Jerjes-Sanchez C, Ramirez-Rivera A, Garcia ML, Arriaga-Nava R, Valencia-Sanchez S, Rosado-Buzzo A, Pierzo JA, Rosas ME. Streptokinase and heparin versus heparin alone in massive pulmonary embolism: a randomized controlled trial. J Thromb Thrombolysis. 1995;2:67–9.

15. Jerjes-Sanchez C, Ramirez-Rivera A, Arriaga-Nava R, Iglesias-Gonzalez S, Gutierrez P, Ibarra-Perez C, Martinez A, Valencia S, Rosado-Buzzo A, Pierzo JA, Rosas E. High dose and short-term streptokinase infusion in patients with pulmonary embolism. Prospective with seven-year follow-up trial. J Thromb Thrombolysis. 2001;12:237–47.
16. Jerjes-Sanchez C, Elizalde GJ, Sandoval JZ, et al. Diagnostico, estratificacion y tratamiento de la tromboembolia pulmonar aguda. Guias y recomendaciones del capitulo de Circulacion Pulmonar de la Sociedad Mexicana de Cardiologia. Arch Cardiol Mex. 2004;74 Suppl 3: S547–85.
17. Foussas SG, Zairis MN, Lyras AG. Early prognostic usefulness of C-reactive protein added to the thrombolysis in myocardial infarction risk score in acute coronary syndromes. Am J Cardiol. 2005;96:533–37.
18. Becattini C, Agnelli G, Salvi A, Grifoni S, Pancladi LG, Enea I, Blasemin F, Campanini M, Ghirarduzzi A, Casazza F, TIPES Study Group. Bolus tenecteplase for right ventricle dysfunction in hemodynamically stable patients with pulmonary embolism. Thromb Res. 2010;125:e82–6.
19. Meyer G, Vicaut E, Danays T, Agnelli G, Becattini C, Beyer-Westendorf J, Bluhmki E, Bouvaist H, Brenner B, Couturaud F, Dellas C, Empen K, Granca A, Galiè N, Geibel A, Goldhaber SZ, Jimenez D, Kozak M, Kupatt C, Kucher N, Lang IM, Lankeit M, Meneveau N, Pacouret G, Palazzini M, Petris A, Pruszczyk P, Rugolotto M, Salvi A, Schellong S, Sebbane M, Sobkowicz B, Stefanovic BS, Thiele H, Torbicki A, Verschuren F, Konstantinides SV, PEITHO Investigators. Fibrinolysis for patients with intermediate-risk pulmonary embolism. N Engl J Med. 2014;370:1402–11.
20. Kline JA, Nordenholz KE, Courtney DM, Kabrhel C, Jones AE, Rondina MT, Diercks DB, Klinger JR, Hernandez J. Treatment of submassive pulmonary embolism with tenecteplase or placebo: cardiopulmonary outcomes at 3 months: multicenter double-blind, placebo-controlled randomized trial. J Thromb Haemost. 2014;12:459–68.
21. Marti C, John G, Konstantinides S, Combescure C, Sanchez O, Lankeit M, Meyer G, Perrier A. Systemic thrombolytic therapy for acute pulmonary embolism: a systematic review and meta-analysis. Eur Heart J. 2014;36(10):605–14. doi:10.1093/eurheartj/ehu218.

Chapter 6
Current Guidelines and Recommendations for Thrombolysis Use in Pulmonary Embolism

Carlos Jerjes-Sánchez

In the era of evidence-based medicine, guidelines and recommendations coming from medical societies aim to present all the relevant evidence on a particular issue in order to help physicians related to weigh the benefits and risks of a particular diagnosis and/or therapeutic approach. Guidelines and recommendations should be helpful in every day clinical decision-making to improve acute patient care.

A great number of guidelines and recommendations on pulmonary embolism (PE) have been published in the last 10 years, by different medical organizations in different countries. The main characteristic has been summarizing and evaluating all available evidence at the time of the writing process with the aim of assisting all physicians (cardiologists, pulmonologists, surgeons, internal medicine, emergency physicians, etc.) related in acute PE patient care. In addition, all of them intent selecting the best therapeutic approaches for a specific PE patient, taking into account the impact or outcome, as well as the risk–benefit ratio [1].

In the last 3 years, the European Society of Cardiology [1], the American Heart Association [2] and the American College of Chest Physicians [3], in America and Europe brought together leading experts in the field. All of these Task Forces performed a comprehensive review of the published evidence diagnosis and management in acute PE patients; additionally a critical evaluation of assessment of the risk–benefit was done. Although in the level of evidence and the strength of recommendation have some variations, all of them have to help physicians to make the better decision in their daily clinical practice. Additionally, all experts included provided disclosure

C. Jerjes-Sánchez, M.D., F.C.C.P., F.A.C.C. (✉)
Sistema Nacional de Investigadores, Nivel II – Clinical Research Director, Instituto de Cardiologia y Medicina Vascular, TEC Salud

Escuela de Medicina, Tecnológico de Monterrey San Pedro Garza Garcia, Nuevo León, Mexico

Unidad de Investigacion Clinica en Medicina SC Monterrey, Nuevo León, Mexico
e-mail: jerjes@prodigy.net.mx

C. Jerjes-Sánchez, *Thrombolysis in Pulmonary Embolism*,
DOI 10.1007/978-3-319-19707-4_6

statements about all relationships identified as real or potential sources of interest conflicts. The Task Force reports were entirely supported by the American Heart Association, the American College of Chest Physicians, and the European Society of Cardiology. Pharmaceutic industry was not involved in either case.

Although, thrombolysis in well-selected patients is an important therapeutic toll, related physicians have to be in warning of its risks, specifically the most feared: intracranial hemorrhage. We would like to emphasize that in spite all clinical evidence that we have, the ultimate judgment to use a specific care for a specific patient has to be performed under the best clinical judgment by the physician in charge.

This chapter will be focusing on the guidelines and recommendations on PE and thrombolysis coming from the most important cardiology societies and experts in the field. In addition, a brief overview on methodology and recommendations level, as well as, evidence level will be presented. Although, all of these Task Forces are available online, readers will have a quick and easy access. A fast-track analysis comparing thrombolytic regimens in terms of efficacy and safety will be available. In addition, considering the first chapter analyzed in extensive pharmacokinetics and pharmacodynamics of fibrinolytics, this part of the text was not included. Considering the relevance of guidelines and recommendations, the text remained practically as was wrote by the panel of experts. If the reader wants to deepen guidelines and recommendations, these are accessible online.

Management of Massive and Submassive Pulmonary Embolism, Iliofemoral Deep Vein Thrombosis, and Chronic Thromboembolic Pulmonary Hypertension: A Scientific Statement from the American Heart Association

In this guidelines and recommendations, the panel of experts considered that venous thromboembolism is serious health problem. In spite of advanced programs on venous thromboembolism prophylaxis, it is responsible for the hospitalization of >250,000 Americans annually and represents a significant risk for morbidity and mortality [2].

Despite all the publication of evidence-based clinical practice guidelines that we have to drive the management in its acute and chronic forms, the physicians in charge frequently are confronted with manifestations of venous thromboembolism in which the data are sparse; in consequence the optimal management is unclear. In particular, the optimal use of advanced therapies for acute venous thromboembolism, including thrombolysis and catheter-based therapies, remains uncertain. This Task Force report addresses the management of massive and submassive pulmonary embolism (PE), iliofemoral deep vein thrombosis, and chronic thromboembolic pulmonary hypertension. The main target was to provide practical advice to clinicians in charge to optimize the management of patients with these severe manifestations of venous thromboembolism [2]. The recommendations for formulating and issuing AHA Guidelines can be found on the AHA Web Site: http://circ.ahajournals.org/content/123/16/1788.full.pdf+html

Methodology

A writing group was established with representation from the Council on Peripheral Vascular Disease and Council on Cardiopulmonary, Critical Care, Perioperative and Resuscitation of the American Heart Association and vetted by American Heart Association leadership. All writing group members were required to disclose all relationships with industry and other entities relevant to the subject. Three areas were considered and each one was led by a member with content expertise in deep venous thrombosis and chronic thromboembolic pulmonary hypertension. Acute PE had as project leader professor Samuel Z. Goldhaber due to his relevant contributions in the field of thrombolysis and risk stratification [2].

The member of writing groups systematically reviewed and summarized the relevant published literature incorporating all of this information into a manuscript with draft recommendations. Differences in opinion were dealt with through a face-to-face meeting and subsequently through electronic and telephone communications. At the end, final document was a reflection of a consensus view of the entire committee. Areas of uncertainty are also noted in hopes that both basic and clinical research will advance knowledge in this area [2].

The evidence levels and class from American Heart Association were adopted (Tables 6.1 and 6.2). External reviewers appointed by the American Heart Association independently reviewed the document. Each recommendation required a confidential vote by the writing group members after external review of the document. Any writing group member with a relationship with industry relevant to the recommendation was recused from the voting on that recommendation [2]. The readers can access the guidelines on the Web Site of American Heart Association: http://circ.ahajournals.org/content/123/16/1788.full.pdf+html

Thrombolysis

Rationality for Thrombolysis Uses Potential Benefits and Harm

The decision to administer a fibrinolytic agent in addition to heparin anticoagulation requires individualized assessment of the balance of benefits versus risks. Potential benefits include more rapid resolution of symptoms (e.g., dyspnea, chest pain, tachycardia, and psychological distress), stabilization of respiratory and cardiovascular

Table 6.1 Levels of evidence—American Heart Association

Level A:	Multiple populations evaluated. Data derived from multiple randomized clinical trials or meta-analyses
Level B:	Limited populations evaluated. Data derived from a single randomized trial or nonrandomized studies
Level C:	Very limited populations evaluated. Only consensus opinion of experts, case studies, or standard of care

Manual for ACC/AHA Guidelines Writing Committees 2015

Table 6.2 Class of evidence—American Heart Association

Class I	Class IIa	Class IIb	Class III No benefit or Class III Harm		
Benefit >>> Risk	Benefit >> Risk	Benefit ≥ Risk		Procedure/test	Treatment
Procedure/treatment SHOULD be performed/administered	Additional studies with focused objectives needed	Additional studies with broad objectives needed; additional registry data would be helpful	COR III: No benefit	Not helpful	No proven benefit
	IT IS REASONABLE to perform procedure/administer treatment	Procedure/treatment MAY BE CONSIDERED	COR III: Harm	Excess cost w/o benefit or harmful	Harmful to patients
• Recommendation that procedure or treatment is useful/effective	• Recommendation in favor of treatment or procedure being useful/effective	• Recommendation's usefulness/efficacy less well established	• Recommendation that procedure or treatment is not useful/effective and may be harmful		
• Sufficient evidence form multiple randomized trials or meta-analyses	• Some conflicting evidence from multiple randomized trials or meta-analyses	• Greater conflicting evidence from multiple randomized trials or meta-analyses	• Sufficient evidence form multiple randomized trials or meta-analyses		
• Recommendation that procedure or treatment is useful/effective	• Recommendation in favor of treatment or procedure being useful/effective	• Recommendation's usefulness/efficacy less well established	• Recommendation that procedure or treatment is not useful/effective and may be harmful		
• Evidence form single randomized trial or nonrandomized studies	• Some conflicting evidence from a single randomized or nonrandomized studies	• Greater conflicting evidence form single randomized trial or nonrandomized studies	• Evidence form single randomized trial or nonrandomized studies		
• Recommendation that procedure or treatment is useful/effective	• Recommendation in favor of treatment or procedure being useful/effective	• Recommendation's usefulness/efficacy less well established	• Recommendation that procedure or treatment is not useful/effective and may be harmful		
• Only expert opinion, case studies, or standard of care	• Only diverging expert opinion, case studies, or standard of care	• Only diverging expert opinion, case studies, or standard of care	• Only expert opinion, case studies, or standard of care		

Manual for ACC/AHA Guidelines Writing Committees 2015

function (hypotension) without need for mechanical ventilation or vasopressor support; in addition, reduction of right ventricular damage, improved exercise tolerance, prevention of PE recurrence, and increased probability of survival have been observed. Potential harm includes disabling or fatal hemorrhage, including intracerebral hemorrhage, and increased risk of minor hemorrhages, resulting in prolongation of hospitalization and need for blood product replacement [2].

Quantitative Assessment of Outcomes

Patients treated with a fibrinolytic agent have faster restoration of lung perfusion. At 24 h, patients treated with heparin have no substantial improvement in pulmonary blood flow, whereas patients treated with adjunctive fibrinolysis manifest a 30–35 % reduction in total perfusion defect. However, by 7 days, blood flow improves similarly (~65–70 % reduction in total defect). Thirteen placebo-controlled randomized trials of fibrinolysis for acute PE have been published, but only a subset evaluated massive PE specifically. These trials included 480 patients randomized to fibrinolysis and 464 randomized to placebo; 6 of the 13 trials studied alteplase, representing 56 % of all patients (no = 504). These six studies used variable infusion regimens. Two studies administered alteplase by bolus intravenous injection (100 mg or 0.6 mg/kg), and four infused 90–100 mg of alteplase intravenously over a 2-h period. Three of the four used concomitant infusion of intravenous unfractionated heparin (1000–1500 U/h). Four studies used intravenous streptokinase, together enrolling 94 patients. All four studies of streptokinase used a bolus dose (250,000–600,000 U) followed by a 100,000 U/h infusion for 12–72 h. Two studies that examined urokinase, published in 1973 and 1988, together enrolled 190 patients [2].

One study randomized 58 patients to receive weight-adjusted single-bolus intravenous tenecteplase (30–50 mg, with a 5-mg increase in dose for every 10 kg of weight from <60 to>90 kg) or placebo. The odds ratios were calculated by use of fixed effects and random effect models. The evidence suggesting that alteplase treatment was associated with a significantly higher rate of hemorrhage than anticoagulation alone, although these events included skin bruising and oozing from puncture sites. Neither recurrent PE nor death was significantly different in the alteplase versus placebo groups [2].

Alteplase was associated with a trend toward decreased recurrent PE. Similar findings have been reported by Wan et al. [4] and Thabut et al. [5] When Wan et al. [4] restricted their analysis to those trials with massive PE, they identified a significant reduction in recurrent PE or death from 19.0 % with heparin alone to 9.4 % with fibrinolysis (odds ratio 0.45, 95 % CI 0.22–0.90) [1].

Number Needed to Treat

Wan et al. [4] in their analysis restricted to trials that included fibrinolysis for massive PE, found the number needed to treat to prevent the composite end point of recurrent PE or death was 10 patients. This end point was not statistically significant when all trials, including those that studied less severe forms of PE, were included [4]. In this analysis, there was no significant increase in major bleeding, but there was a significant increase in no major bleeding; the number needed to harm was 8 [4]. On the other hand, Thabut et al. [5], using data from all trials regardless of PE severity but before the publication of the largest randomized trial to date, estimated the number needed to harm at 17.

Impact of Fibrinolysis on Submassive Pulmonary Embolism

At least four registries have documented the outcomes of PE patients (MAPPET [6], ICOPER [7], RIETE [8] and EMPEROR [9]). The data coming from these registries suggest a trend toward a decrease in all-cause mortality from PE, especially massive PE in those patients treated with fibrinolysis. The 30-day mortality rate directly attributed to PE in normotensive patients in the recently completed EMPEROR registry was 0.9 % (95 % CI 0–1.6). Data from these registries indicate that the short-term mortality rate directly attributable to submassive PE treated with heparin anticoagulation is probably <3.0 %. The implication is that even if adjunctive fibrinolytic therapy has extremely high efficacy, for example, a 30 % relative reduction in mortality, the effect size on mortality due to submassive PE is probably <1 %. Thus, secondary adverse outcomes such as persistent right ventricular dysfunction, chronic thromboembolic pulmonary hypertension, and impaired quality of life represent appropriate surrogate goals of treatment [2].

Impact of Fibrinolysis on Intermediate Outcomes

Among PE patients, to determine whether adjunctive fibrinolytic therapy can effectively reduce the outcome of dyspnea and exercise intolerance caused by persistent pulmonary hypertension (World Health Organization, WHO Group 4 pulmonary hypertension); it is first necessary to examine the incidence of persistently elevated right ventricular systolic pressure or pulmonary arterial pressure, measured 6 or more months after acute PE. The current literature includes only four studies that report baseline and follow-up right ventricular systolic pressure or pulmonary arterial pressures by use of pulmonary arterial catheter or Doppler echocardiography [10–13]. These data suggest that compared with heparin alone, heparin plus fibrinolysis yields a significant favorable change in right ventricular systolic pressure and pulmonary arterial pressure incident between the time of diagnosis and follow-up [2].

The largest study, accounting for 162 of the 205 patients, was the only one that was prospectively designed to assess outcomes for all survivors at 6 months [13]. All patients were normotensive at the time of enrollment. Follow-up included Doppler echocardiographic estimation of the right ventricular systolic pressure, a 6-minute walk test, and New York Heart Association (NYHA) classification. The study protocol in that report recommended addition of alteplase (0.6 mg/kg infused over 2 h) for patients who experienced hemodynamic deterioration, defined as hypotension, cardiac arrest, or respiratory failure requiring mechanical ventilation.

Among the 144 patients who received heparin only, 39 (27 %) demonstrated an increase in right ventricular systolic pressure at 6-month follow-up, and 18 (46 %) of these 39 patients had either dyspnea at rest (NYHA classification more than II) or exercise intolerance (6-minute walk distance <330 m). The mean 6-minute walk distance was 364 m for the alteplase group versus 334 m for the heparin-only patients. No patient treated with adjunctive alteplase demonstrated an increase in right ventricular systolic pressure at 6-month follow-up, which suggests that thrombolytic therapy may have the benefit of decreasing the incidence of chronic thromboembolic pulmonary hypertension [13].

Contraindications to Fibrinolysis

Because of small sample sizes and heterogeneity, the clinical trials provide limited guidance in establishing contraindications to the use of fibrinolytic agents in PE. Contraindications must therefore be extrapolated from author experience and from guidelines for ST-elevation myocardial infarction patients. Absolute and relative contraindications are showed in Table 6.3. Recent surgery, depending on the territory involved, and minor injuries, including minor head trauma due to syncope, are not necessarily barriers to fibrinolysis. The clinician is in the best position to judge the relative merits of fibrinolysis on a case-by-case basis [2].

Synthesis of Data into a Treatment Algorithm

Low-risk PE patients have an unfavorable risk–benefit ratio with fibrinolysis. Patients with PE that causes hypotension probably do benefit from fibrinolysis. Management of submassive PE crosses the zone of equipoise, requiring the clinician to use clinical judgment. Two criteria can be used to assist in determining whether a patient is more likely to benefit from fibrinolysis: (1) Evidence of present or developing circulatory or respiratory insufficiency; or (2) evidence of moderate to severe RV injury [2].

Evidence of circulatory failure includes any episode of hypotension or a persistent shock index (heart rate in beats per minute divided by systolic blood pressure in millimeters of mercury) >1. The definition of respiratory insufficiency may include hypoxemia, defined as a pulse oximetry reading <95 % when the patient is breathing room air and clinical judgment that the patient appears to be in respiratory distress. Alternatively, respiratory distress can be quantified by the numeric Borg score, which assesses the severity of dyspnea from 0 to 10 (0 = no dyspnea and 10 = sensation of choking to death); fewer than 10 % of patients with acute PE report a Borg score >8 at the time of diagnosis [2].

Evidence of moderate to severe right ventricular injury may be derived from Doppler echocardiography that demonstrates any degree of right ventricular hypokinesis, McConnell's sign (a distinct regional pattern of right ventricular dysfunction with akinesis of the mid-free-wall but normal motion at the apex), interventricular septal shift or bowing, or an estimated right ventricular systolic pressure >40 mmHg.

Table 6.3 Risk factors for bleeding with and without contraindications to use of thrombolytic therapy from AHA, ACCP and ESC guidelines

	American Heart Association, 2011	American College of Chest Physicians, 2012	European Society of Cardiology, 2014
Major contraindications	Any prior intracranial hemorrhage	Structural intracranial disease	Hemorrhagic stroke or stroke of unknown origin at any time
	Structural intracranial cerebrovascular disease	Previous intracranial hemorrhage	Ischemic stroke in the preceding 6 months
	Malignant intracranial neoplasm	Ischemic stroke within 3 months	Central nervous system damage or neoplasms
	Ischemic stroke within 3 months	Active bleeding	Recent major trauma/surgery/head injury in the preceding 3 weeks
	Suspected aortic dissection	Recent brain or spinal surgery	Gastrointestinal bleeding within the last month
	Active bleeding or bleeding diathesis	Recent head trauma with fracture or brain injury	Known bleeding risk
	Recent surgery significant closed-head or facial trauma with XR evidence of bony fracture or brain injury	Bleeding diathesis	
Relative contraindications	Age >75 years	Systolic BP>180 mmHg	Transient ischemic attack in the preceding 6 months
	Current use of anticoagulation	Diastolic BP>110 mmHg	Oral anticoagulant therapy
	Pregnancy	Recent bleeding (non intracranial)	Pregnancy, or within 1 week postpartum
	Noncompressible vascular punctures	Recent surgery	Noncompressible puncture site
	Traumatic or prolonged cardiopulmonary resuscitation (>10 min)	Recent invasive procedure	Traumatic resuscitation
	Recent internal bleeding (within 2–4 weeks)	Ischemic stroke more that 3 months previously	Refractory hypertension (systolic blood pressure >180 mmHg)
	Chronic, severe and poorly controlled hypertension	Anticoagulation (e.g., VKA therapy)	Advanced liver disease
	Systolic BP>180 mmHg	Traumatic cardiopulmonary resuscitation	Infective endocarditis
	Diastolic BP>110 mmHg	Pericarditis or pericardial fluid	Active peptic ulcer
	Dementia	Diabetic retinopathy	
	Remote ischemic stroke (>3 months)	Pregnancy	
	Major surgery within 3 weeks	Age >75 years	
		Low body weight (e.g., <60 kg)	
		Female sex	
		Black race	

Table 6.4 Fibrinolytic regimens recommended by the American Heart Association, American College of Chest Physicians and European Society of Cardiology

Thrombolytic agent	American Heart Association, 2011	American College of Chest Physicians, 2012	European Society of Cardiology, 2014
Streptokinase	250,000-IU IV bolus followed by 100,000-IU/h infusion for 12–24 h	25,000-IU IV bolus over 15 min by 100,000 IU for 12 h	250,000 IU as a loading dose over 30 min, followed by 100,000 IU/h over 12–24 h Accelerated regimen: 1.5 million IU over 2 h
Urokinase	4400-IU/kg bolus, followed by 4400-IU/kg'h for 12–24 h	4400 IU/kg, bolus followed by 2200–4400 IU/kg/h for 12 h	4400 IU/kg as a loading dose over 10 min, followed by 4400 IU/kg/h over 12–24 h Accelerated regimen: 3,000,000 IU over 2 h
rt-PA	Alteplase: 100-mg IV infusion over 2 h	0.6 mg/kg over 15 min or 100 mg over 2 h	100 mg over 2 h; or 0.6 mg/kg over 15 min (maximum dose 50 mg)

IU international units, *rt-PA* recombinant human tissue-plasminogen activator

Biomarker evidence of moderate to severe right ventricular injury includes major elevation of troponin measurement or brain natriuretic peptides. A limitation of this approach is that these variables are generally presented as dichotomous, and there are no universally agreed on thresholds for minor or major abnormalities. Practical judgment of the bedside physician is required [2].

This panel of experts recommends fibrinolytic administration by peripheral intravenous catheter (Table 6.4). FDA-recommended infusion dose of alteplase at 100 mg as a continuous infusion over 2 h. The FDA recommends withholding anticoagulation during the 2-h infusion period. Two ongoing randomized controlled trials will help address the controversial question about which patients with submassive PE will benefit from fibrinolysis. Both trials use tenecteplase as the fibrinolytic, an agent that is not approved by the FDA for treatment of PE. The larger trial (the Pulmonary EmbolIsm THrOmbolysis Study, PEITHO) [14] and the trial (Tenecteplase Or Placebo: Cardiopulmonary Outcomes At 3 Months, TOPCOAT) [15].

Recommendations for Fibrinolysis for Acute Pulmonary Embolism

1. Fibrinolysis is reasonable for patients with massive acute PE and acceptable risk of bleeding complications (Class IIa; Level of Evidence B).
2. Fibrinolysis may be considered for patients with submassive acute PE judged to have clinical evidence of adverse prognosis (new hemodynamic instability, worsening respiratory insufficiency, severe right ventricular dysfunction, or major myocardial necrosis) and low risk of bleeding complications (Class IIb; Level of Evidence C).

3. Fibrinolysis is not recommended for patients with low-risk PE (Class III; Level of Evidence B) or submassive acute PE with minor right ventricular dysfunction, minor myocardial necrosis, and no clinical worsening (Class III; Level of Evidence B).
4. Fibrinolysis is not recommended for undifferentiated cardiac arrest (Class III; Level of Evidence B) [1].

Antithrombotic Therapy for Venous Thromboembolism Disease: Antithrombotic Therapy and Prevention of Thrombosis, 9th Ed: American College of Chest Physicians Evidence-Based Clinical Practice Guidelines

Methodology

The methodology used for the Antithrombotic Therapy and Prevention of Thrombosis, 9th ed: American College of Chest Physicians Evidence-Based Clinical Practice Guidelines (AT9), incorporates current evidence-based approaches to the appraisal and synthesis of evidence and to the formulation of clinical practice recommendations. The process thus ensures explicit, transparent, evidence-based clinical practice guidelines [16].

The objective of AT9 was to optimize patient's important health outcomes and the processes of care for patients who have experienced or are at risk for thrombotic events. The targeted users of these guidelines are healthcare providers in both primary and specialty care who assist patients in making treatment choices that optimize benefits, minimize harms and burdens, and are consistent with patient values and preferences [16].

Clinical areas were designated as articles, and a methodologist without important intellectual or financial conflicts of interest led a panel for each article. Only panel members without significant conflicts of interest participated in making recommendations. Panelists specified the population, intervention and alternative, and outcomes for each clinical question and defined criteria for eligible studies. Panelists and an independent evidence-based practice center executed systematic searches for relevant studies and evaluated the evidence, and where resources and evidence permitted, they created standardized tables that present the quality of the evidence and key results in a transparent fashion [16].

One or more recommendations relate to each specific clinical question, and each recommendation was clearly linked to the underlying body of evidence. Judgments regarding the quality of evidence and strength of recommendations were based on approaches developed by the Grades of Recommendations, Assessment, Development, and Evaluation Working Group. Panel members constructed scenarios describing relevant health states and rated the disutility associated with these states based on an additional systematic review of evidence regarding patient values and preferences for antithrombotic therapy. These ratings guided value and preference decisions underlying the recommendations. Each topic panel identified questions in which resource allocation issues were particularly important and, for these issues, experts in economic analysis provided additional searches and guidance [16].

AT9 methodology reflects the current science of evidence-based clinical practice guideline development, with reliance on high-quality systematic reviews, a standardized process for quality assessment of individual studies and the body of evidence, an explicit process for translating the evidence into recommendations, disclosure of financial as well as intellectual conflicts of interest followed by management of disclosed conflicts, and extensive peer review [16]. A summary of the methodology can be seen in Table 6.5. Additionally, the ACCP recommendations based on evidence quality are shown in Table 6.6.

Presentation as Deep Venous Thrombosis or Pulmonary Embolism

In addressing deep venous thrombosis, the panel first reviews studies that included (1) only patients who presented with symptomatic deep venous thrombosis or (2) patients who presented with deep venous thrombosis or PE (i.e., meeting the broader criterion of venous thromboembolism). For the PE components, the experts reviewed studies (and subgroups within studies) that required patients to have presented with symptomatic PE (who may also have had symptoms of deep venous thrombosis) [3].

For this reason and because more patients with venous thromboembolism present with symptoms of deep venous thrombosis alone than with symptoms of PE (including those who also have symptoms of deep venous thrombosis), the deep venous thrombosis section deals with a larger body of evidence than the PE section. In the evaluation of anticoagulant therapy, there are a number of justifications for inclusion of patients who present with deep venous thrombosis and PE in the same study, and for extrapolating evidence obtained in patients with one presentation of venous thromboembolism (e.g., deep venous thrombosis) to the other presentation (e.g., PE) [3].

First, a majority of patients with symptomatic deep venous thrombosis also have PE (symptomatic or asymptomatic), and a majority of those with symptomatic PE also have deep venous thrombosis DVT (symptomatic or asymptomatic). Second, clinical trials of anticoagulant therapy have yielded similar estimates for efficacy and safety in patients with deep venous thrombosis alone, in those with both deep venous thrombosis and PE, and in those with only PE. Third, the risk of recurrence appears to be similar after PE and after proximal deep venous thrombosis [3].

Consequently, the results of all studies of deep venous thrombosis have been considered when formulating recommendations for short- and long-term anticoagulation of proximal deep venous thrombosis and PE, and these recommendations are essentially the same for proximal deep venous thrombosis or PE. There are, however, some important differences between patients who present with PE and those who present with DVT that justify separate consideration of some aspects of the treatment of PE [3].

Table 6.5 Methodology for the development of antithrombotic therapy and prevention of thrombosis guidelines ACCP

Objectives	Process
Composition and selection of topic panel members	The ACCP Executive Committee selected panel members for each article based on their previous experience with guideline development and in particular with methods developed by GRADE working group. All were approved after review of their conflict of interest disclosures. Each topic panel also included a frontline physician who were charged with the following: proposing important real-world clinical questions on the prevention, diagnosis, and treatment of thrombosis and reviewing the draft manuscripts and recommendations to assess the usability of the guidelines and the feasibility of implementation of AT9 recommendations
Evidence review	The thrombosis expert on the EC along with deputy editors defined the scope of the clinical questions that each article would address, based on relevant population, alternative management strategies and outcomes (population, intervention, comparator, and outcome [PICO] format). Each clinical question provided the framework for formulating study inclusion and exclusion criteria guided the search for relevant evidence; systematic reviews and original studies. Panels typically restricted included studies to RCTs for intervention questions but included observational studies when there was paucity of RCT data addressing an intervention and for questions of risk assessment
Assessing studies and summarizing evidence	The AT9 group developed and applied uniform criteria for evaluating the risk of bias associated with individual RCTs and observational studies (cohort studies with concurrent controls, cohort studies with historical controls, case–control studies, or case series) on the criteria recommended by the Cochrane Collaboration
Values and preferences	Through a systematic review of the literature bearing on patient values and preferences regarding antithrombotic therapy. Also conducted a values rating exercise on patient scenarios, the mean values of these ratings guided the trade-offs between thrombotic and bleeding events and, thus, the determination of strong versus weak recommendations
Resource use issues	The group restricted economic evaluation to recommendations, which it was plausible that resource use considerations might change the direction or strength of the recommendation and in which high-quality economic evaluations were available
Disclosing and managing conflicts of interest	All panelists were required to disclose both financial conflicts of interest, such a receipt of founds for consulting with industry, and intellectual conflicts of interest, such as publication of original data bearing directly on a recommendation. Financial and intellectual interests were classified as primary and secondary (more serious and less serious respectively). Panel members with primary conflicts related to a particular recommendation did not participate in the final deliberations that led to the decision regarding the direction or strength of a recommendation, nor did they vote on recommendations for which they were primarily conflicted. Panelists with primary conflicts could, however, participate in discussions and offer their opinions on interpretations of the evidence
Finalizing the recommendations	Following approaches recommended by the GRADE working group the formulation of recommendations considered the balance between the desirable and undesirable consequences of an intervention; the quality of evidence; the variability in patient values and preferences; and, on occasion, resource use issues. The recommendations were graded as strong when desirable effects were much greater than undesirable effects or vice versa
Review by ACCP and external reviewers	The ACCP HSP Committee established a process for the thorough review of all ACCP evidence-based clinical practice guidelines. After final review by the AT9 Executive Committee, the guidelines underwent review by the Cardiovascular and Pulmonary Vascular Networks of the ACCP, the HSP Committee, and the ACCP Board of Regents. The ACCP HSP Committee established a process for the thorough review of all ACCP evidence-based clinical practice guidelines. After final review by the AT9 EC, the guidelines underwent review by the Cardiovascular and Pulmonary Vascular Networks of the ACCP, the HSP Committee, and the ACCP Board of Regents. Finally, the Editor in Chief of *CHEST* read and forwarded the manuscripts for independent, external peer review prior to acceptance for publication. No recommendations or assessments of the quality of the evidence could be changed without the express approval of the topic panel members, AT9 EC, HSP Committee, and ACCP Board of Regents

Table 6.6 ACCP recommendations based on evidence quality

	Grade	1: Strong recommendation	2: Weak recommendation
Quality of evidence	A: High-quality	1a: Strong recommendation based on high-quality evidence	2a: Weak recommendation based on high-quality evidence
	B: Moderate-quality	1b: Strong recommendation based on moderate-quality evidence	2b: Weak recommendation based on moderate-quality evidence
	C: Low-quality	1c: Strong recommendation based on low-quality evidence	2c: Weak recommendation based on low-quality evidence

First, the risk of early death (within 1 month) from venous thromboembolism due to either the initial acute episode or recurrent venous thromboembolism is much greater after presenting with PE than after deep venous thrombosis; this difference may justify more aggressive initial treatment of PE (e.g., thrombolytic therapy, insertion of an inferior vena cava filter, more intensive anticoagulant therapy) compared with deep venous thrombosis [3].

Second, recurrent episodes of venous thromboembolism are about three times as likely to be PE after an initial PE than after an initial deep venous thrombosis (i.e., about 60 % after a PE versus 20 % after a deep venous thrombosis); this difference may justify more aggressive, or more prolonged, long-term therapy [3].

Third, the long-term sequelae of PE are cardiorespiratory impairment, especially due to pulmonary hypertension, rather than prothrombotic syndrome of the legs or arms. These differences are most important for recommendations about the use of thrombus removal procedures (e.g., thrombolytic therapy) in patients who present with deep venous thrombosis and PE [3]. Guidelines and recommendations from American College of Chest Physicians are on journal Chest: http://www.chestnet.org/Guidelines-and-Resources/Guidelines-and-Consensus-Statements/Antithrombotic-Guidelines-9th-Ed.

Systemic Thrombolytic Therapy for Pulmonary Embolism

Systemic Thrombolytic Therapy Versus Anticoagulation

Alone for PE: Randomized trials have established that, at 24 h, thrombolytic therapy improves (1) pulmonary artery hemodynamic measurements (e.g., mean pulmonary artery pressure improvement, 4.4 mmHg; 95 % CI, 2 4.6–4.2), (2) arteriovenous oxygen (difference of 2 0.3 [2 0.4–2 0.2]), (3) pulmonary perfusion (50 % early improvement in perfusion scan, OR, 3.8; 95 % CI, 0.9–15.7), and (4) echocardiographic assessment (OR for improved right ventricular wall movement, 3.1; 95 % CI, 1.5–6.3) [3].

Thrombolytic therapy, however, does not appear to reduce the extent of residual thrombosis. It is uncertain whether the benefits of more rapid resolution of PE outweigh the risk of increased bleeding associated with thrombolytic therapy. In patients with PE, severity of presentation is expected to depend on the extent of embolism (i.e., degree of pulmonary artery obstruction) and the presence and severity of chronic cardiopulmonary impairment. Patients with the most severe presentations who have the highest risk of dying from an acute PE have the most to gain from thrombolysis [3].

Prognosis in Patients with Acute Pulmonary Embolism

Of patients who are diagnosed with PE and start treatment, ~5 % die of the initial PE or another PE within the next 7 days. However, although the risk of dying of PE differs markedly among patients, no validated risk prediction tool is available. Risk of dying of PE is estimated to be ~70 % if cardiopulmonary arrest occurs (~1 % of patients at presentation), 30 % if there is shock requiring inotropic support (~5 % of patients), and ~2 % in patients who are not hypotensive [3].

In patients with normal systemic arterial pressure, prognosis can also differ, depending on (1) clinical evaluation, (2) cardiac biomarkers such as troponin or brain natriuretic peptide, and (3) assessment of right ventricular size and function [3].

Clinical evaluation involves assessment of general appearance, blood pressure, heart rate, respiratory rate, temperature, pulse oximetry, and signs of right ventricular dysfunction (e.g., distended jugular veins, tricuspid regurgitation, accentuated P_2). Clues on the electrocardiogram include right bundle branch block, S_1 Q_3 T_3, and T-wave inversion in leads V1 through V4. Elevation of cardiac troponins indicates right ventricular microinfarction, and echocardiography may show right ventricular hypokinesis; both are risk factors for early mortality and are associated with a worse outcome when they occur together. Right ventricular enlargement on the CT pulmonary angiogram, (right ventricular diameter ≥90 % than the left ventricular diameter) may also be an independent risk factor for death and nonfatal complications [3].

Risk of Bleeding with Thrombolytic Therapy

The panel of experts did not identify any validated risk prediction tool for bleeding with thrombolytic therapy in patients with PE. However, they assumed that the assessment of bleeding risk with thrombolytic therapy is similar in patients with PE and with ST-elevation myocardial infarction. Table 6.3 lists risk factors for bleeding with thrombolytic therapy, categorized as major and relative contraindications.

Trials Evaluating Thrombolytic Therapy in Patients with Acute Pulmonary Embolism

Considering the evidence coming from the findings of thirteen randomized control trials comparing thrombolytic therapy with anticoagulant therapy; additionally, an important number of meta-analyses of these studies, the evidence suggests that thrombolysis may be associated with a reduction in mortality and recurrent PE and is associated with an increase in major bleeding, as has been established in patients with myocardial infarction [3].

The quality of evidence regarding mortality and recurrent PE is low because of the risk of bias, serious imprecision and suspected publication bias. A previous meta-analysis that categorized studies as either including, or not including, patients with cardiopulmonary compromise, suggested that thrombolytic therapy reduced the composite outcome of death and recurrent PE in studies that included the sickest patients [2]. However, the data available from these studies are not sufficiently detailed to enable a subgroup analysis evaluating outcomes in patients with hemodynamic compromise or other markers of heightened risk of death (e.g., right ventricular dysfunction) [3].

Balancing Benefits and Harms of Thrombolytic Therapy

In patients who present with PE and hypotension (e.g., systolic pressure blood pressure <90 mmHg or a documented drop in systolic blood pressure >40 mmHg with evidence of poor perfusion), especially if they have a low risk of bleeding, even modest efficacy of thrombolytic therapy is likely to reduce deaths from PE more than it would increase fatal bleeds and nonfatal intracranial bleeds [3].

The ultimate judgment of the entire AT9 panel was to issue a weak recommendation for patients with PE and hypotension given the uncertainty of the benefit. In most patients with PE, given the certain risks of bleeding and less-certain benefits, thrombolysis is likely to be harmful. Selected patients without hypotension may benefit from thrombolysis because their initial clinical presentation or clinical course after starting anticoagulant therapy suggests that they are at high risk of dying. There is no explicit clinical prediction rule that identifies this subgroup of patients. AT9 panel suggests that such patients are identified predominantly by clinical evidence of instability (e.g., a decrease in systolic BP that still remains >90 mmHg, tachycardia, elevated jugular venous pressure, clinical evidence of poor tissue perfusion, hypoxemia) and failure to improve on anticoagulant therapy [3].

As noted previously, laboratory (e.g., troponin, brain natriuretic peptide), electrocardiogram, echocardiography, and CT evidence of right ventricular dysfunction or enlargement, can supplement the clinical evaluation of instability; however, they are not sufficiently predictive to serve as indications for thrombolytic therapy and it is not recommended for routine use [3].

Recommendations for Thrombolytic Therapy

In patients with acute PE associated with hypotension (e.g., systolic blood pressure <90 mmHg) who do not have a high risk of bleeding, the panel of experts suggests systemically administered thrombolytic therapy over no such therapy (Grade 2C) [3].

In most patients with acute PE not associated with hypotension, we recommend against systemically administered thrombolytic therapy (Grade 1C) [3].

In selected patients with acute PE not associated with hypotension and with a low risk of bleeding whose initial clinical presentation or clinical course after starting anticoagulant therapy suggests a high risk of developing hypotension, we suggest administration of thrombolytic therapy (Grade 2C) [3].

Systemic Thrombolytic Therapy Regimen for Pulmonary Embolism

Twelve randomized trials (total of 938 patients) have compared the rate of thrombus resolution achieved with various intravenous thrombolytic regimens. These regimens included urokinase given over 2 or 12 h; streptokinase given over 2, 12, or 24 h; and recombinant human tissue-type plasminogen activator (rt-PA) given over 15 min or 2 h, reteplase in two boluses 30 min apart, and desmoteplase in three different doses as a bolus. An additional study compared IV with pulmonary artery catheter administration of rt-PA (50 mg over 2 h) [3].

The results of studies that compared different approaches to thrombolysis in patients with PE (noted previously) suggest that (1) prolonged infusions of thrombolytic agents (e.g., >12 h) are associated with higher rates of bleeding (2) 2-h infusions achieve more rapid clot lysis than 12- or 24 h infusions; (3) when a high-concentration 2-h infusion of thrombolysis is administered, there is no clear difference in the efficacy or safety of rt-PA versus streptokinase; (4) bolus rt-PA regimens (e.g., ~50 mg in ≤15 min) appears to be as effective and safe as a 2-h infusion of 100 mg of rt-PA; and (5) infusion of rt-PA directly into a pulmonary artery as opposed to a peripheral vein does not accelerate thrombolysis but does cause more frequent bleeding at the catheter insertion site (there was no attempt to infuse rt-PA directly into or to mechanically disrupt the thrombus in this study from 1988) [3].

When a lytic agent is appropriate for PE, current evidence supports that thrombolytic therapy should be infused into a peripheral vein over ≤2 h. At a dose of 100 mg over 2-h, rt-PA is currently the most widely used and evaluated regimen. In patients with imminent or actual cardiac arrest, bolus infusion of thrombolytic therapy is indicated. The quality of evidence for comparisons of systemic thrombolytic agents and regimens (e.g., different doses or durations of infusion) is low based on very serious imprecision and risk of bias. In addition, there is substantial potential for publication bias. Based on this evidence, the experts provide only weak recommendations for all comparisons of thrombolytic agents and regimens in the short-term treatment of PE [3]. The thrombolytic regimens recommended by the American College of Chest Physicians, as well as, absolute and relative contraindications are set in Tables 6.3 and 6.4.

Recommendations for Thrombolytic Regimen

In patients with acute PE, when a thrombolytic agent is used, the experts suggest short infusion times (e.g., a 2-h infusion) over prolonged infusion times (e.g., a 24-h infusion) (Grade 2C) [3].

In patients with acute PE, when a thrombolytic agent is used, the panel of experts suggests administration through a peripheral vein over a pulmonary artery catheter (Grade 2C) [3].

2014 ESC Guidelines on the Diagnosis and Management of Acute Pulmonary Embolism: The Task Force for the Diagnosis and Management of Acute Pulmonary Embolism of the European Society of Cardiology Endorsed by the European Respiratory Society

Methodology

The European Society of Cardiology guidelines and recommendations represent the official position of this Cardiology Society on diagnosis and management of acute pulmonary embolism (PE). Members of this Task Force were selected considering their expertise in PE patient care. Selected experts in the field undertook a comprehensive review of the published evidence for management (including diagnosis, treatment, prevention, and rehabilitation) of a given condition according to European Society of Cardiology Committee for Practice Guidelines policy [1].

A critical evaluation of diagnostic and therapeutic procedures was performed including assessment of the risk–benefit ratio. Estimates of expected health outcomes for larger populations were included, where data exist. The level of evidence and the strength of recommendation of particular management options were weighed and graded according to predefined scales (Tables 6.7 and 6.8) [1].

The experts of the writing and reviewing panels filled in declarations of interest forms, which might be perceived as real or potential sources of conflicts of interest. Any changes in declarations of interest that arise during the writing period must be notified to the European Society of Cardiology and updated. The Task Force received its entire financial support from the European Society of Cardiology without any involvement from healthcare industry [1].

The European Society of Cardiology Committee for Practice Guidelines supervises and coordinates the preparation of new Guidelines produced by Task Forces, expert groups, or consensus panels. The Committee is also responsible for the endorsement process of these Guidelines. The European Society of Cardiology Guidelines undergoes extensive review by the Committee for Practice Guidelines and external experts. After appropriate revisions it is approved by all the experts involved in the Task Force [1].

Table 6.7 Classes of recommendation European Society of Cardiology

Classes of recommendation	Class I	Class II	Class IIa	Class IIb	Class III
Definition	Evidence and/or general agreement that a given treatment or procedure is beneficial, useful, effective	Conflicting evidence and/or a divergence of opinion about the usefulness/efficacy of the given treatment or procedure	Weight of evidence/opinion is in favor of usefulness/efficacy	Usefulness/efficacy is less well established by evidence/opinion	Evidence or general agreement that the given treatment or procedure is not useful/effective, and in some cases may be harmful
Suggested wording to use	Is recommended/is indicated		Should be considered	May be considered	Is not recommended

Table 6.8 ESC levels of evidence

Level A	Data derived from multiple randomized clinical trials or meta-analyses
Level B	Data derived from a single randomized clinical trial or large nonrandomized studies
Level C	Consensus of opinion of the experts and/ or small studies, retrospective studies, registries

The finalized document was approved by the Committee for Practice Guidelines for publication in the European Heart Journal. It was developed after careful consideration of the scientific and medical knowledge and the evidence available at the time of their dating. The task of developing European Society of Cardiology Guidelines covers not only the integration of the most recent research, but also the creation of educational tools and implementation programs for the recommendations [1]. The recommendations for formulating and issuing European Society of Cardiology Guidelines can be found on ESC Web Site: http://www.escardio.org/guidelinessurveys/esc-guidelines/about/Pages/ruleswriting.aspx [1].

The first Guidelines and recommendations on clinical management of PE from European Society of Cardiology were published in the years 2000 and 2008. Many recommendations have retained or reinforced their validity; however, new data has extended or modified our knowledge in respect of optimal diagnosis, assessment and treatment of patients with PE. The most clinically relevant new aspects of this 2014 version as compared with its previous version published in 2008 relate to: (1) Recently identified predisposing factors for venous thromboembolism, (2) simplification of clinical prediction rules, (3) age-adjusted D-dimer cut-offs, (4) subsegmental PE, (5) incidental, clinically unsuspected PE, (6) advanced risk stratification of intermediate-risk PE, (7) initiation of treatment with vitamin K antagonists, (8) treatment and secondary prophylaxis of venous thromboembolism with the new direct oral anticoagulants, (9) efficacy and safety of reperfusion treatment for patients at intermediate risk, (10) early discharge and home (outpatient) treatment of PE, (11) current diagnosis and treatment of chronic thromboembolic pulmonary hypertension, (12) formal recommendations for the management of PE in pregnancy and in patients with cancer [1].

Thrombolytic Treatment

Thrombolysis in acute PE patients restores pulmonary perfusion more rapidly than anticoagulation with unfractionated heparin alone. The early resolution of pulmonary obstruction leads to a prompt reduction in pulmonary artery pressure and resistance, with a concomitant improvement in right ventricular function. The hemodynamic benefits of thrombolysis are confined to the first few days; in survivors, differences are no longer apparent at 1 week after treatment. The thrombolytic regimens for PE and the contraindications are shown in Tables 6.3 and 6.4. Accelerated regimens administered over 2-h are preferable to prolonged infusions of first-generation thrombolytic agents over 12–24 h. Reteplase and desmoteplase have been tested against recombinant human tissue-type plasminogen activator (rt-PA) in acute PE, with similar results in terms of hemodynamic parameters [1].

Tenecteplase was tested against placebo in patients with intermediate-risk PE. At present, none of these agents is approved for use in PE. Unfractionated heparin infusion should be stopped during administration of streptokinase or urokinase; it can be continued during rt-PA infusion. In patients receiving low-molecular weight-heparin or fondaparinux at the time that thrombolysis is initiated, infusion of unfractionated heparin should be delayed until 12 h after the last low-molecular weight-heparin injection (given twice daily), or until 24 h after the last low-molecular weight-heparin or fondaparinux injection (given once daily) [1].

Given the bleeding risks associated with thrombolysis and the possibility that it may become necessary to immediately discontinue or reverse the anticoagulant effect of heparin, it appears reasonable to continue anticoagulation with unfractionated heparin for several hours after the end of thrombolytic treatment before switching to low-molecular weight-heparin or fondaparinux [1].

Overall, 90 % of patients appear to respond favorably to thrombolysis, as judged by clinical and echocardiographic improvement within 36 h. The greatest benefit is observed when treatment is initiated within 48 h of symptom onset, but thrombolysis can still be useful in patients who have had symptoms for 6–14 days. A review of randomized trials performed before 2004 indicated that thrombolysis might be associated with a reduction in mortality or recurrent PE in high-risk patients who present with hemodynamic instability [1].

In a recent epidemiological report, in-hospital mortality attributable to PE was lower in unstable patients who received thrombolytic therapy, compared with those who did not (RR 0.20; 95 % CI 0.19–0.22; $p<0.0001$). Most contraindications to thrombolysis should be considered relative in patients with life-threatening, high-risk PE. In the absence of hemodynamic compromise at presentation, the clinical benefits of thrombolysis have remained controversial for many years. In a randomized comparison of heparin versus alteplase in 256 normotensive patients with acute PE and evidence of right ventricular dysfunction or pulmonary hypertension—obtained by clinical examination, echocardiography, or right heart catheterization—thrombolytic treatment (mainly secondary thrombolysis) reduced the incidence of escalation to emergency treatment (from 24.6 % to 10.2 %; $p=0.004$), without affecting mortality [1].

More recently, the Pulmonary Embolism Thrombolysis (PEITHO) trial was published [14]. This was a multicenter, randomized, double-blind comparison of thrombolysis with a single weight-adapted intravenous bolus of tenecteplase plus heparin versus placebo plus heparin. Patients with acute PE were eligible for the study if they had right ventricular dysfunction, confirmed by echocardiography or CT angiography, and myocardial injury confirmed by a positive troponin I or -*T* test.

A total of 1006 patients were enrolled. The primary efficacy outcome, a composite of all-cause death or hemodynamic decompensation/collapse within 7 days of randomization, was significantly reduced with tenecteplase (2.6 % versus 5.6 % in the placebo group; $p=0.015$; OR 0.44; 95 % CI 0.23–0.88). The benefit of thrombolysis was mainly driven by a significant reduction in the rate of hemodynamic collapse (1.6 % versus 5.0 %; $p=0.002$); all cause 7-day mortality was low: 1 % in the tenecteplase group and 2 % in the placebo group ($p=0.43$). In another randomized study comparing low-molecular weight-heparin alone versus low-molecular weight-heparin plus an intravenous bolus of tenecteplase in intermediate-risk PE, patients treated with tenecteplase had fewer adverse outcomes, better functional capacity, and greater quality of life at 3 months [1, 14].

Thrombolytic treatment carries a risk of major bleeding, including intracranial hemorrhage (Table 6.3). Analysis of pooled data from trials using various thrombolytic agents and regimens reported intracranial bleeding rates between 1.9 % and 2.2 %. Increasing age and the presence of comorbidities has been associated with a higher risk of bleeding complications. The PEITHO trial showed a 2 % incidence of hemorrhagic stroke after thrombolytic treatment with tenecteplase (versus 0.2 % in the placebo arm) in patients with intermediate–high-risk PE. Major nonintracranial bleeding events were also increased in the tenecteplase group, compared with placebo (6.3 % versus 1.5 %; $p<0.001$) [1].

These results underline the need to improve the safety of thrombolytic treatment in patients at increased risk of intracranial or other life-threatening bleeding. A strategy using reduced-dose rt-PA appeared to be safe in the setting of "moderate" PE in a study that included 121 patients, 319 and another trial on 118 patients with hemodynamic instability or "massive pulmonary obstruction" reported similar results. An alternative approach may consist of local, catheter-delivered, ultrasound-assisted thrombolysis using small doses of a thrombolytic agent. In patients with mobile right heart thrombi, the therapeutic benefits of thrombolysis remain controversial. Good results were reported in some series, but in other reports short-term mortality exceeded 20 % despite thrombolysis [1].

Therapeutic Strategies

Pulmonary embolism with shock or hypotension (high-risk pulmonary embolism) patients with PE presenting with shock or hypotension are at high risk of in-hospital death, particularly during the first few hours after admission. Besides hemodynamic and respiratory support, intravenous unfractionated heparin should be administered to these patients as the preferred mode of initial anticoagulation, as low-molecular weight-heparin or fondaparinux have not been tested in the setting of hypotension and shock [1].

Primary reperfusion treatment, particularly systemic thrombolysis, is the treatment of choice for patients with high-risk PE. In patients with contraindications to thrombolysis—and in those in whom thrombolysis has failed to improve the hemodynamic status—surgical embolectomy is recommended if surgical expertise and resources are available. As an alternative to surgery, percutaneous catheter-directed treatment should be considered if expertise with this method and the appropriate resources are available on site. In these cases, treatment decisions should be made by an interdisciplinary team involving a thoracic surgeon or interventional cardiologist, as appropriate [1].

Pulmonary embolism without shock or hypotension (intermediate- or low-risk pulmonary embolism): For most cases of acute PE without hemodynamic compromise, low-molecular weight-heparin or fondaparinux, given subcutaneously at weight-adjusted doses without monitoring, is the treatment of choice unless there is severe renal dysfunction. Patients not suffering from shock or hypotension require further risk stratification after the diagnosis of PE has been confirmed. In these patients, risk assessment should begin with a validated clinical score, preferably the Pulmonary Embolism Severity Index or simplified Pulmonary Embolism Severity Index [1].

Low-risk patients in the Pulmonary Embolism Severity Index Class I or II, and probably those with simplified Pulmonary Embolism Severity Index of 0, should be considered for early discharge and outpatient treatment, if this appears feasible based on the patient's anticipated compliance as well as his/her family and social background. For all other patients, assessment of right ventricular function by echocardiography (or CT angiography) and cardiac troponin testing should be considered. Based on the results of a recently published randomized trial [14], and as explained in the section on prognostic assessment, patients with acute PE, an echocardiogram or CT scan indicating RV dysfunction, and a positive cardiac troponin test belong to an intermediate high-risk group [1].

Full-dose systemic thrombolytic therapy, given as primary reperfusion therapy, can prevent potentially life-threatening hemodynamic decompensation or collapse in these patients, but this benefit is counterbalanced by a high risk of hemorrhagic stroke or major nonintracranial bleeding [14]. Accordingly, systemic thrombolysis is not routinely recommended as primary treatment for patients with intermediate–high-risk PE, but should be considered if clinical signs of hemodynamic decompensation appear. Surgical pulmonary embolectomy or percutaneous catheter-directed treatment may be considered as alternative, "rescue" procedures for patients with intermediate–high-risk PE, in whom hemodynamic decompensation appears imminent and the anticipated bleeding risk under systemic thrombolysis is high [1].

Other laboratory markers, such as brain natriuretic peptide, NT-pro-brain natriuretic peptide and heart-type fatty acid-binding protein, have also been shown to possess additive prognostic value to clinical and imaging parameters in cohort studies; their potential therapeutic implications have not yet been investigated in prospective trials. Normotensive patients in the Pulmonary Embolism Severity Index Class III or higher, or simplified Pulmonary Embolism Severity Index of at least 1, in whom the echocardiogram (or CT angiogram) or the cardiac troponin test—or both—are normal, belong to an intermediate–low-risk group. Anticoagulation is indicated. Existing evidence does not support primary reperfusion treatment. There is no evidence to suggest that bed rest has any beneficial effect on these patients' clinical outcome [1].

Areas of Uncertainty

Although a large number of recent cohort studies have helped to further refine risk stratification in non-high-risk patients with confirmed PE, the clinical implications of prognostic assessment—and in particular the therapeutic strategy for patients at intermediate high risk—warrant further investigation. It will be necessary to elaborate on (i) whether reduced-dose intravenous thrombolysis is indeed safe and effective and (ii) whether catheter-directed treatment can evolve to become a widely available (and affordable) alternative option. The results of the completed large phase III trials on the use of new oral anticoagulants in the treatment of PE and secondary prevention of VTE appear convincing and confirm that the breakthrough in anticoagulation therapy has extended to include VTE. Nevertheless, the accumulation of clinical experience with these dru under "real-world" conditions will have to proceed at a prudent pace. Finally, further management trials are necessary to "crystallize" the criteria that might permit early discharge and home treatment of low-risk patients with acute PE [1].

References

1. Konstantinides SV, Torbicki A, Agnelli G, Danchin N, Fitzmaurice D, Galie N, Gibbs JSR, Huisman MV, Humbert M, Kucher N, Lang I, Lankeit M, Lekakis J, Maack C, Mayer E, Meneveau N, Perrier A, Pruszczyk P, Rasmussen LH, Schindler TH, Svitil P, Noordegraaf AV, Zamorano JL, Zompatori M. 2014 ESC guidelines on the diagnosis and management of acute pulmonary embolism. The Task Force for the Diagnosis and Management of Acute Pulmonary Embolism of the European Society of Cardiology (ESC). Eur Heart J. 2014;35:3033–80. doi:10.1093/eurheartj/ehu283.
2. Jaff MR, McMurtry MS, Archer SL, Cushman M, Goldenberg NA, Goldhaber SZ, Jenkins JS, Kline JA, Michaels AD, Thistlethwaite P, Vedantham S, White RJ, Zierler BK, on behalf of the American Heart Association Council on Cardiopulmonary, Critical Care, Perioperative and Resuscitation, Council on Peripheral Vascular Disease, and Council on Arteriosclerosis, Thrombosis and Vascular Biology. Management of massive and submassive pulmonary embolism, iliofemoral deep vein thrombosis, and chronic thromboembolic pulmonary hypertension: a scientific statement from the American Heart Association. Circulation. 2011;123:1788–830. doi:10.1161/CIR.0b013e318214914f.
3. Kearon C, Akl EA, Comerota AJ, Prandoni P, Bounameaux H, Goldhaber SZ, Nelson ME, Wells PS, Gould MK, Dentali F, Crowther M, Kahn SR. Antithrombotic therapy for VTE disease: antithrombotic therapy and prevention of thrombosis, 9th ed: American College of Chest Physicians evidence-based clinical practice guidelines. Chest. 2012;141(2 Suppl):e419S–94S.
4. Wan S, Quinlan DJ, Agnelli G, Eikelboom JW. Thrombolysis compared with heparin for the initial treatment of pulmonary embolism: a metaanalysis of the randomized controlled trials. Circulation. 2004;110:744–9.
5. Thabut G, Thabut D, Myers RP, Bernard-Chabert B, Marrash-Chahla R, Mal H, Fournier M. Thrombolytic therapy of pulmonary embolism: a meta-analysis. J Am Coll Cardiol. 2002;40:1660–7.
6. Kasper W, Konstantinides S, Geibel A, Olschewski M, Heinrich F, Grosser KD, Rauber K, Iversen S, Redecker M, Kienast J. Management strategies and determinants of outcome in acute major pulmonary embolism: results of a multicenter registry. J Am Coll Cardiol. 1997;30:1165–71.
7. Goldhaber SZ, Visani L, De Rosa M. Acute pulmonary embolism: clinical outcomes in the International Cooperative Pulmonary Embolism Registry (ICOPER). Lancet. 1999;353:1386–9.
8. Laporte S, Mismetti P, Décousus H, Uresandi F, Otero R, Lobo JL, Monreal M, RIETE Investigators. Clinical predictors for fatal pulmonary embolism in 15,520 patients with venous

thromboembolism: findings from the Registro Informatizado de la Enfermedad Trombo-Embolica venosa (RIETE) Registry. Circulation. 2008;117:1711–6.
9. Schreiber D, Lin B, Liu G, Briese B, Hiestand B, Slatter D, Kline J, Pollack C. Variation in therapy and outcomes in massive pulmonary embolism from the Emergency Medicine Pulmonary Embolism in the Real World Registry (EMPEROR). Acad Emerg Med. 2009; 16(S77).
10. De Soyza ND, Murphy ML. Persistent post-embolic pulmonary hypertension. Chest. 1972;62: 665–8.
11. Schwarz F, Stehr H, Zimmermann R, Manthey J, Kübler W. Sustained improvement of pulmonary hemodynamics in patients at rest and during exercise after thrombolytic treatment of massive pulmonary embolism. Circulation. 1985;71:117–23.
12. Sharma GV, Folland ED, McIntyre KM, Sasahara AA. Long-term benefit of thrombolytic therapy in patients with pulmonary embolism. Vasc Med. 2000;5:91–5.
13. Kline JA, Steuerwald MT, Marchick MR, Hernandez-Nino J, Rose GA. Prospective evaluation of right ventricular function and functional status 6 months after acute submassive pulmonary embolism: frequency of persistent or subsequent elevation in estimated pulmonary artery pressure. Chest. 2009;136:1202–10.
14. Meyer G, Vicaut E, Danays T, Agnelli G, Becattini C, Beyer-Westendorf J, Bluhmki E, Bouvaist H, Brenner B, Couturaud F, Dellas C, Empen K, Granca A, Galiè N, Geibel A, Goldhaber SZ, Jimenez D, Kozak M, Kupatt C, Kucher N, Lang IM, Lankeit M, Meneveau N, Pacouret G, Palazzini M, Petris A, Pruszczyk P, Rugolotto M, Salvi A, Schellong S, Sebbane M, Sobkowicz B, Stefanovic BS, Thiele H, Torbicki A, Verschuren F, Konstantinides SV, PEITHO Investigators. Fibrinolysis for patients with intermediate-risk pulmonary embolism. N Engl J Med. 2014;370:1402–11.
15. Kline JA, Nordenholz KE, Courtney DM, Kabrhel C, Jones AE, Rondina MT, Diercks DB, Klinger JR, Hernandez J. Treatment of submassive pulmonary embolism with tenecteplase or placebo: cardiopulmonary outcomes at 3 months: multicenter double-blind, placebo-controlled randomized trial. J Thromb Haemost. 2014;12:459–68.
16. Guyatt GH, Norris SL, Schulman S, Hirsh J, Eckman MH, Akl EA, Crowther M, Vandvik PO, Eikelboom JW, McDonagh MS, Lewis ZS, Gutterman DD, Cook DJ, Schünemann HJ. Methodology for the development of antithrombotic therapy and prevention of thrombosis guidelines antithrombotic therapy and prevention of thrombosis, 9th ed: American College of Chest Physicians Evidence-Based Clinical Practice Guidelines. Chest. 2012;141(2 Suppl):e53S–70S.

Chapter 7
Thrombolysis in Pulmonary Embolism

Carlos Jerjes-Sánchez

Historic Perspective

The Beginning of High Dose and Short-Term Streptokinase Infusion

In 1993, we reported the first successful massive pulmonary embolism (PE) case submitted to high dose (1,500,000 IU) and short-term (1 h) streptokinase infusion by peripheral vein [1]. The patient was a 65-year-old woman with no prior cardiac or pulmonary disease. She had a history of moderate smoking, obesity, and hypertension. Patient was asymptomatic and with normal life until July 1, 1992 when suddenly had chest pain associated to dyspnea. She was admitted to emergency room with severe chest pain and respiratory failure. On admission, with respiratory rate 38/min, blood pressure 150/100 mmHg, and heart rate 150/min. Clinical examination showed jugular distention, S3 right sound and increased second pulmonary sound. No symptoms or signs of deep venous thrombosis were identified. Electrocardiogram showed sinusal tachycardia, right axis deviation, new right bundle branch block, aVR ST-elevation and right ventricular overload and ST depression in V2, V3, V4, and V6 leads. Chest X-ray findings were irrelevant. Blood gases showed severe hypoxemia. V/Q lung scan had high probability for PE. Transthoracic echocardiogram showed right ventricular end diastolic diameter/left ventricular end diastolic diameter ratio >2:1, right ventricular diameter >35 mm, without regional or global right ventricular hypokinesis [1].

C. Jerjes-Sánchez, M.D., F.C.C.P., F.A.C.C. (✉)
Sistema Nacional de Investigadores, Nivel II – Clinical Research Director,
Instituto de Cardiologia y Medicina Vascular, TEC Salud

Escuela de Medicina, Tecnológico de Monterrey San Pedro Garza Garcia,
Nuevo León, Mexico

Unidad de Investigacion Clinica en Medicina SC Monterrey, Nuevo León, Mexico
e-mail: jerjes@prodigy.net.mx

C. Jerjes-Sánchez, *Thrombolysis in Pulmonary Embolism*,
DOI 10.1007/978-3-319-19707-4_7

The clinical condition suddenly worsening, respiratory failure increase and patient had sustained hypotension (60/20 mmHg); diagnosis of unprovoked massive PE with obstructive shock was established and we started anticoagulation with 10,000 U bolus of unfractionated heparin. Considering the clinical condition thrombolysis was started with 1,500,000 IU of streptokinase by peripheral vein. Clinical condition improved in the next 30 min, blood pressure returned to normality, on electrocardiogram heart rate decreased to 100/min and right ventricular overload signs disappeared, and blood gases showed normoxemia. Patient had excellent in-hospital outcome without major or minor bleeding complications and was discharged asymptomatic, with a normal transthoracic echocardiogram and pulmonary scan perfusion, and on oral anticoagulation treatment [1].

This was the first report in world literature in which streptokinase at high dose and rapid infusion was effective and safe in a massive PE patient. Previously, this streptokinase regimen has been used in hundreds of thousands of ST-elevation myocardial infarction patients with excellent results. We elected this thrombolytic regimen based on: our previous experience in ST-elevation myocardial infarction patients, previous evidence using 3,000,000 IU of streptokinase in PE patients [2], and finally, on streptokinase thrombolysis mechanisms. This fibrinolytic agent induces fibrinolytic system activation with subsequent thrombolysis through a biphasic reaction; in the first phase streptokinase binds plasminogen to form streptokinase-plasminogen activator; in a second phase, this activator with a limited proteolytic activity, plasminogen, converts to the powerful proteolytic enzyme, plasmin, which dissolves fibrin on thrombus structure, with subsequent thrombolysis. Depending on streptokinase dose, exogenous or endogenous lysis can be induced. With a reduced streptokinase dose, exogenous lysis is characterized for limited activator formation, plasmin high concentration, surface lysis, and as consequence the possibility of bleeding complications increases. With high streptokinase dose it is possible to obtain extensive activator formation with more efficient lysis reducing bleeding risk. Additionally, the main target in PE patient submitted to thrombolysis will be to achieve a fast "pharmacologic embolectomy" to reduce acute pulmonary hypertension and right ventricular dysfunction. This could be obtained using high dose in short-term streptokinase infusion [1].

This case also supports the echocardiogram role in emergency room department and the possible relevance of electrocardiogram as indirect indicator of reperfusion. Considering this result, the necessity to prove high dose in short-term streptokinase infusion in terms of efficacy and safety through randomized control trial was mandatory.

Right Ventricular Myocardial Infarction Secondary to Massive Pulmonary Embolism

In 1995, our group published the first case with right ventricular myocardial infarction in the setting of massive pulmonary embolism in Mexico and Latin America [3].

The patient was a 60-year-old male with no prior cardiac or pulmonary disease. He was asymptomatic and with normal life until June 9, 1992, when he developed sudden redness, edema, and pain in left leg. Erysipelas and cellulitis was diagnosed and patient was hospitalized receiving antibiotics and NSAIDs. No thrombus prophylaxis was started. In-hospital, he remained stable until June 18, when he suddenly had severe chest pain, dyspnea, and hypotension (80/50 mmHg). An electrocardiogram showed sinusal tachycardia, right axis deviation, ST-elevation aVR, and in V1 qR with ST-elevation, with ST depression in DI and aVL leads; also right ventricular overload and ST depression in V2, V3, V4, and V6 anterior leads, this was interpreted as acute atrial and right ventricular dilatation with right ventricular overload secondary to PE [3].

Considering the persistence of this clinical condition, patient was transferred to Cardiology Hospital at National Medical Center. Patient arrived 4 h after starting severe respiratory failure symptoms, with blood pressure of 80/40 mmHg and heart rate of 120/min. Clinical examination showed jugular distention, S3 right sound and diminished intensity heart sounds. A new electrocardiogram showed sinusal tachycardia, largets right axis deviation and ST-elevation from V1 to V4; right unipolar leads (v4R) also showed ST-elevation. These findings were considered as an expression of right ventricular myocardial infarction [3]. Given this cardiogenic shock state he was treated with tracheal intubation and mechanical ventilation. Chest X-ray showed bilateral oligohemia, right pulmonary artery dilatation, and elevated right diaphragm. Blood gases showed severe hypoxemia (45 mmHg). A transthoracic echocardiogram revealed right ventricular dilatation with severe global hypokinesis. Considering the critical condition and despite the time of onset symptoms, rescue thrombolysis with 1,500,000 IU intravenous streptokinase in one-hour was administered. After thrombolysis transthoracic echocardiogram showed that although pulmonary arterial hypertension improved, severe global hypokinesis remained. Patient died in cardiogenic shock 3 h later [3].

Necropsy study proved massive PE by 80 % an occlusive thrombus in right pulmonary artery. Right heart was dilatated and microscopic and macroscopic findings of subendocardial right ventricular myocardial infarction were identified. Left and right coronary had 40 and 50 % of atheroma obstruction. No thrombus or rupture plaque, neither left ventricle ischemia was observed [3].

In massive PE, under clinical and experimental conditions, right ventricular dysfunction secondary to subendocardial or subepicardial right ventricular ischemia is the main determinant factor to cardiopulmonary failure, hypoxemia, cardiogenic shock and mortality. If the ischemic cascade is not interrupted this event could lead to right ventricular infarction. This complication was described by Dack and cols. for the first time in 1949 [4]. In the setting of massive or submassive PE acute right ventricular myocardial infarction could explain in part, that clinical manifestations, electrocardiogram findings and clinical instability are not only the simple expression of right ventricular pressure overload, and real mechanisms of acute ischemia have to be considered [3].

This case showed the relationship between massive PE and right ventricle myocardial infarction as a determinant factor for mortality. The hemodynamic and

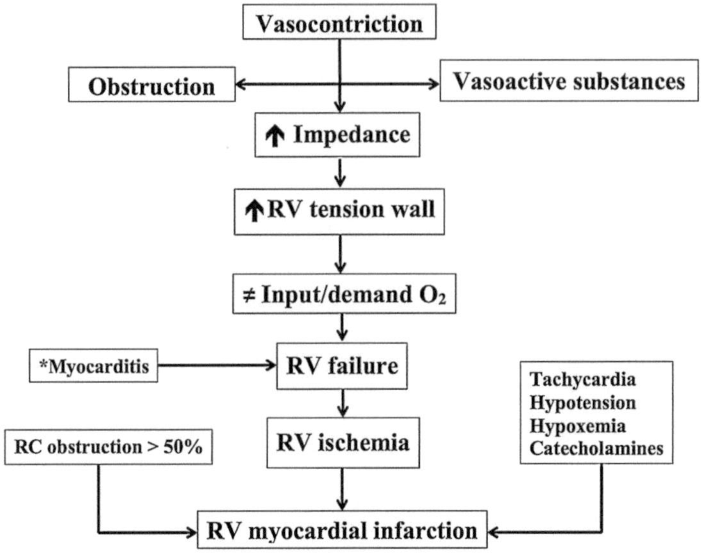

Fig. 7.1 Modified of C Jerjes Sanchez y *cols*. Ischemic cascade that are generated from a massive PE over the right ventricle, and the phenomena that can increase or reduce the degree of ischemia. Myocarditis as an important trigger to RV failure; and potential importance of greater obstruction of 50 % of the corresponding coronary artery. *Begieneman MVP, *et al.* Pulmonary embolism causes endomyocarditis in the human heart. Heart 2008; 94:450-456

cardiovascular responses to massive PE are set in Fig. 7.1. Following this model, in this way, all submassive or massive PE patients will have right ventricular myocardial infarction as complication. However, independent variables could modify the outcome of myocardial ischemia as: pulmonary and/or coronary artery hyperreactivity, degree of coronary resistances, coronary dominant pattern, and collateral circulation presence. Implications of these mechanisms could be: first, in the presence of critical right coronary disease, right ventricular ischemia, and necrosis could be established more quickly, and second, a right coronary dominant pattern could extend right ventricular ischemia to left ventricle [3].

In our case, transthoracic echocardiogram was an important tool in diagnosis and stratification. Considering the age, clinical presentation, and ST dynamic changes on electrocardiograms, a suspicion of acute coronary syndrome was considered. However, transthoracic echocardiogram showed right ventricular dysfunction with severe global hypokinesis excluding this possibility. Severe right ventricular dysfunction could explain the lack of correlation between pulmonary artery pressure and pulmonary resistance. Electrocardiogram in this context could be another important tool in the setting of PE risk, not only as an early indicator of pulmonary reperfusion, also through ST dynamic changes high-risk PE could be identified [3]. Necessarily, we need to change our traditional way to analyzing electrocardiogram changes; persistent or transitory ST-elevation or depression have to be considered as severe myocardial ischemia expression and jeopardized right ventricular mass.

Both conditions required a fast-track therapeutic approach to establish a thrombus lysis to preserve right ventricular viability, through reducing right ventricular dysfunction avoiding right ventricular myocardial infarction, a mortality determinant.

Both cases were the beginning of the series of studies that tested the safety and effectiveness of high dose in short-term (one-hour) streptokinase infusion.

Streptokinase and Heparin Versus Heparin Alone in Massive Pulmonary Embolism: A Randomized Controlled Trial

Study No. 1

Background

In 1977, streptokinase was approved by the FDA for the treatment of PE (250,000 IU/30 min and then 100,000 IU/h/24 h). Recently, we reported the successful use of 1,500,000 IU of streptokinase over 1 h in one patient with massive PE and cardiogenic shock [1]. We subsequently undertook a trial of eight patients with PE who were randomized to high dose, short infusion of streptokinase followed by heparin versus heparin alone. When all four heparin alone patients died compared with none in the streptokinase group, we terminated the trial [5].

Methodology

Inclusion criteria: (a) patients aged 15 years or more; (b) previously healthy; (c) PE diagnosis sustained by high clinical suspicion (one or more major risk factors and clinical, ECG, chest X-ray, blood gas findings; (d) PE proven by: high probability V/Q lung scan, suggestive echocardiogram, or DVT (5) by radiovenogram; (e) massive PE defined: >9 obstructed segments on V/Q lung scan with or without cardiogenic shock (systolic blood pressure <90 mmHg); (f) <9 obstructed segments on V/Q lung scan but with right ventricular dysfunction and or extensive DVT; g) symptoms or signs of PE within 14 days after onset symptoms [5].

Exclusion criteria: (a) previous PE; (b) patients with <3 segmental defects on V/Q lung scan, with normal echocardiogram and without DVT; (c) absolute contraindication for thrombolytic therapy: active or recent hemorrhage, intracranial disease, head trauma, neurologic or major surgery within previous 6 weeks, or any concurrent condition considered to limit survival to a few months [5].

Patients were randomized to streptokinase followed by heparin or to heparin alone.

Streptokinase group: received 1,500,000 IU of streptokinase over 1 h by peripheral vein, followed by a bolus of 10,000 U of heparin and then a constant infusion of 1000 U/h of heparin titrated to PTT of 2–2.5 times control. Heparin group: followed the same regimen, without streptokinase. In the survivors of the acute phase, on the fifth day, heparin was overlapped with coumadin and was stopped on day 7. Patients were kept on coumadin, aiming for an INR between 2.0 and 3.0 for 3 months or more, depending on the presence of major risk factors [5].

V/Q Lung scans were performed in anterior, posterior, and lateral and oblique views. Echocardiograms required measurements of right and left ventricular size and motion, ejection fraction, abnormal septal position, paradoxical systolic motion, tricuspid, and/or pulmonary regurgitation. Parasternal long axis, apical four chambers, and subcostal four chambers view were performed. Pulmonary arterial pressure was determined with the modified Bernoulli formula. Static and dynamic venograms with 99 technetium-labeled albumin macroaggregates were performed.

Results

Eight patients were enrolled, four in each group, all with massive PE and cardiogenic shock. The mortality in the streptokinase group was 0 % compared to 100 % ($p=0.02$) in the heparin group. Therefore, after discussion with the ethics committee, the trial was terminated [5].

The characteristic of this study, main target, fibrinolytic regimens and hospital type is shown in Table 7.1. In Table 7.2, all demographic variables related with age, acute and chronic inflammation, as well as, acute venous thrombosis incidence and triggers were described. In Table 7.3, it is possible to observe the main variables related with clinical, echocardiographic, and VQ lung scan findings. Mortality and recurrence incidence, residual thrombus and rescue therapeutic approach are shown in Table 7.4. Table 7.5 was designed to fibrinolytic regimens, adjunctive treatment, and bleeding complications. Also, 289 patients with proven PE treated in almost 20 years period have been included.

Table 7.1 Studies characteristics of 289 patients with proven pulmonary embolisms

Variable	1992	1992–1994	1996–2002	2002–2004	2009–2011
Number of patients	8	40	131	80	30
Randomized	Yes	No	No	Yes	No
Controlled	UFH	No	NBP with or without RVH	UFH	No
Open	Yes	Yes	Yes	Yes	Yes
Multicenter trial	No	No	No	Yes	No
Objective	Efficacy	Safety	NBP with or without RVH	Evolution	Security
60 min regimen	1,500,000 UI SK	1,500,000 UI SK	1,500,000 UI SK	100 mg rt-PA, alteplase	TNK-t-PA/ 10 s mg/kg
Hospital	Cardiology	Cardiology	Cardiology	Cardiology/ Community	Cardiology

UFH unfractionated heparin, *NBP* normal blood pressure, *RVH* right ventricular hypokinesis, *SK* streptokinase, *rt-PA* recombinant human tissue-type plasminogen activator = alteplase, *TNK-t-PA* tenecteplase-tissue-type plasminogen activator

Table 7.2 Demographic characteristics for 289 patients with pulmonary embolism

Variable	1992	1992–1994	1996–2002	2002–2004	2009–2011
Number of patients	8 = *N*	40 = %	131 = %	80 = %	30 = %
Age/gender female	51 ± 23/1 %	47 ± 15/25 %	61 ± 18/41 %	52 ± 16/56 %	58 ± 6/73 %
Health	100 (%)	100	37	34	33
Age >65	1	–	34	34	53
Chronic inflamación	8	48	74	83	83
Acute deep venous thrombosis	0	85	23	80	44
Triggers: stasis	8	85	48	73	26
Acute inflamación	–	–	68	55	44

Table 7.3 Clinical, echocardiographic, and VQ lung scan findings in 289 patients with pulmonary embolism

Variable	1992	1992–1994	1996–2002	2002–2004	2009–2011
Number of patients	8 = *N*	40 = %	131 = %	80 = %	30 = %
High-risk PET	8	100	100	100	100
Dyspnea and/or angina	7/8	83/80	79/86	85/73	93/59
Third sound right ventricular	8	95	92	96	97
Cardiogenic shock	8	40	Low BP 28	16	3
RVD (mm)	40.5 ± 2.8	40.7 ± 2.5	39.8 ± 3.70	43.9 ± 4.4	39 ± 4.3
RV/LV ≥ 2:1	8	100	100	100	100
RVHK %	8	67	47	75	86
PSD before thrombolysis	–	9.69 ± 1.16 (29)	9.35 ± 3.42 (79)	10.7 ± 1.7 (32)	12 ± 4.2 (17)

RVD right ventricular diameter, *RV/LV* right ventricular end diastolic diameter/left ventricular end diastolic diameter ratio, *RVHK* right ventricular hypokinesis, *PSD* perfusion segmental defects

Table 7.4 Cardiovascular adverse events and therapeutic rescue approaches

Variable	1992	1992–1994	1996–2002	2002–2004	2009–2011
60 min regimen	SK 1,500,000	SK 1,500,000	SK 1,500,000	rt-PA 100 mg	TNK-t-PA/10 seg mg/kg
Number of patients	8 = *N*	40 = %	131 = %	80 = %	30 = %
Mortality	T 0/4 H *p* = 0.02	12	28/61 RVHK	T 3–25 H	13
Recurrence	0	18	11	T10–H 20	3
Rescue thrombolysis	0	10	5	10	0
Rethrombolysis	0	–	7	0	0
Residual thrombus	2	18	26	10	7
P. pulmonary intervention	0	–	16	5	7
Surgical embolectomy	0	–	2	0	0

SK streptokinase, *rt-PA* recombinant human tissue-type plasminogen activator, *TNK-t-PA* Tenecteplase-tissue-type plasminogen activator, *T* thrombolysis, *H* heparin, *RVHK* right ventricular hypokinesis, *P* percutaneous

Table 7.5 Fibrinolytic regimen bolus, adjunctive treatment and bleeding complication findings in 289 patients with pulmonary embolism

Variable	1992	1992–1994	1996–2002	2002–2004	2009–2011
60 min regimen	SK 1,500,000	SK 1,500,000	SK 1,500,000	rT-PA 100 mg	TNK-t-PA/10 s mg/kg
Number of patients	8	40	131	80	30
Bolus	No	No	No	20 mg <65 years 15 mg >65 years	Yes
Unfractionated heparin	Bolus 10,000/1000/h	Bolus 10,000/1000/h	Bolus 5000/1000/h	Bolus 60 U/kg or 12 U/kg	Bolus 60 U/kg or 12 U/kg
Low-molecular-weight heparin	No	No	No	1 mg/kg/12 h 24–48 h/7 days	1 mg/kg/12 h 24–48 h/7 days
Intracranial hemorrhage (%)	0	0	2	0	0
Major hemorrhage (%)	0	2	8	8	3
Minor hemorrhage (%)	0	0	5	5	10

SK streptokinase, *rt-PA* recombinant human tissue-type plasminogen activator, *TNK-t-PA* Tenecteplase-tissue-type plasminogen activator

These eight patients had similar baseline characteristics, except in time elapsed from onset of symptoms of the first event of PE before randomization, which occurred by chance. Patients in streptokinase group arrived to the Emergency Department from 1 to 4 h after onset symptoms of PE, whereas patients in heparin group had a first PE in other hospitals. In this first pulmonary event, they had minor PE by 1, 2, 2 and 3 occluded segments on V/Q lung scan, with hemodynamic stability, without any evidence of acute pulmonary arterial hypertension and with therapeutic PTTs [5].

There, they were asymptomatic and suddenly had recurrences of massive PE, with severe respiratory failure and were transferred to our hospital 2–4 h after onset symptoms of a new event. The time elapsed from onset of cardiogenic shock was comparable in both groups. All patients had similar clinical characteristics and echocardiographic abnormalities. The patients who were randomized to receive streptokinase plus heparin improved their clinical and echocardiographic findings in the first hour after treatment. The V/Q lungs scan postthrombolytic therapy showed 3, 4, 4, and 5 segments perfusion defects and DVT were proved [5].

All patients in heparin group died despite endotracheal intubation, mechanical ventilation, and Swan-Ganz catheterization. Necropsy was performed in three patients, all had massive PE and, both macroscopically and histologically, the presence of right ventricle acute myocardial infarction, two were subendocardial and one transmural, in all cases without significant coronary arterial obstruction. The four patients who lived were discharged in good conditions. After 2 years follow-up, all are in functional class I, without pulmonary arterial hypertension, and without recurrent PE [5].

Lessons Learned for This Study

We present the first randomized clinical trial that demonstrates a decreased mortality rate with thrombolysis compared with heparin alone among patients with massive PE [5].

Because of their grave clinical condition, in the acute phase the diagnosis of PE was sustained by high clinical suspicion and bedside echocardiogram only. Later, diagnosis of PE was confirmed by means of high probability V/Q lung scans and proven DVT on streptokinase group and through high probability V/Q lung scan in two patients of heparin group and by necropsy in three of them. On admission, the baseline clinical and echocardiographic data showed severe right ventricular dysfunction and cardiogenic shock. However, after treatment, the patients who received streptokinase plus heparin had earlier reversal of hemodynamic disturbances than patients who received only heparin, who deteriorated and died [5].

We did not observe major or minor hemorrhagic complications possibly due to the patient's young age, because the streptokinase was used through a peripheral vein, and because of a diagnostic strategy which avoided vascular puncture [5].

The role of echocardiography was to establish bedside diagnosis of massive PE, to ascertain the severity of pulmonary arterial hypertension, and to document abnormalities of motion and geometry of the right ventricle. The findings in the necropsy studies have been previously reported [3] and suggest that right ventricular myocardial infarction could cause irreversible right ventricular dysfunction and mortality [5].

The patients who received thrombolysis had reductions in pulmonary arterial hypertension, right ventricular dysfunction, and preservation of ventricular myocardial viability. Rapid reversal of right ventricular failure, noted previously in recombinant human tissue-type plasminogen activator, alteplase patients who compared with heparin alone patients, is the likely mechanism that prevented death from acute PE [5].

There were two limitations of study: (1) small sample size, and (2) gross imbalance in the onset of the first PE, however, at that moment, patients in heparin group did not have right ventricular dysfunction. The observations from this randomized controlled clinical trial indicate that among patients with massive PE and cardiogenic shock, prompt administration of thrombolytic therapy can be lifesaving compared with heparin alone [5].

Additionally, the results reproduce in terms of safety and effectivity, our previous clinical observations [1, 3] with the streptokinase regimen proposed. Furthermore, in-hospital results were extended in 2-year follow-up in which no recurrence, no PE mortality was observed. This study has been criticized for two reasons: first, because patients in heparin group had had a first PE in other hospitals inducing gross imbalance in onset of the first PE. However, they had basal echocardiogram evaluations proving normal right ventricular function; second, the small sample size; if the study had not been suspended it is possible a major number of patients with acute PE could have been saved. However, for our clinical research group, four patients with PE and severe right ventricular dysfunction on heparin alone who died compared with four streptokinase patients who alive, was sufficient to suspend the clinical trial. Additionally, three new right ventricular myocardial infarction cases were identified.

High Dose and Short-Term Thrombolytic Regimen in Pulmonary Embolism Patients: Prospective with 7-Year Follow-Up Trial

Study No. 2

Background

Thrombolysis in PE accelerates reversal of right ventricular dysfunction and reduces recurrent PE rate and mortality, among proper selected patients. Infusions of short duration and high concentration act most rapidly and enhance safety. The sole investigation demonstrating that thrombolysis reduces mortality from PE has been our previous randomized controlled trial, in which 1,500,000 IU in one-hour streptokinase infusion followed by heparin compares with heparin alone improved survival in patients with massive PE, severe right ventricular dysfunction and cardiogenic shock [5]. Nevertheless, it was a small trial and more evidence needs to consider this accessible thrombolytic regimen as an effective and safety alternative.

In addition, there is little evidence that assesses the long-term benefits of thrombolytic therapy after initial PE event [6].

Now, we present the results of a subsequent prospective trial in 40 consecutive new patients with PE, in whom a high dose and short-term streptokinase regimen through peripheral vein reversed acute pulmonary arterial hypertension, clinical and echocardiographic evidence of right ventricular dysfunction and improved pulmonary perfusion without increasing hemorrhagic complications. In a 7-year follow-up, evidence suggests that this streptokinase regimen preserves functional class, without recurrence or chronic pulmonary arterial hypertension [6].

Methodology

In our previous randomized controlled trial [5], originally we intended to enroll 40 patients, however, the study had early stopped for ethical reasons after the first 8 patients had dramatic differences in terms of mortality ($p=0.02$). This result provides reasonably strong evidence to design a new prospective, noncomparative, open label with a long follow-up trial [6].

Primary end points: In acute phase, baseline and post thrombolytic characteristics were analyzed to know the efficacy and safety of a high dose and short-term streptokinase infusion in terms of pulmonary arterial hypertension, right ventricular dysfunction, perfusion abnormalities, recurrence, mortality, and hemorrhagic complications. In long-term follow-up, we assessed functional class, recurrence, chronic pulmonary arterial hypertension, postthrombotic-syndrome and mortality.

Secondary end point: Identify right ventricular hypokinesis as major risk factor to recurrence and mortality [6].

Patients were considered for the study if they had: (a) age 15 years or more, (b) previously healthy, (c) clinical suspicion of PE: one or more major risk factors (prolonged bed rest, major surgery, obesity, trauma, puerperium, smoking, estrogens, and long travel) and clinical (sudden dyspnea, angina-like pain, S3 gallop, syncope, shock or cardiac arrest), ECG (new ST segment depression or T wave inversion in leads V1–V4, new right bundle branch block or new right axis deviation), chest X-ray, (band atelectasis, focal oligemia, pulmonary artery enlargement, elevated hemidiaphragm) blood gas (hypoxemia and hypocapnia) findings, (d) PE proven (high clinical suspicion plus suggestive echocardiogram), plus high probability V/Q lung scan and deep venous thrombosis by radiovenogram, (e) massive PE defined as >9 obstructed segments on V/Q lung scan with cardiogenic shock (systolic blood pressure <90 mmHg), (f) large PE defined as >7 obstructed segments on V/Q lung scan without cardiogenic shock with or without right ventricular dysfunction and/or extensive deep venous thrombosis, (g) patients referred within 14 days after onset of symptoms [6].

Conditions to excluded patients: (a) previous PE, (b) V/Q lung scan with normal, near normal or medium perfusion abnormalities without right ventricular dysfunction and without extensive deep venous thrombosis, (c) absolute contraindication for thrombolytic therapy as active or recent hemorrhage, intracranial disease, head trauma, neurologic or major surgery within previous 6 weeks, or any concurrent condition limiting survival to a few months [6].

All patients received a bolus of 10,000 U of heparin and then 1,500,000 IU of streptokinase over one-hour by peripheral vein, followed by a constant infusion of 1000 U/h of heparin titrated to PTT of 2–2.5 times control. In the survivors of the acute phase, on the first to third day, heparin was overlapped with coumadin and was stopped on day 7. The patients were kept on coumadin, aiming for an INR between 2.0 and 3.0 for 6 months or more, depending on the presence of major risk factors [6].

All patients with high clinical suspicion of PE (major risk factors, clinical manifestations, and chest X-ray, ECG and blood gases) were under a 24-h "fast-track" echocardiography evaluation and treatment within the Emergency Department. Patients with clinical, ECG and echocardiographic findings of severe pulmonary arterial hypertension and right ventricular dysfunction with normal blood pressure (impending hemodynamic instability) [7] or cardiogenic shock, were considered at highest risk and an experienced physician administered thrombolytic therapy by peripheral vein, as soon as possible [6].

These were the only patients in whom V/Q lung scan was performed after starting treatment. Twenty-four hours after thrombolytic therapy, all patients had lung scan evaluation and deep venous thrombosis search. When severe pulmonary arterial hypertension and right ventricular dysfunction were excluded, lung scan was performed before starting streptokinase regimen [6].

Baseline, 1, 24 h, at discharge and follow-up echocardiograms were done. The echocardiographic examination and interpretation were performed before and after starting thrombolytic therapy by one experienced echocardiographer. Qualitative evaluation: (a) right ventricular end diastolic diameter/left ventricular end diastolic diameter ratio (RVEDD/LVEDD) was considered normal when LVEDD was larger than RVEDD and abnormal if RVEDD was equal or larger than LVEDD [6].

Right ventricular wall abnormalities were assessed as follows: normal, moderate regional hypokinesis, severe regional hypokinesis, regional akinesis, global hypokinesis, (b) left ventricular motion, (c) abnormal septal position, (d) paradoxical systolic motion, (e) loss of inspiratory collapse of the inferior cava vein. The qualitative evaluation of right ventricular wall motion was considered as follows: Quantitative evaluation: (a) pulmonary artery systolic pressure determined with the modified Bernoulli formula, (b) measurements of right and left ventricular size, (c) ejection fraction, (d) tricuspid and pulmonary regurgitation, (e) right ventricular wall thickness. Echocardiography was standardized using the apical four chambers, parasternal long and short axis. When these positions were not appropriate, a subcostal four-chamber view was used [6].

Baseline, 24 h and at discharge perfusion scan with intravenously injected 99mTC/DTPA in anterior, posterior, lateral and oblique views were performed. Ventilation lung scan was done with 99mTC/MAA aerosol inhalation. The scans were scored through a segmental method that includes all views. A search for deep venous thrombosis with static and dynamic venograms with 99 technetium-labeled albumin macroaggregates was performed. One experienced nuclear medicine specialist analyzed all studies [6].

Analysis of efficacy: Baseline and 24 h clinical evaluation included: clinical, ECG, chest X-ray, PaO_2, pulmonary arterial hypertension improvement. Pre- and post-treatment lung scans and echocardiograms were analyzed regarding perfusion abnormalities, pulmonary artery systolic pressure, and right ventricular dysfunction behavior. In-patient recurrence and mortality were evaluated. Follow-up evaluation included functional class, recurrent PE, chronic pulmonary arterial hypertension, post-postthrombotic syndrome, and mortality [6].

Major hemorrhages were defined as: stroke (confirmed by computed tomography), hematomas >5 cm, prolonged external bleeding at puncture site, oral or gastrointestinal bleeding, hematuria or another bleeding with concomitant hypotension that required treatment with intravenous fluids, blood transfusion, surgical control, discontinuation of thrombolytic regimen, decrease >15 % points in hematocrit or >5 g/dL in hemoglobin. Minor hemorrhage was defined as: decrease between 10 and 15 % points in hematocrit or 3–5 g/dL in hemoglobin reduction [6].

All surviving patients were educated regarding symptoms and signs of recurrent PE after hospital discharge and had follow-up by the Principal Investigator (CJS). All patients had monthly visit, during the first 3 months and then every 3 months. In each visit clinical and echocardiographic evaluations were done. V/Q lung scan and venogram were performed at the third month and every 6 months up to January 1996. Then, direct telephone contact follow-up was done until September 1999 [6].

Results

From February 1992 until April 1994, 40 consecutive patients with high clinical suspicion and highest risk PE (right ventricular dysfunction and normal blood pressure—impending hemodynamic instability—and cardiogenic shock) were enrolled. In all, PE was proved by high probability V/Q lung scan and necropsy (four patients). In 33 patients, long follow-up was obtained. Patients were young predominantly females. All patients had a recent acute PE event, diagnosed through a noninvasive workup strategy; 60 % of the patients had normal blood pressure and 40 % had cardiogenic shock. At beginning, all patients had severe acute pulmonary arterial hypertension and in 29 patients baseline V/Q lung scan showed extensive perfusion abnormalities (Table 7.6) [6].

As has been previously proved, 11 ill patients received streptokinase regimen without V/Q lung scan. In the next 24 h all patients had a high probability V/Q lung scan. Right ventricular hypokinesis on echocardiography was recognized in a high percent of the patients. Patients referred between 10 and 14 days after onset symptoms received heparin in secondary hospitals. After patients arrival in the Emergency Department, mean time to starting streptokinase infusion was 1.88 ± 0.71 (range 45 min to 3 h) [6].

Streptokinase efficacy. Pre- and postthrombolytic improvement on severe acute right ventricular dysfunction, perfusion abnormalities, and pulmonary arterial hypertension through clinical, V/Q lung scan and echocardiography baseline and 24 h assessment is shown in Table 7.6.

Table 7.6 Baseline characteristics of patients and assessment streptokinase regimen

Variable	Streptokinase 1,500,000 IU/1 h infusion	
	n = 40	%
Age (years)	47.3 ± 15.3	
Female	25	62
Male	15	37
Deep venous thrombosis	34	85
Prolonged bed rest	18	45
Obesity	13	32
Lower extremity trauma	11	27
Puerperium	7	17
Smoking	6	15
Estrogen	6	15
Surgery	5	12
Long travel in sitting position	4	10
Onset symptoms (days)		
0–5	34	85
6–10	4	10
11–14	2	5
Diagnostic workup		
ECG	40	100
Echocardiogram	40	100
Lung scan	40	100
Radionuclide venogram	40	100
Normal blood pressure	24	60
Cardiogenic shock	16	40
Pulmonary artery systolic pressure	60.37 ± 6.43	
No. of segmental perfusion defects	9.69 ± 1.16	
Right ventricular hypokinesia	28	67

In the acute phase, five patients died (12 %), all had severe pulmonary arterial hypertension and severe right ventricle dysfunction. Four had cardiogenic shock and a remarkable characteristic was a longer time between onset symptoms and starting thrombolysis (mean 40.60 ± 33.13, range 12–79 h) regarding 35 patients who survived (mean 1.88 ± 0.71, range 45 min to 3 h). After treatment, all of these patients died within 72 h [6].

Three patients suffering cardiogenic shock improved after thrombolysis, however, they had early recurrence in the next hours, hemodynamic instability and died. Two of them received nonsuccessful rescue thrombolysis with the same regimen due to nonaccess to another thrombolytic regimen or surgical embolectomy. Three other patients had recurrence, two had critically ill conditions and successful rescue thrombolysis was performed. In another patient, recurrent left upper lung PE was observed on V/Q lung scan after successful streptokinase regimen. Neither signs nor symptoms were identified and possible fragmentation, thrombosis, or silent PE was considered [6].

The diagnosis of recurrent PE was established through high clinical suspicion and new evidence of pulmonary arterial hypertension and right ventricular dysfunction and/or new perfusion abnormalities on V/Q lung scan. The streptokinase role on the lysis of lower extremity thrombi and recurrent PE event cannot be excluded [6]. Postmortem study was performed in four patients, in which massive PE with right ventricle subendocardial acute myocardial infarction and normal coronary arteries were proved. CK-MB or troponin measurements were not done [6].

When patients who died were compared with patients who survived, right ventricular global hypokinesis was identified as independent risk factor for mortality before thrombolytic therapy ($p<0.0001$). Risk factors for mortality after thrombolytic therapy were: 6 h or over between onset symptoms and streptokinase regimen ($p=0.02$), severe and sustained systolic pulmonary arterial hypertension ($p=0.001$) in association with right ventricular hypokinesis ($p=0.001$), hypoxemia ($p=0.02$) and right ventricular acute myocardial infarction ($p<0.0001$). Right ventricular hypokinesis on echocardiography ($p=0.02$) was the only independent risk factor for recurrence [6].

Only one major hemorrhage was identified (2 %). A 66-year old woman arrived with massive PE, severe acute right ventricular dysfunction, cardiogenic shock and tracheal intubation and mechanical ventilation were considered. The patient had oral hemorrhage secondary to traumatic intubation and received 2 U of packed red blood cells. She received mechanical ventilation more than 48 h and was eventually discharged. In this trial, no intracranial hemorrhage was observed. Four patients (10 %) had immediate reactions characterized by transient hypotension, two of them had skin rashes and rigors. The streptokinase infusions were never stopped, and improvement was obtained with intravenous fluids. (250 mL in 30 min) In patients with allergic reactions, intravenous diphenhydramine (0.5–1 g) and intravenous hydrocortisone (100 mg) were effective [6].

Transthoracic echocardiogram was performed and was considered technically adequate in 100 % of the cases; however, none of the patients had COPD or comorbid obesity. Right and left ventricular abnormalities were often present in patients with acute PE. Right ventricular wall motion abnormalities recognized were: (a) right ventricular hyperkinesia (base, mid-right ventricular free wall and apex) (12/40), (b) moderate or severe regional hypokinesis (24/40), and (c) severe global hypokinesis (4/40). The qualitative RVEDD/LVEDD analysis showed an abnormal ratio in all patients, being 2:1 in 36 patients (12 with hyperkinesia alone and 24 with hypokinesis) and >2:1 in four patients (global hypokinesis). All had similar degree of pulmonary arterial hypertension and in 29 patients in which lung scans were performed, there were extensive perfusion abnormalities. Only one patient had a right ventricular thrombus in-transit and none had right ventricular hypertrophy [6].

After thrombolytic therapy, despite clinical, pulmonary artery systolic pressure and perfusion abnormalities improvement, nine patients had persistent right ventricle regional hypokinesis. In four, these wall motion abnormalities persisted for the next 3 or 4 months and then right ventricular function normalized. In the other five patients, right ventricular hypokinesis was a remarkable characteristic in the follow-up and the possibility of right ventricle acute myocardial infarction was considered. In two, coronary angiography was performed, and no coronary lesions were detected [6].

In 35 patients that survived acute phase, a follow-up was achieved in 33 patients (94 %). During the follow-up period, six patients were lost for a few months and later on four were recovered. In the two lost patients, 1 year and 15 days follow-up was obtained. In 33 patients, mean follow-up was 5.32±2.57 (range 5 years, 1 month to 7 years, 7 months). All patients were asymptomatic, without recurrent PE, chronic pulmonary arterial hypertension or death. In the later years, four patients had postthrombotic syndrome [6].

Lessons Learned from This Study

These data suggesting that with major or massive PE, a short-term streptokinase infusion plus heparin establishes rapid reversal of pulmonary arterial hypertension and right ventricular heart failure without increasing hemorrhagic complications. The evidence obtained in a 7-year follow-up ascertains that this streptokinase regimen could avoid cardiovascular adverse events. These findings support our previous results [1, 3, 5].

In high-risk PE patients, the efficacy of streptokinase in high concentration over a brief time period was proved. These data suggest a pathophysiology modification, possibly through a reduction of large clot burden breaking the cardiac complex mechanisms of death. Recently, a French trial in PE low-risk patients utilized 1,500,000 IU streptokinase in 2 h and proved effective to reduce total pulmonary resistance [8]. In German trial, other acute myocardial infarction thrombolytic regimen, (double reteplase bolus) in patients with massive PE, appeared to be at least as effective for reducing pulmonary vascular resistance as a traditional 2-h alteplase infusion [9].

Baseline and persistent severe right ventricular hypokinesis emerge as an independent risk factor for recurrence and mortality. When patients who survived were compared with patients who died other mortality risk factors included late and failed thrombolysis, sustained and severe pulmonary hypertension, and relentless hypoxemia and right ventricular acute myocardial infarction. Extreme right ventricular dysfunction recognized on echocardiography had a close relationship with right ventricular acute myocardial infarction at necropsy, suggesting myocardial cell injury as the principal mechanism for explaining right wall motion abnormalities. The high mortality in patients with late, nonreversible and lethal right ventricular dysfunction state requires broadening thrombolysis criteria in the setting of early right ventricular dysfunction states [6].

In PE trials, as in this trial, no intracranial hemorrhage with streptokinase using was observed. The noninvasive design and younger age of patients were favorable factors to prevent major hemorrhagic complications. Furthermore, no risk factors for this feared complication (increased age >70 years, thrombolytic agent administered over a prolonged period, catheterization, diastolic hypertension, prior brain vascular, multiple venous punction, and chronic hypertension disease) were identified. Minor complications of streptokinase were easily controlled [6].

Right ventricular hypokinesis and its close relationship with mortality and recurrence, as well as echocardiographic characteristics of acute myocardial infarction, late and early recovery of regional right ventricular wall motion abnormalities were consistent with the existing literature. In acute phase and in the follow-up, echocardiography was an important and sensitive tool providing diagnostic, functional, and prognostic information. This nonexpensive and accessible implement was an excellent indirect reperfusion marker. In addition, it provides unique insight into the pathophysiology of PE and provides an objective and modern concept of "acute cor pulmonale," extending our clinical sensitivity beyond the usual and subjective clinical and blood pressure stratification: "hemodynamic stability" or "clinical stability." As has been previously observed in a 1-year follow-up, a sustained pulmonary artery systolic pressure >50 mmHg after thrombolytic therapy was a remarkable marker of adverse outcome. A nonexpected echocardiography finding was right ventricular hyperkinesis without hypokinesis, at present time a possible mechanism for this finding, could be an early right ventricular dysfunction state [6].

The present data demonstrate the outcome in a 7-year follow-up. This high dose and short duration streptokinase infusion possibly avoids adverse cardiovascular events. This good prognosis is comparable with our previous experience, however, those studies were limited to few patients with only 2- and 3-year follow-up [5, 10]. Previously, only one trial with similar follow-up had a comparable outcome. In a substudy of Urokinase Pulmonary Embolism and Urokinase–Streptokinase Pulmonary Embolism Trials, thrombolytic therapy appears to decrease thromboembolic events, maintains pulmonary reserve, and may prevent the development of pulmonary hypertension [11]. In another previous study with 5-year survival analysis, in which only 47 % received thrombolytic therapy, mortality rate was associated with underlying disease [12]. In our long-term favorable outcome, younger age, none of the comorbid conditions, particularly occult malignant disease, 6 months effective anticoagulation and a close contact avoiding risk factors to deep venous thrombosis were determinant [6].

Study advantages were: Participating physicians had more than 10 years experience in management of PE, thus facilitating the decision to proceed with thrombolysis. In addition, a short time window to onset of symptoms and a fast track to starting thrombolysis in Emergency Department limited the period of right ventricular dysfunction. The abnormal RVEDD/LVEDD ratio 1.0 or greater considered in this study characterize a high-risk group of patients. Considering that there is not a clear definition of right ventricular dysfunction, this qualitative stratification avoids low-risk patients [6].

Limitations of this study were: The relatively young age of our patient population undoubtedly underestimates the overall risks of major hemorrhagic complications and overestimates the beneficial. High-risk patients were excluded (previous PE, heart failure, ischemic heart disease), to obtain a better analysis of pulmonary perfusion and the right ventricular function behavior. This report was based upon an open-label and observational design.

Finally, contemporary PE thrombolysis regimen (FDA and non-FDA approved) includes high concentration of drugs administered over a brief duration (rt-PA 100 mg/2 h, urokinase 3,000,000 U/2 h, streptokinase 1,500,000 IU/2 h and reteplase, 10 U separated by 30 min). High dose and short-term streptokinase infusion (1,500,000 IU/1 h) that has been used successfully in tens of thousands of myocardial infarction patients, has been the only thrombolysis regimen that reduces mortality in PE [5].

These data may provide necessary evidence to consider this accessible and inexpensive streptokinase regimen as effective and safe alternative in patients with right ventricular dysfunction, normal blood pressure and cardiogenic shock. In addition, our results add new evidence to few follow-up studies to assess the long-term benefits of thrombolytic therapy in patients with PE.

Lastly, our data indicated that among properly selected high-risk PE patients, short-term streptokinase infusion is effective and safe.

In-Hospital and Long-Term Outcome in Pulmonary Embolism Patients Submitted to Thrombolysis

Study No. 3

Background

Currently right ventricular hypokinesis (RVH) is a mortality risk marker, in pulmonary embolism (PE); it identifies submassive or high-risk PE and stratifies patients to thrombolysis [13–15]. This therapeutic approach improves clinical outcome [6, 8, 9, 12–15] and reduces mortality in patients with severe right ventricular dysfunction [5]. However it is not known whether the use of FT improves the in-hospital and follow-up outcome in patients with RVH and clinical stability. Previously, in PE with severe pulmonary arterial hypertension, without RVH and normal blood pressure, we observed a better outcome compared with RVH patients [6]. Considering this evidence, we hypothesized that thrombolysis use in an early stage of right ventricular dysfunction could reduce cardiovascular adverse events, thus improving outcome. We prospectively tested this hypothesis in a controlled study with in-hospital and long-term follow-up in PE patients submitted to thrombolysis.

Methodology

This was a prospective, controlled, open label, with a long-term follow-up in one center trial. Objective: to know whether thrombolysis in PE patients without RVH and normal blood pressure reduces major adverse cardiovascular events and improves in-hospital and long-term outcome compared to RVH patients. Groups: patients with and without RVH.

Inclusion criteria: (a) proved PE, (b) high-risk, (c) normal BP, (d) transthoracic and/or transesophageal echocardiography with signs of severe RVD, (e) referred within 14 days after onset of symptoms, (f) ≥15 years. Exclusion criteria: (a) cardiogenic shock or hypotension secondary to PE, (b) severe chronic pulmonary arterial hypertension, (c) absolute contraindication for FT such as active or recent major hemorrhage, intracranial hemorrhage, head trauma, neurologic or major surgery within previous 6 weeks, uncontrolled hypertension or noncompressible site venous puncture, (d) any concurrent condition limiting short-term survival.

Stratification and therapeutic approach have been previously published [5, 6], in brief, patients with clinical stability or impending clinical instability [7] were under fast-track stratification and diagnosis, including bedside echocardiogram; then, an experienced physician administered FT within the first 30–90 min after the patient arrived to Emergency Care Department. Twenty-four hours after all patients had clinical, VQ/lung scan, echocardiographic evaluation and deep venous thrombosis search.

In nonsuccess thrombolysis patients, rescue thrombolysis, rethrombolysis, or percutaneous pulmonary intervention were considered. After FT, when central pulmonary thrombus was detected by V/Q lung scan, angiography or transesophageal echocardiography [16] a percutaneous pulmonary intervention (catheter fragmentation plus fibrinolysis in situ or balloon angioplasty) was considered.

After providing informed consent, all patients received a bolus of 5000 or 10,000 U of unfractionated heparin and then 1,500,000 IU of streptokinase over 1 h by a peripheral vein, followed by a continuous infusion of 1000 U/h of heparin titrated to a PTT of 2–2.5 times control. In survivors of the acute phase, on the first day, heparin was overlapped with warfarin and was stopped when two consecutive therapeutic INR (2.0–3.0) were obtained. The patients were kept on warfarin for 6 months or more, depending on risk factors.

Baseline, 24 h, at discharge and follow-up echocardiograms were done. The transthoracic and transesophageal echocardiography examination and interpretation were performed before and after starting FT by one experienced echocardiographer. Echocardiographic signs of severe right ventricular dysfunction were: right ventricular dilatation 35 mm, RVEDD $\geq$ 2:1 than LVEDD ratio, severe pulmonary arterial systolic pressure $\geq$50 mmHg (calculated by tricuspid regurgitation velocity, gradient was calculated with modified Bernoulli's formula).

Qualitative right ventricular wall motion abnormalities were assessed as follows: without hypokinesis, regional hypokinesis, or global hypokinesis. Left ventricular motion, right ventricular wall thickness, abnormal septal position, paradoxical systolic motion, and loss of inspiratory collapse of the inferior cava vein were analyzed. Transthoracic echocardiography was performed according to the American Society of Echocardiography recommendations [17]. However, apical four chambers view was used to evaluate right ventricular/left ventricular ratio and right ventricular wall motion. When transthoracic acoustic window was suboptimal or when thrombus in-transit was suspected, a transesophageal echocardiography was performed to assess the right ventricular function and to search for thrombus in the main pulmonary artery or its proximal branches.

All surviving patients were educated on symptoms and signs of recurrent PE as well as on warfarin use, and had follow-up by the Principal Investigator (CJS). All patients had monthly visits during the first 6 months and then every 3 months if oral anticoagulation was stopped. In each 3 month office visit, clinic and echocardiographic evaluations were done; V/Q lung scan and lower extremity venous ultrasonography were performed every 6 months the first 5 years and then every year. Patients under long-term oral anticoagulation had medical monthly visit including INR. Office visit contact follow-up was done until December 2013.

Definitions

Proved PE: by high probability V/Q lung scans, pulmonary angiography or necropsy. Secondary or provoked PE: characterize events that occurred in the presence of obvious provoking factors (surgery, trauma, etc.). Idiopathic or unprovoked PE: event in absence of classic provoking factors. Normal blood pressure: diastolic: 60–90 mmHg; systolic: 100–150 mmHg.

High-risk PE: a definition was proposed including at least two clinical and electrocardiogram variables, as well as full echocardiogram findings. Clinical: sudden or persistent dyspnea plus ischemic-like chest pain and/or syncope, (b) S3 gallop, (c) pulse oxymetry <95 %. Electrocardiogram: (a) new ECG signs of right ventricular strain, (new right bundle branch block or right axis deviation), (b) qR in V1, (c) transitory or persistent ST-elevation >1 mm in leads V1, V2, and V3, (d) transient or persistent ST depression >1 mm in leads V1, V2, and V3 or over, (e) T wave inversion in leads V1–V4. Echocardiogram: (a) RVEDD/LVEDD ≥ 2:1, (b) with or without regional or global RVH, (c) right ventricular diameter ≥35 mm, (d) systolic pulmonary arterial pressure ≥50 mmHg [5, 6].

Major adverse cardiovascular events: mortality, recurrence, cardiogenic shock, and cardiac arrest. Mortality secondary to PE: in acute phase secondary to cardiogenic shock or ventricular arrhythmia with echocardiography findings of pulmonary arterial hypertension and right ventricular dysfunction [5, 6, 18]. Recurrent PE: proved new PE (new perfusion lung scan defect) in-hospital or in the follow-up with or without clinical instability [5, 6, 18]. Recurrent deep vein thrombosis: diagnosed by ultrasonography, a new noncompressible venous segment in the proximal veins, an increase of 4 mm. or more in thrombus diameter with compression or an increase of 1–4 mm in diameter combined with an extension of at least 4 cm in length [5, 6].

Rethrombolysis: after successful thrombolysis (clinical and echocardiographic improvement) a new fibrinolytic regimen due to in-hospital PE recurrence with right ventricular dysfunction. Rescue thrombolysis: a second fibrinolytic regimen immediately administered to patients with nonsuccess thrombolysis and persistent or worsening clinical instability and right ventricular dysfunction.

Major hemorrhage: stroke (confirmed by computed tomography), hematoma >5 cm, prolonged external bleeding at puncture site, oral or gastrointestinal bleeding, hematuria or another bleeding with concomitant hypotension that required treatment with intravenous fluids, blood transfusion, surgical control, discontinuation of FT regimen, decrease >15 % points in hematocrit or >5 g/dL in hemoglobin [5, 6]. Minor hemorrhage: 10–15 % decrease in hematocrit or 3–5 g/dL in hemoglobin reduction [5, 6].

Reperfusion criteria: clinical, electrocardiogram, echocardiogram, and V/Q lung scan improvement after FT regimen compared with baseline state. Postthrombotic syndrome: swelling, pain, purpura, skin pigmentation, eczematoid dermatitis, pruritus, ulceration, and cellulitis. Chronic pulmonary arterial hypertension: mean pulmonary arterial pressure ≥25 mmHg through right heart catheterization with pulmonary capillary wedge pressure <15 mmHg and a pulmonary vascular resistance of <3 Wood units.

Results

From January 1996 until May 2002, 131 patients with full inclusion criteria and proven PE were enrolled. Among them, 61 had RVH and 70 did not. PE was proved by V/Q lung scan and follow-up was obtained until December 2013 in all patients. Considering our risk definition, V/Q lung scan and echocardiographic findings, all patients had high-risk, extensive PE, and severe pulmonary arterial hypertension and right ventricular remodeling (Table 7.7).

Demographic characteristics are shown in Table 7.7. RVH patients were older and both groups had a similar gender ratio. Among previously healthy patients, in those with previous deep venous thromboembolism, chronic endothelial dysfunction and inflammation risk factors had similar incidence. In both groups, acute medical infections occurred around index event [19] in a higher proportion than "classic" conditions involving stasis and coagulation cascade and platelet activation (Tables 7.7 and 7.8).

Over 70 % of the patients had PE index event at home characterized by dyspnea and ischemic-like chest pain, without history of hospitalization, cancer, minor or major surgery, trauma, fracture or estrogens use. In all patients dyspnea was a remarkable finding, presenting at rest in 47 % and during exertion in 51 % of RVH patients; in the opposite group dyspnea had similar characteristics, 53 % at rest and 49 % during exertion. RVH group had higher incidence of syncope, low borderline "normal" blood pressure, late arrival, right ventricular dilatation and thrombus in-transit than the opposite group (Table 7.7).

Table 7.7 Assessment of streptokinase regimen

Variable	Pre $n=40$	Post $n=40$	p Value
Dyspnea	33	5	<0.001
Angina-like pain	32	1	<0.001
S3 gallop	38	2	<0.001
Shock	16	3	0.001
Respiratory rate	35.40±6.07	23.17±5.25	<0.0001
Heart rate	123.57±13.85	89.45±13.83	<0.0001
DBP	73.50±20.19	76.66±14.38	0.2224
PaO_2	50.15±10.62	62.55±10.64	<0.0001
Perfusion defects (29 patients)	9.69±1.16	3±1.41	<0.0001
Echocardiography findings			
PASP	60.37±6.43	32.12±7.72	<0.0001
RVD	40.72±2.51	32.80±3.68	<0.0001
LVD	26.57±5.77	44.57±6.46	<0.0001
RV hypokinesia	28	14	<0.0005
Ejection fraction	40.82±11.61	49.85±10.51	<0.0001
ASP	37	16	<0.001
PSM	36	6	<0.001

DBP diastolic blood pressure, *PASP* pulmonary arterial systolic pressure, *RVD* right ventricle diameter, *LVD* left ventricle diameter, *ASP* abnormal septal position, *PSM* paradoxical systolic motion

Table 7.8 Demographic characteristics

Variable	With RVH $n=61$(%)	Without RVH $n=70$ (%)	p Value
Age (years ± SD)	61 ± 17.5	52 ± 16.2	0.002
Age range (years)	28–89	26–86	
Female	37/60	41/59	0.94
Male	24/39	29/41	
Previous cardiovascular state			
Healthy	26/43	23/33	0.33
History of PE or DVT	16/26	14/20	0.52
Risk factors related with chronic endothelial dysfunction and inflammation			
Increasing age >65 years	20/33	25/36	0.86
Obesity	18/30	21/30	0.89
Smoking	17/28	18/26	0.93
Hypertension	15/25	14/20	0.67
Diabetes	13/21	16/23	0.84
Triggers			
Acute medical infections	35/49	47/51	0.33
Immobility	13/21	15/21	0.84
Trauma	2/3	2/3	0.62
Orthopedic surgery	6/10	6/9	0.95
General surgery	4/7	3/4	0.85
CABG	2/3	3/4	0.87
Urologic surgery	1/2	1/1	0.53
Molecular thrombophilia	1/2	2/3	0.90
Clinical presentation			
Index event at home	47/77	50/71	0.84
Dyspnea	49/80	55/78	0.97
Ischemic-like chest pain	52/85	61/87	0.95
Syncope	11/18	0/0	0.0006
Right ventricular third sound	57/93	63/90	0.69
Blood pressure			
Systolic blood pressure	106 ± 4.41	130 ± 11.44	<0.0001
Diastolic blood pressure	66 ± 3.86	82 ± 6.36	<0.0001
Onset symptoms (h)			
0–24	0/0	48/69	<0.0001
24–72	22/36	17/24	0.20
>72	39/64	5/7	<0.0001
ECG findings			
ST depression	51/83	56/80	0.97
T wave inversion	50/81	56/80	0.97
qR V_1	20/32	25/36	0.86
ST-elevation	19/31	22/31	0.89
Echocardiographic and lung scan			
Right ventricular diameter	42.65 ± 3.78	39.80 ± 3.70	0.001
PASP	57 ± 5.4	56 ± 3.2	0.001
Thrombus in-transit	6/10	0/0	0.01
No. of SPD	8.7 ± 4.2	9.3 ± 3.4	0.44

CABG coronary artery bypasses graft, *RVD* right ventricular dysfunction, *PASP* pulmonary artery systolic pressure, *SPD* segmental perfusion defects

Table 7.9 Infections associated to PE index event

Acute infections	With RVH $n=35$(%)	Without RVH $n=47$ (%)
Bronchitis	8/22	9/19
Pneumonia	6/17	8/17
COPD exacerbation	5/14	6/12
Gastrointestinal	5/14	5/11
Urinary	4/11	6/12
Upper respiratory tract	3/8	5/11
Prostate	3/8	4/9
Cholecystitis	1/3	4/9

Main characteristics in patients without RVH were better BP levels and early arrival after onset symptoms. Based on echocardiographic and lung scan findings both groups had severe RVD, acute pulmonary arterial hypertension and extensive PE. Table 7.9 summarizes the in-hospital and follow-up outcome and bleeding complications rate. Higher incidence of major adverse cardiovascular events and non-successful thrombolysis was a characteristic in RVH patients. In addition, more thrombus resistance expressed by residual thrombosis, and by the requirement of pharmacological and/or mechanical rescue strategies were observed in these patients (Table 7.10).

Bleeding complications: although there was not statistical significance among major and minor events, a trend for more events was observed in RVH patients. Femoral hemorrhage in patients under pulmonary percutaneous intervention was the main cause of bleeding. Only one case of intracranial hemorrhage was observed.

Follow-up: six patients with RVH and 7 without were lost (9 and 10 %, PNS). Mortality secondary to PE was low in both groups. Nevertheless, patients with RVH had the highest incidence of arterial vascular thrombosis and high mortality trend secondary to acute vascular syndrome (coronary, carotid, cerebral, and aortic). Postthrombotic syndrome was a serious long-term complication in both groups. In a long-term follow-up only one case with chronic thromboembolic pulmonary hypertension was identified (2 %).

Lessons Learned from This Study

Three important findings were observed in this study. First, among PE patients with normal blood pressure, thrombolysis use in an early right ventricular dysfunction stage improved in-hospital outcome compared with RVH patients. Second, clinical characteristics showed another link among acute infections [18], traditional atherothrombosis risk factors [19–25], and PE, suggesting that inflammation has a role in triggering such events. Third, the longer follow-up in PE patients submitted to FT—to our best knowledge—, shows low recurrence, mortality related, and chronic thromboembolic pulmonary arterial hypertension incidence.

Table 7.10 In-hospital mortality, adverse events and follow-up

Characteristic	With RVH $n=61$(%)	Without RVH $n=70$ (%)	p Value
In-hospital			
Mortality	17/28	0/0	<0.0001
Recurrence	10/16	4/6	0.09
Cardiac arrest	9/15	0/0	0.002
Asymptomatic recurrent PE	6/10	6/9	0.95
Successful fibrinolytic therapy	41/67	70/100	<0.0001
Residual thrombosis	16/26	5/7	0.006
Rethrombosis	8/13	1/1	0.02
Rescue thrombolysis	6/10	0/0	0.02
PPI	16/26	5/7	0.006
Surgery embolectomy	1/2	0/0	
Bleeding complications			
Major hemorrhage	7/12	4/6	0.38
Lung	1/2	2/3	0.90
Gastrointestinal	2/3	0/0	0.41
Venous puncture	3/5	2/3	0.87
Intracranial	1/2	0/0	0.94
Minor hemorrhage	5/8	2/3	0.33
Venous puncture	5/8	2/3	0.33
Follow-up			
Mortality			
Secondary to PE	2/3	0/0	0.41
Acute vascular syndrome	7/11	4/6	0.38
Another vascular thrombosis	12/20	2/3	0.004
Postthrombotic syndrome	15/25	16/23	0.97
Chronic PAH	0/0	1/2	0.94

PPI percutaneous pulmonary intervention, *PAH* pulmonary arterial hypertension

Currently, in spite of the identification of RVH and structural injury, thrombolysis use in normotensive patients is controversial. The rationality for its use in the setting of normal blood pressure and right ventricular dysfunction comes from experimental and human models [26], and pathophysiological mechanisms [27]. This suggests that its use in an early state of right ventricular dysfunction, could break complex mechanisms of ventricular damage, initial subendocardial ischemia, structural injury, and inflammatory response [26, 27], avoiding RVH, an independent risk factor for recurrence and mortality [5, 6, 10, 12, 28–33].

Regarding clinical presentation, although all patients had blood pressure in normal ranges, in those with RVH, blood pressure levels were found in significant lower range (Table 7.7), suggesting a major degree of right ventricular dysfunction with a compensated systemic perfusion (neurohormonal, adrenergic and vasopressin system activity). Clinicians have to be in warning in patients with this characteristic.

The need to improve risk stratification though more sensitive neurohormonal activity and/or ischemia biomarkers is one of the greatest contemporaneous challenges [34, 35].

In the setting of similar PE extension and pulmonary arterial hypertension severity, the only significant clinical difference in RVH patients was time between onset symptoms and thrombolysis use, suggesting ischemia time as the main RVH mechanism [28]. However, age-related increased RV myocardial stiffness [36], coronary artery disease or less right ventricular microvessels [37] could have an additional role.

Additionally, thrombolysis success and residual thrombosis could be time-depending as has been demonstrated in another model of vascular thrombosis [38]. Therefore, time as adjunctive treatment has to be considered in PE patients with these characteristics. Previously, high dose and short-term streptokinase infusion in a broad clinical spectrum of PE patients [1, 3, 5, 6] has been efficient and safe [1, 3, 5, 6]. In this study older patients were enrolled and similar safe in terms of intracranial hemorrhage was observed.

In spite of the same noninvasive diagnosis approach a trend towards high bleeding complications was observed [5, 6]. Several factors could explain these findings, elderly patients with comorbidities were included, more invasive procedures were performed and unfractionated heparin regimen not designed as an adjunctive treatment to thrombolysis was used. Considering our previous results [5, 6] and although there is not a universal consensus, thrombolysis has been the standard of care in PE patients with RVH and normal blood pressure in the last years in our center.

Another significant finding was the high incidence of idiopathic PE linked with chronic and acute inflammation factors. The "atypical" clinical profile in our patients included index event at home, aged >50 years, atherothrombosis risk factors, previous acute infections, and dyspnea at exertion plus ischemic-like chest pain. Emergency physicians should be warned and not limit their thinking to "typical" PE (chronic or incurable disease, hospitalization, cancer, major surgery, bed-bound, etcetera) presentation, which could lead to misdiagnosis of acute coronary syndromes. Our results add new evidence to previous observations from EMPEROR registry [39]; there, another "atypical" PE presentation including male Caucasian and African American young employed independent individuals living with dyspnea at exertion was described. Also, the increased incidence of PE in male gender could be another confounding factor [40, 41].

Our results provide another link between inflammation and PE and support previous [19–21] and current clinical and molecular evidence [22–26] suggesting a close relationship among atherothrombosis risk factors and venous thrombosis [19]. In both groups, a dominant clinical characteristic was the presence of risk factors related with chronic and acute inflammation around index event, conditions that could induce cytokines expression and regulation of inflammatory response. In this model of low pressure segment circulation thrombosis [42], it is possible that interleukin-6 [22, 23] induces coagulation cascade activation through tissue factor, fibrinogen, factor VIII, and von Willebrand factor expression. These factors could increase platelet aggregation, sensitivity to thrombin, and both endothelial activation and endothelial cell damage. It has also been reported that interleukin-6 lowers the concentration of the natural inhibitors of hemostasis such as antithrombin and protein S [43], as well as, thrombomodulin, a natural anticoagulant [44].

On the other hand, acute infections induce white-cell activation, dehydration, and bed rest [18] as collateral thrombosis mechanisms. It is important to recognize that inflammatory and thrombotic pathways share common signaling pathways and that inflammatory responses promote activation of the clotting cascade and stimulate platelet activation [44]. Considering all these evidence linking inflammation with PE [19–28] it is possible to propose that new risk factors should be added to the list of venous thromboembolism precipitants [19] particularly in high-risk elderly population.

In this group with age-dependent alterations of hemostasis and endothelial dysfunction inducing thrombosis [45], high infection incidence, and home immobility are the rules, so nonpharmacological (diet, vaccines) [46] and pharmacological primary prevention (statins) strategies have to be considered [18, 24–26]· It is unknown whether, low-molecular weight heparin or new anticoagulants have a role in this population. Considering all of this evidence, it is possible that "unprovoked" or "idiopathic" PE term has to be reconsidered.

Several important findings are coming from the longer follow-up in PE patients submitted to FT. Lower recurrence and mortality related could be attributed to the close contact and expertise of physicians involved, as well as, continuous patient training on disease and oral anticoagulants use. The incidence of chronic thromboembolic pulmonary arterial hypertension observed was 2 %, similar to previously reported (4 % [47] and 1 % [48]) in patients in whose FT was underused (11 % [48], 8 % [49]). However, a trend to reduce the frequency of chronic thromboembolic pulmonary hypertension (1 of 131 vs. 7 of 223) [49] was observed.

This finding suggests that thrombolysis plus oral anticoagulation could reduce the frequency of chronic thromboembolic pulmonary hypertension in patients with first event of acute PE improving the outcome [50, 51]. In addition, this study broadens current knowledge about whether routine echocardiographic evaluation after acute PE may help to identify early stage of chronic thromboembolic pulmonary arterial hypertension [51]. Early after acute PE was resolved, patient had normal echocardiogram, absent symptoms, and no residual thrombus on ultrasound.

In the follow-up, after a long "honeymoon" period, echocardiogram was an important tool to identify early stage of pulmonary arterial hypertension through mild RV remodeling and abnormal pulmonary systolic pressure. It is possible that in the follow-up of extensive PE with or without RVH, under thrombolysis or not, such testing every 3 or 6 months may lead to an early pulmonary arterial hypertension suspicion.

This strategy could improve management and outcome, avoiding detection in advanced stages. Postthrombotic syndrome was a serious long-term complication and its incidence increased (27 %) regarding our previous (4 %) observations [6]. This evidence establishes a unique opportunity to assess current clinical practice and outcome in PE patients and contributes to implementing quality assessment processes. It is possible that systemic thrombolysis was effective in some patients but not in others, suggesting the need of an early deep venous thrombosis search in order to offer catheter lab or endovascular center access for early mechanical, pharmacomechanical FT and/or surgical venous thrombectomy [51].

The study limitations are: open label, nonrandomized and non-mortality study; biomarkers of ventricular dysfunction, and cellular injury were not available. No test to directly or indirectly prove inflammation state was done and it was not possible to identify seasonal patterns of influenza infection. We did not include a control group in our analysis of potential triggers of thrombosis. Therefore, statements made regarding potential triggers could not be tested, and this part of our analysis should be seen as merely explorative. None test to excluded molecular thrombophilia was done. Finally, although wall motion abnormalities were analyzed by echocardiography it is not possible to rule out poor right ventricular ejection fraction in these patients [51].

Thrombolysis by peripheral vein in PE patients with normal blood pressure and without RVH improved in-hospital outcome compared with RVH patients. In a long-term follow-up, although its use may reduce chronic thromboembolic pulmonary arterial hypertension, it did not improve postthrombotic syndrome incidence. A blind, randomized control trial with significant sample to reproduce our results is mandatory.

one-hour Recombinant Human Tissue-Type Plasminogen Activator, Alteplase Infusion Compared with Unfractionated Heparin

Study No. 4

The main characteristics of this study were analyzed in deep in Chap. 5, in brief: The role of enoxaparin and weight-adjusted unfractionated heparin as adjunct to fibrinolytic therapy in pulmonary embolism is unknown.

In a prospective, open label, controlled multicenter trial, 80 patients with high-risk pulmonary embolism were enrolled. Forty patients received recombinant human tissue-type plasminogen activator, alteplase infusion plus weight-adjusted unfractionated heparin (24–48 h) and then enoxaparin (7 days). In control group unfractionated heparin standard regimen was used. There were no differences on pulmonary embolism extension, ($p = 0.63$) and right ventricular hypokinesis (0.07) in both groups. In terms of in-hospital survival ($p = 0.009$), escalation treatment ($p < 0.001$) and in-hospital stay ($p < 0.001$) patients who received recombinant human tissue-type plasminogen activator, alteplase had better outcome than opposite group. In a 30 ($p < 0.001$) and 90 ($p < 0.001$) days follow-up pulmonary perfusion was improved in patients who received enoxaparin versus heparin alone without increasing major bleeding complications.

Lessons Learned from This Study

The results of this control trial suggest that PE patients with right ventricular dysfunction, the recombinant human tissue-type plasminogen activator, alteplase improve in-hospital and follow-up outcome compared with unfractionated heparin alone. The intravenous anticoagulation strategy used was effective and safe [52].

Tenecteplase-Tissue-Type Plasminogen Activator Registry in High-Risk Pulmonary Embolism

Study No. 5

Thrombolysis with alteplase or streptokinase in 1 h improved mortality and outcome in well-selected PE patients. A new fibrin-specific fibrinolytic third generation, tenecteplase-tissue-type plasminogen activator (TNK-t-PA) with a better pharmacologic and pharmacokinetic profile emerges as an interesting therapeutic alternative.

TNK-t-PA profile has been analyzed in Chap. 2, in brief: It has been improved in terms of immunogenicity, half-life, fibrin specificity, plasminogen activation, activation of fibrinogen linked to plasminogen, limited activity of fibrinogen and plasminogen; as well as resistance of plasminogen activator inhibitor-1, paradoxical procoagulant effect, and no depletion of α_2-antiplasmin compared with first and second generation fibrinolytics. Additionally, 10 or 5 s bolus facilitates thrombolysis administration. Considering all of these advantages, TNK-t-PA is close to be considered as "ideal" fibrinolytic agent.

We conducted a prospective registry from one center with 6 months follow-up. The main objective was to determine the outcome of patients with high-risk PE carried fibrinolytic therapy with TNK-t-PA. The methodology has been published previously [52], in brief: Inclusion criteria: aged >15 years, high-risk PE, proved PE, patients referred within 14 days after onset of symptoms. Exclusion criteria: history of severe chronic pulmonary arterial hypertension, absolute contraindication for thrombolysis, and any concurrent condition limiting short-term survival.

Stratification, Thrombolysis, and Diagnosis Workup

Risk stratification and diagnosis approach were the same used in the last years all patients with high clinical suspicion of PE (major risk factors, clinical manifestations, chest X-ray, electrocardiogram and oximetry) were under a one-hour "fast-track" echocardiography evaluation and treatment within the Emergency Department. In patients with high-risk PE with clinical stability, impeding instability or instability an experienced physician administered thrombolysis by peripheral vein as soon as possible reproducing ST-elevation myocardial infarction strategy to reduce ischemia and right ventricular dysfunction time. Patients with impeding instability or instability were the only in whom V/Q lung scan or CT angiography was performed after starting treatment. When severe right ventricular wall motion abnormalities were excluded lung scan or CT angiography was performed before starting thrombolysis. After fibrinolytic regimen, all patients had clinical, electrocardiogram and echocardiographic evaluation. If there was nonsuccess thrombolysis or in-hospital recurrence, rescue thrombolysis, rethrombolysis or percutaneous pulmonary intervention were considered. Twenty-four to 72 h after thrombolysis all patients had tests to assess pulmonary circulation and deep venous thrombosis search [52].

Pharmacologic regimen: All patients were assigned to weight-adjusted intravenous unfractionated heparin received a bolus of 60 U/kg 15 (maximum 4000 U) and then a 10 s bolus of TNK-t-PA based on weight patient: <60 kg, 6000 U (30 mg) in 6 mL; >60 to <70 kg, 7000 U (35 mg) in 7 mL; >70 to <80 kg, 8000 U (40 mg) in 8 mL; >80 to <90, 9000 U (45 mg) in 90 mL; >90 kg, 10,000 U (50 mg) in 10 mL.

After a constant heparin infusion (12 U/kg/h, maximum 1000 U/h) adjusted to maintain an activated partial thromboplastin time of 50–70 s for 24–48 h was started. Then, the first subcutaneous dose of 1 mg/kg of enoxaparin was applied. To achieve sustained anticoagulation, this subcutaneous dose was repeated every 12 h until hospital discharge for a maximum of 7 days. In control group UH standard regimen was used: bolus of 5000 or 10,000 U followed by a constant infusion of 1000 U/h of heparin titrated to APTT of 2–2.5 times control by 7 days. In all survivor patients, on the first day to third day, heparin was overlapped with warfarin. The patients were kept on warfarin, aiming for an INR between 2.0 and 3.0 for 6 months or more, depending on the presence of major risk factors.

V/Q lung scans: Baseline, 24 h and at discharge, and 30 and 90 days perfusion scan in anterior, posterior, lateral and oblique views were performed. Ventilation lung scan was done. Echocardiograms: Baseline, 1 h, 24 h, at discharge and follow-up echocardiograms were done. The echocardiographic examination and interpretation were performed before and after starting thrombolysis. Qualitative: right ventricular end diastolic diameter, regional and global hypokinesis, paradoxical septal motion, loss of inspiratory collapse or the inferior cava vein. Quantitative evaluation: pulmonary artery systolic pressure determined with the modified Bernoulli formula, measurements of right and left ventricular size, ejection fraction, tricuspid and pulmonary regurgitation and right ventricular wall thickness. Echocardiography was standardized using the apical four chambers, parasternal long and short axis. When these positions were not appropriate, a subcostal four-chamber view was used [52].

Analysis of efficacy: Baseline and 24 h clinical evaluation included: clinical, electrocardiogram, chest X-ray, oximetry, pulmonary arterial hypertension and right ventricular dysfunction improvement. Pre- and posttreatment lung scans and echocardiograms were analyzed regarding perfusion abnormalities, pulmonary arterial systolic pressure, and right ventricular dysfunction behavior. In-patient mortality, recurrence, treatment escalation, duration of in-hospital stay was evaluated.

Follow-up evaluation included functional class, recurrent PE, chronic pulmonary arterial hypertension, postthrombotic syndrome and mortality. Follow-up: visits at 30, 90, and 180 days and then every 2 months until 6 months. In the two subsequent visits ECG, TTE, V/Q lung scan or any other test assessing pulmonary circulation were done. At the end visit only electrocardiogram and transthoracic echocardiogram were performed [52].

Definitions

High-risk PE was based on three variables of clinical, electrocardiogram and echocardiogram categories were required at least. Clinical: (a) sudden or persistent dyspnea plus chest pain and or syncope, (b) S3 gallop, (c) hypoxemia, (d) hypotension, (e) shock, (f) cardiac arrest 13. Electrocardiogram: (a) new ECG signs of right ventricular strain, (new right bundle branch block or right axis deviation), (b) qR in V1, (c) transitory or persistent ST-elevation >1 mm in leads V1, V2, and V3, (d) transitory or persistent ST depression >1 mm in leads V1, V2, and V3 or over, (e) T wave inversion in leads V1–V4 13. Echocardiogram: (a) right ventricular end diastolic diameter/left ventricular end diastolic diameter ratio (RVEDD/LVEDD) >2:1, (b) regional or global right ventricular hypokinesis, (c) right ventricular diameter >35 mm, c systolic pulmonary arterial pressure >50 mmHg [52].

In this registry, D-Dimer, troponin expression and brain natriuretic peptide type-B were for first time used. The same previous definitions as right ventricular hypokinesis, PE proved, mortality secondary to PE, major adverse cardiovascular events, global mortality, treatment escalation, recurrent PE, and deep venous thrombosis, reperfusion criteria, rethrombolysis and rescue thrombolysis were used. Also major hemorrhage and minor hemorrhages were considered too [52].

From 2009 to 2011, 30 patients with full inclusion criteria were enrolled. Age 58.62±6 years, female 73 %. Cardiovascular risk factors: age >60 years 53 %, obesity 55 %, smoking 59 %, hypertension 53 %, diabetes mellitus 53 %, dyslipidemia 55 %, Triggers: infection 43 %, immobility 18 %, travel 9 %, hospitalization 9 %, molecular thrombophilia 9 %, oral anticonception 9 %, bed rest 6 %, cancer 6 %, abnormal ejection fraction <40 % 3 %. Clinical presentation: Dyspnea 93 %, like-ischemic chest pain 59 %, syncope 40 %, and cardiogenic shock 3 %. Clinical examination: third sound right ventricular 97 %, decreased pulmonary second sound 93 %, heart rate 114.16±11.5/min., systolic blood pressure 105±22.7 mmHg, diastolic blood pressure 70±16.7 mmHg, oxygen saturation 87.6±6.25 %.

Thorax radiograph: Westermark sign 93 %, elevated right diaphragm 78 %, right pulmonary artery dilatation 65 %. The electrocardiographic findings were sinus tachycardia 100 %, acute pulmonary hypertension 90 %, qRV1 62 %, ST-transitory elevation leads V1–V4 40 %, T inversion in leads V1–V6 62 % and inferior leads 62 %, ST depression leads V1–V4. Echocardiographic findings: right ventricular diameter 39±4.3, pulmonary arterial systolic pressure 54.8±6.0, RVEDD/LVEDD>2:1 100 %, tricuspid regurgitation 90 %, right ventricular hypokinesis

90 % and McConnell sign 731 %, patent foramen ovale 18 %, in-transit thrombus 18 %. Diagnosis by V/Q lung scan 90 %, perfusion defects 12 ± 4.2.

Laboratory and biomarkers: Leukocytosis, 56 %, elevated fibrinogen 96 % hyperglycemia 128.7 ± 35.0 mg/dL, abnormal serum creatinine 46 %; Brain natriuretic peptide type-B: 581 ± 254 pg/mL; D-dimer: 5711 ± 819 ng/mL; and troponin expression in only 7 patients, 0.06 ± 0.03 (0.06–0.13) ng/mL. At discharge: D-dimer 505 ± 1063 and brain natriuretic peptide 110 ± 158.

All patients received TNK-t-PA, 1 patient 25 mg, 1 patient 30 mg, 13 patients 40 mg, other 3 45 mg and 14 patients 50 mg. Time-onset symptoms-to door 128.55 ± 10 h and time-door-to needle 111.6 ± 10 min. After thrombolysis, reperfusion criteria were improved on: heart rate 79.6 ± 12/min., systolic blood pressure 118.6 ± 8.3 mmHg, diastolic blood pressure 74.5 ± 8.22 mmHg, oxygen saturation 98.5 ± 2.5 %; on echocardiogram pulmonary arterial systolic pressure 34.6 ± 4.3 and right ventricular diastolic diameter 31.8 ± 4.3. In-transit thrombus 0. In-hospital stay 7.1 ± 2.83

Major adverse cardiovascular events: Mortality 13 %, recurrence 3 %, residual thrombus and percutaneous pulmonary intervention 7 % respectively. Intracranial hemorrhage 0 %, major hemorrhages 3 %, and minor bleeding 10 %. In a 6-month follow-up no mortality or recurrence related with PE was identified. In addition no bleeding complications were registered.

Lessons Learned from This Study

Until our knowledge, this is the first registry with tenecteplase in Latin-American population with an acute PE event. Overall, this study shows the real clinical practice in Emergency Department from a Cardiology hospital. Additionally, three important findings were observed in this prospective registry: first, the same doses used in ST-elevation myocardial infarction patients plus unfractionated heparin low dose as a bridge to low-molecular weight heparin was safe; second, TNK-t-PA improves in-hospital and follow-up outcome, and third, despite that all patients had severe right ventricular dysfunction and extensive lung thrombus, a minority had troponin expression.

In PEITHO study, important and favorable findings to support thrombolysis use in clinical stable patients were observed, however all were counterbalanced by a high incidence of bleeding complications [53]. Although, in this prospective registry the incidence of bleeding complications was low, it could be attributed to weight-adjusted dose of intravenous unfractionated heparin recommended in ST-elevation myocardial infarction guidelines, This unfractionated heparins dosing was associated with absence of intracranial hemorrhage as was observed with one-hour alteplase infusion [52].

The main advantages of using it as “bridge” before starting enoxaparin are: short half-life, hepatic clearance, effective antidote, and available test to know the activity. In this period, it is possible to stratify renal function to starting low or standard enoxaparin dose reducing bleeding complications. After the high-risk period for bleeding complications low-molecular-weight heparin improves and simplifies the traditional anticoagulation approach through easier administration, sustained anticoagulation and an enhanced antithrombotic effect [52]. Additionally with this strategy, a short in-hospital stay was achieved with recurrence rate reduction and subsequent impact in-hospital costs. However it is important to consider the expertise of physicians in chart, natural selection to choose low-risk patients to thrombolysis and not older patients could be another explanation.

Although effectivity was not the main target of the registry, TNK-t-PA dosed on weight patient was effective to improve in-hospital and 6-month outcome in high-risk PE patients. Ten second TNK-t-PA bolus not only was practical and simple to use but also improves clinical and echocardiogram criteria reperfusion. The last three important TNK-t-PA randomized control trials compared with heparin improve mortality and or reducing scaled treatment [53–55]. Another important finding was in-transit thrombus resolution, suggesting that faster TNK-t-PA thrombolytic effect could be translated to clinical practice.

Finally, despite severe right ventricular dysfunction by echocardiogram and brain natriuretic peptide type-B, only a minority had troponin expression. Considering that in PEITHO study only patients with expression of this biomarker were considered with high-risk PE, two important considerations emerge; first a high number of patients with clinical stability and severe right ventricular dysfunction are misclassified and second the necessity of early ischemic biomarkers are mandatory.

Clinical Implications

We are presenting 289 patients with proved extensive PE associated with extensive severe acute pulmonary arterial hypertension and right ventricular dysfunction, in which a high dose in short-term thrombolysis infusion by peripheral vein was effective and safe. The main characteristics of these patients are shown in Tables 7.1, 7.2, 7.3, 7.4, and 7.5. Patients were attended in cardiology hospitals and physicians involved had experience in thrombolysis and anticoagulant treatment in different cardiovascular clinical situations.

The majority of the patients were young associated with chronic or acute inflammation factors. All of them had extensive PE (Table 7.3) considering the number of perfusion segmental defects identified in VQ lung scan. Furthermore, on echocardiogram all patients had severe right ventricular dilatation. This data confirm severe right ventricular dilatation in all patients included.

In our series, mortality and bleeding complications had low incidence (Tables 7.4 and 7.5). A possible explanation included age, fast-track thrombolysis in Emergency Department, no venous puncture, and short-term thrombolysis infusion. In spite of these results, when a recombinant human tissue-type plasminogen activator, alteplase was used in a multicenter trial [18], less recurrence and necessity of rescue procedures were observed (Table 7.4).

In a prospective registry TNK-t-PA was safe when unfractionated heparin dose recommended in ST-elevation myocardial infarction patients was used. Pharmacologic and pharmacokinetic characteristics were translated to clinical practice improving in-hospital and 6-month follow-up.

Although, we do not have a head-to-head study, a second- and third-generation fibrinolytics could be a better option in PE patients with extensive pulmonary affection and severe right ventricular dysfunction.

References

1. Jerjes-Sánchez C, Ramírez RA, Arriaga NR, Pimentel MG. Dosis altas e infusión rápida de estreptoquinasa para el tratamiento de tromboembolia pulmonar masiva. Arch Inst Cardiol Mex. 1993;63:227–34.
2. Ozbeck C, Sen S, Frank S, Dyckmans J, Schieffer H. Rapid high dose streptokinase in severe pulmonary embolism. Lancet. 1989;334:229–30.
3. Jerjes-Sanchez C, Gutierrez-Fajardo P, Ramirez-Rivera A, Garcia ML, Hernández CHG. Infarto agudo del ventrículo derecho secundario a tromboembolia pulmonar masiva. Arch Inst Cardiol Mex. 1995;65:65–73.
4. Dack S, Master AM, Horn H, Grishman A, Field LE. Acute coronary insufficiency due to pulmonary embolism. Am J Med. 1949;7:464–77.
5. Jerjes-Sanchez C, Ramirez-Rivera A, Garcia ML, Arriaga-Nava R, Valencia-Sanchez S, Rosado-Buzzo A, Pierzo JA, Rosas ME. Streptokinase and heparin versus heparin alone in massive pulmonary embolism: a randomized controlled trial. J Thromb Thrombolysis. 1995;2:67–9.
6. Jerjes-Sanchez C, Ramirez-Rivera A, Arriaga-Nava R, Iglesias-Gonzalez S, Gutierrez P, Ibarra-Perez C, Martinez A, Valencia S, Rosado-Buzzo A, Pierzo JA, Rosas E. High dose and short-term streptokinase infusion in patients with pulmonary embolism. Prospective with seven-year follow-up trial. J Thromb Thrombolysis. 2001;12:237–47.
7. Goldhaber SZ. Thrombolysis in pulmonary embolism: a debatable indication. Thromb Haemost. 2001;86:444–51.
8. Meneveau N, Schiele F, Metz D, Valette B, Attali P, Vuillemenot A. Comparative efficacy of a two-hour regimen of streptokinase versus alteplase in acute massive pulmonary embolism: Immediate clinical and hemodynamic outcome and one-year follow-up. J Am Coll Cardiol. 1998;31:1057–63.
9. Tebbe U, Graf A, Kamke W, Zahn R, Forycki F, Kratzsch G, Günther B. Hemodynamic effects of double-bolus reteplase versus alteplase infusion in massive pulmonary embolism. Am Heart J. 1999;138:39–44.
10. Ramirez-Rivera A, Gutierrez-Fajardo P, Jerjes-Sanchez C, Hernandez-Chavez G. Acute right myocardial infarction without significant obstructive coronary lesions secondary to massive pulmonary embolism. Chest. 1993;104:80S.
11. Sharma GVRK, Folland ED, McIntyre KM, Sasahara AA. Long-term benefit of thrombolytic therapy in patients with pulmonary embolism. Vasc Med. 2000;5:91–5.
12. Riveiro A, Lindmarker P, Johnsson H, Juhlin-Dannfelt A, Jorfeldt L. Pulmonary embolism: one year follow-up with echocardiography Doppler and five-year survival analysis. Circulation. 1999;99:1325–30.
13. Konstantinides S, Geibel A, Heusel G, Heinrich F, Kasper W. Heparin plus alteplase compared with heparin alone in patients with submassive pulmonary embolism. N Engl J Med. 2002;347:1143–50.
14. Meneveau N, Mingb LP, Seronde MF, Mersina N, Schielea F, Caulfield F, Bernard Y, Bassand JP. In-hospital and long-term outcome after sub-massive and massive pulmonary embolism submitted to thrombolytic therapy. Eur Heart J. 2003;24:1447–54.

15. Goldhaber SZ, Come PC, Lee RT, Brauwald LT, Parker JA, Haire WD, Feldstein ML, Miller M, Toltzis R, Smith JL, Taveira de Silva AM, Mogtader A, McDonough TJ. Alteplase versus heparin in acute pulmonary embolism; randomized trial assessing right-ventricular function and pulmonary perfusion. Lancet. 1993;341:507–11.
16. Podbregar M, Krivec B, Voga G. Impact of morphologic characteristics of central pulmonary thromboemboli in massive pulmonary embolism. Chest. 2002;122:973–9.
17. Recommendations for a standardized report for adult transthoracic echocardiography: a report from the American Society of Echocardiography's Nomenclature and Standards Committee and Task Force for a Standardized Echocardiography Report. JASE. 2002;15:275–90.
18. Smeeth L, Cook C, Thomas S, Hall AJ, Hubbard R, Vallance P. Risk of deep vein thrombosis and pulmonary embolism after acute infection in a community setting. Lancet. 2006;367: 1075–9.
19. Jerjes-Sanchez C. Venous and arterial thrombosis. A continuum spectrum of the same disease? Eur Heart J. 2005;26:1–2.
20. Prandoni P, Bilora F, Marchiori A, Bernardi E, Peitrobeli F, Lensing AWA, Prins MH, Girolami A. An association between atherosclerosis and venous thrombosis. N Engl J Med. 2003;348:1435–41.
21. Becattini C, Agnelli G, Prandoni P, Silingardi M, Salvi R, Taliani MR, Poggio R, de Imberti D, Ageno W, Pogliani E, Porro F, Casazza F. A prospective study on cardiovascular events after acute pulmonary embolism. Eur Heart J. 2005;26:77–83.
22. Libby P, Crea F. Clinical implications of inflammation for cardiovascular primary prevention. Eur Heart J. 2010;31:777–83.
23. Libby P, Ridker PM, Hansson GK, for the Leducq Transatlantic Network on Atherothrombosis. Inflammation in atherosclerosis: from pathophysiology to practice. J Am Coll Cardiol. 2009;54:2129–38.
24. Glynn RJ, Danielson E, Fonseca FA, Genest J, Gotto Jr AM, Kastelein JJ, Koenig W, Libby P, Lorenzatti AJ, MacFadyen JG, Nordestgaard BG, Shepherd J, Willerson JT, Ridker PM. A randomized trial of rosuvastatin in the prevention of venous thromboembolism. N Engl J Med. 2009;360:1851–61.
25. Piazza G, Goldhaber ZS. Venous thromboembolism and atherothrombosis. An integrated approach. Circulation. 2010;121:2146–50.
26. Goldhaber ZS. Risk factors for venous thromboembolism. J Am Coll Cardiol. 2010;56:1–7.
27. Stevinson BG, Hernandez-Nino J, Rose G, Kline JA. Echocardiographic and functional cardiopulmonary problems 6 months after first-time pulmonary embolism in previously healthy patients. Eur Heart J. 2007;28:2517–24.
28. Lualdi JC, Goldhaber SZ. Right ventricular dysfunction after acute pulmonary embolism: pathophysiologic factors, detection, and therapeutic implications. Am Heart J. 1995;130:1276–82.
29. Kucher N, Rossi E, De Rosa M, Goldhaber SZ. Prognostic role of echocardiography among patients with acute pulmonary embolism and a systolic arterial pressure of 90 mm hg or higher. Arch Intern Med. 2005;165:1777–81.
30. Grifoni S, Vanni S, Magazzini S, Olivotto I, Conti A, Zanobetti M. Association of persistent right ventricular dysfunction at hospital discharge after acute pulmonary embolism with recurrent thromboembolic events. Arch Intern Med. 2006;166:2151–6.
31. Goldhaber SZ. Assessing the prognosis of acute pulmonary embolism. Chest. 2008;133:334–6.
32. Riveiro A, Lindmarker P, Juhlin-Dannfelt A, Johnson H, Jorfeldt L. Echocardiography Doppler in pulmonary embolism: right ventricular dysfunction as predictor of mortality. Am Heart J. 1997;134:479–87.
33. Kasper W, Konstantinides S, Geibel A. Prognostic significance of right ventricular afterload stress detected by echocardiography in patients with clinical suspected pulmonary embolism. Heart. 1997;77:346–9.
34. Dellas C, Puls M, Lankeit M, Schäfer K, Cuny M, Berner M, Hasenfuss G, Konstantinides S. Elevated heart-type fatty acid-binding protein levels on admission predict an adverse outcome in normotensive patients with acute pulmonary embolism. J Am Coll Cardiol. 2010;55: 2150–7.

35. Lankeit M, Friesen D, Aschoff J, Dellas C, Hansefub G, Katus H, Konstantinides S, Giannitis E. Highly sensitive troponin T assay in normotensive patients with acute pulmonary embolism. Eur Heart J. 2010;31:1836–44.
36. Borlaug BA, Paulus WJ. Heart failure with preserved ejection fraction: pathophysiology, diagnosis and treatment. Eur Heart J. 2011;32:670–9.
37. Bogaard HJ, Natarajan R, Henderson SC, Long CS, Kraskauskas D, Smithson L, Ockaili R, McCord JM, Voelkel NF. Chronic pulmonary artery pressure elevation is insufficient to explain right heart failure. Circulation. 2009;120:1951–60.
38. Silvain J, Collet JP, Nagaswami C, Beygui F, Edmondson KE, Bellemain-Appaix A, Cayla G, Pena A, Brugier D, Barthelemy O, Montalescot G, Weisel JW. Composition of coronary thrombus in acute myocardial infarction. J Am Coll Cardiol. 2011;57:1359–67.
39. Pollack CV, Schreiber D, Goldhaber SZ, Slattery D, Fanikos J, O'Neil BJ, Thompson JR, Hiestand B, Briese BA, Pendleton RC, Miller CD, Kline JA. Clinical characteristics, management, and outcomes of patients diagnosed with acute pulmonary embolism in the emergency department: initial report of EMPEROR (Multicenter Emergency Medicine Pulmonary Embolism in the Real World Registry). J Am Coll Cardiol. 2011;57:700–6.
40. Laporte S, Mismetti P, Décousus H, Uresandi F, Otero R, Lobo JL, Monreal M, from the RIETE Investigators. Clinical predictors for fatal pulmonary embolism in 15 520 patients with venous thromboembolism findings from the Registro Informatizado de la Enfermedad Trombo Embolica venosa (RIETE) Registry. Circulation. 2008;117:1711–6.
41. Steffel J, Braunwald E. Novel oral anticoagulants: focus on stroke prevention and treatment of venous thrombo-embolism. Eur Heart J. 2011;32:1968–76.
42. Kaski JC, Arrebola-Moreno AL. Inflammation and thrombosis in atrial fibrillation. Rev Esp Cardiol. 2011;64:551–3.
43. Gurbel PA, Tantry US. Antiplatelet and anticoagulants agents in heart failure. J Am Coll Cardiol FH. 2014;2:1–15.
44. Croce K, Libby P. Intertwining of thrombosis and inflammation in atherosclerosis. Curr Opin Hematol. 2007;14:55–61.
45. Capodanno D, Angiolillo DJ. Antithrombotic therapy in the elderly. J Am Coll Cardiol. 2010;56:1683–92.
46. Phrommintikul A, Kuanprasert S, Wongcharoen W, Kanjanavanit R, Chaiwarith R, Sukonthasarn A. Influenza vaccination reduces cardiovascular events in patients with acute coronary syndrome. Eur Heart J. 2011;32:1730–5.
47. Pengo V, Lensing AWA, Prins MH, Marchiori A, Davidson BL, Tiozzo F, Albanese P, Biasiolo A, Pegoraro C, Iliceto S, Prandoni P, For the Thromboembolic Pulmonary Arterial Hypertension Group. Incidence of chronic thromboembolic pulmonary arterial hypertension after pulmonary embolism. N Engl J Med. 2004;350:2257–64.
48. Becattini C, Agnelli G, Pesavento R, Siingardi M, Poggio R, Taliani MR, Ageno W. Incidence of chronic thromboembolic pulmonary arterial hypertension after a first episode of pulmonary embolism. Chest. 2006;130:172–5.
49. Kline JA, Steuerwald MT, Marchichk M, Hernandez-Nino J, Rose GA. Prospective evaluation of right ventricular function and functional status six months after acute submassive pulmonary embolism. Frequency of persistent or subsequent elevation in estimated pulmonary artery pressure. Chest. 2009;136:1202–10.
50. Piazza G, Goldhaber SZ. Chronic thromboembolic pulmonary hypertension. N Engl J Med. 2011;364:351–60.
51. A scientific statement from American Heart Association. Management of massive and submassive pulmonary embolism, ileofemoral deep venous thrombosis and chronic thromboembolic pulmonary hypertension. Circulation. 2011. doi:10.1161/CIR.0b012e318214914f.
52. Jerjes-Sanchez C, Villarreal-Umaña S, Ramirez-Rivera A, Garcia-Sosa A, Canseco LM, Archondo T, Reyes E, Garza A, Arriaga R, Castillo F, Jasso O, Garcia H, Bermudez M, Hernández JM, Garcia J, Martinez P, Rangel F, Gutierrez J, Comparan A. Improving adjunctive treatment in pulmonary embolism and fibrinolytic therapy. The role of enoxaparin and weight-adjusted unfractionated heparin. J Thromb Thrombolysis. 2009;27:154–62.

53. Meyer G, Vicaut E, Danays T, Agnelli G, Becattini C, Beyer-Westendorf J, Bluhmki E, Bouvaist H, Brenner B, Couturaud F, Dellas C, Empen K, Granca A, Galiè N, Geibel A, Goldhaber SZ, Jimenez D, Kozak M, Kupatt C, Kucher N, Lang IM, Lankeit M, Meneveau N, Pacouret G, Palazzini M, Petris A, Pruszczyk P, Rugolotto M, Salvi A, Schellong S, Sebbane M, Sobkowicz B, Stefanovic BS, Thiele H, Torbicki A, Verschuren F, Konstantinides SV, PEITHO Investigators. Fibrinolysis for patients with intermediate-risk pulmonary embolism. N Engl J Med. 2014;370:1402–11.
54. Kline JA, Nordenholz KE, Courtney DM, Kabrhel C, Jones AE, Rondina MT, Diercks DB, Klinger JR, Hernandez J. Treatment of submassive pulmonary embolism with tenecteplase or placebo: cardiopulmonary outcomes at 3 months: multicenter double-blind, placebo-controlled randomized trial. J Thromb Haemost. 2014;12:459–68.
55. Becattini C, Agnelli G, Salvi A, Grifoni S, Pancladi LG, Enea I, Blasemin F, Campanini M, Ghirarduzzi A, Casazza F, TIPES Study Group. Bolus tenecteplase for right ventricle dysfunction in hemodynamically stable patients with pulmonary embolism. Thromb Res. 2010;125:e82–6.

Chapter 8
Thrombolysis in Special Situations

Carlos Jerjes-Sánchez and Anabel Garcia-Sosa

Thrombolysis In-Transit Thrombus Patients

In-transit thrombus: blood thrombus located inside right cavities of the heart, sometimes free-floating, or sometimes trapped in a foramen ovale.

This entity represents an occasional finding that astounds physicians during echocardiographic assessment and stratification in pulmonary embolism (PE) suspected patients. In-transit thrombus has been described as an image that can take many forms and sizes, that can even been motile, and sometimes remembers left ventricular masses or those described in deep venous thrombosis. Although at present time, the exact mechanism producing in-transit thrombus is unknown, several hypothesis have been proposed [1]: (a) During the developing of venous thromboembolic disease, thrombus formed inside the deep venous system is freed and travels up to the right heart to reach the pulmonary circulation, resulting in different occlusion grades and a myriad of symptoms; (b) thrombus is formed in situ caused by structural defects or intracardiac devices.

Recently, the presence of inflammatory cells and myocytolysis related with intracavitary thrombi in the left and right ventricle of patients who died because of PE as a presumed new source of ventricular dysfunction was described [2]. Myocarditis was considered based on Dallas criteria (aggregation of inflammatory cells in the

C. Jerjes-Sánchez, M.D., F.C.C.P., F.A.C.C. (✉)
Sistema Nacional de Investigadores, Nivel II – Clinical Research Director,
Instituto de Cardiologia y Medicina Vascular, TEC Salud

Escuela de Medicina, Tecnológico de Monterrey San Pedro Garza Garcia, Nuevo León, Mexico

Unidad de Investigacion Clinica en Medicina SC Monterrey, Nuevo León, Mexico
e-mail: jerjes@prodigy.net.mx

A. Garcia-Sosa, M.D.
Department of Emergency Room, Hospital de Cardiologia No. 34,
Instituto Mexicano del Seguro Social, Monterrey, Nuevo Leon, Mexico
e-mail: anabel.garcia@udicem.org

C. Jerjes-Sánchez, *Thrombolysis in Pulmonary Embolism*,
DOI 10.1007/978-3-319-19707-4_8

myocardium coinciding with areas of myocytolysis). These findings were not observed in no-PE and pulmonary arterial hypertension patients. Compared with controls extravascular foci of aggregates of lymphocytes, neutrophilic granulocytes and macrophages were found dispersed in the right and left ventricle, coinciding with areas of myocytolysis, indicating myocarditis in acute PE patients. Considering previous observations, myocardial inflammation has to be considered as another possible mechanism participating in the setting of thrombus in situ on right ventricular wall or in another cardiac structure.

Echocardiography has improved in-transit thrombus diagnosis since it is not expensive, noninvasive, available, and an objective method to search for intracardiac masses; unfortunately it is not used as frequently as it should. Echocardiogram provides critical information related to physiologic changes occurring during PE. This accessible tool also helps us to establish risk, drive therapy, and evaluate treatment response, and to exclude intracardiac thrombus or patent foramen ovale [3–8]. Recently, the European Cooperative Study on the clinical significance of right heart thrombi [1] reported the echocardiographic evaluation of 119 patients with PE and right heart thrombi, who were classified into three groups; type A: the most frequent, thrombus acquires a serpent or worm form, it is highly mobile, thin, long, and mostly changing (Fig. 8.1); type B: mostly nonmotile, it can assume left heart thrombus form, and it is never seen with a worm form (Fig. 8.2); type C: it is neither type A nor type B, it does not have a worm form, but is highly mobile, and it could remember a myxoma (Figs. 8.3 and 8.4). This classification is clinically relevant considering its close relationship with embolic events and/or the potentially embolic source (deep venous thrombosis), being the major risk factor for these events thrombus mobility and worm-shaped thrombus (Table 8.1).

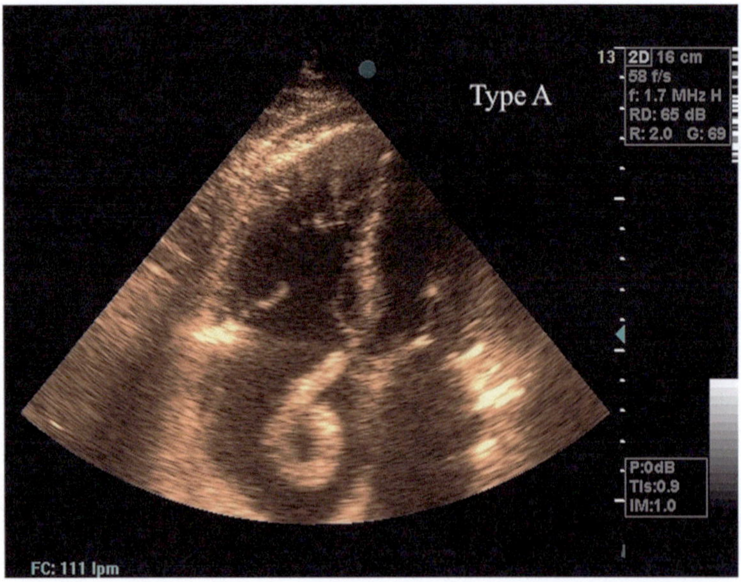

Fig. 8.1

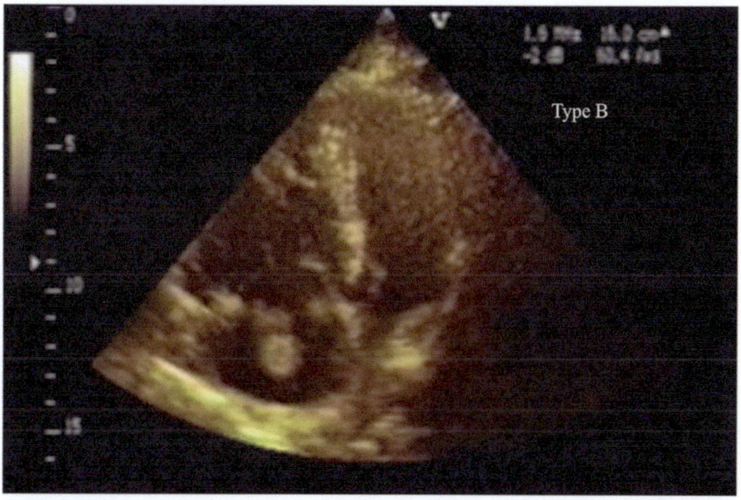

Fig. 8.2

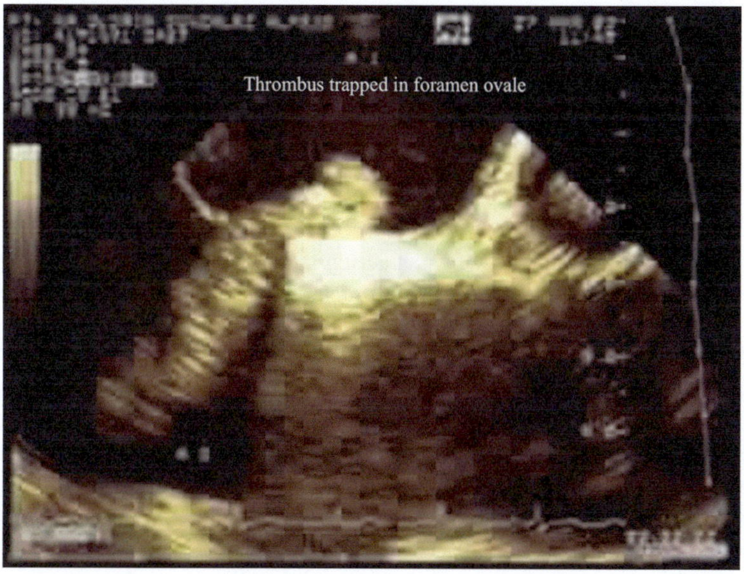

Fig. 8.3

In-transit thrombus incidence is unknown, but in a subanalysis from ICOPER registry [6] among 1135 patients studied with echocardiogram, 4 % had in-transit thrombus; Pierre-Justin and Pierard [9] reported 4 % incidence and Chartier et al. [10] found 8.2 %. In a prevalence study in Switzerland among 23,796 autopsies in general population, intracardiac thrombus prevalence was 7.2 % and 2.2 % had

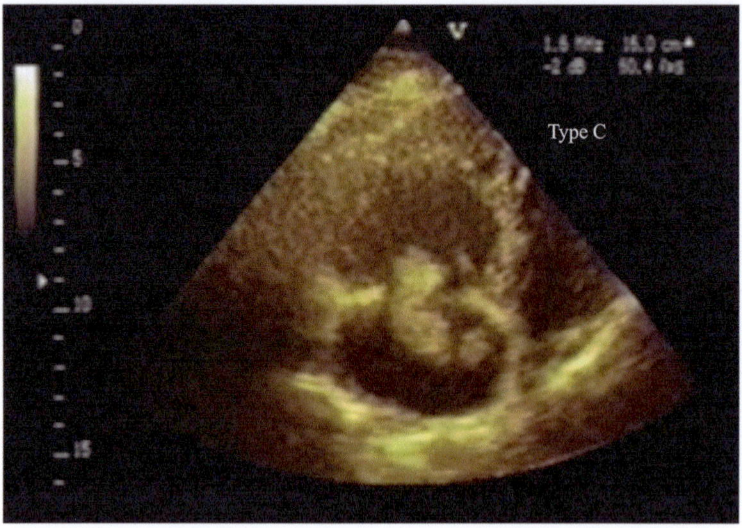

Fig. 8.4

Table 8.1 Association between in-transit thrombus and embolic events

	Type	Number of patients	Associated to DVT (%)	Associated to PE (%)
Kronik et al. (1989)	A	48	63	98
	B	57	25	40
	C	14	36	62

right heart cavities thrombus [4]. Considering the evidence coming from ICOPER study [5], PE patients with in-transit thrombus had more hemodynamic compromise, hypotension, syncope [10], right ventricular hypokinesis, higher troponin levels [11], twice more heart failure level, and more frequent right bundle branch block, compared with patients without in-transit thrombus.

In addition, all mortality cause at 14 days and 3 months among PE patients were higher in those with in-transit thrombus (21 % versus 11 %, and 29 % versus 16 %, respectively). Chartier et al. [10] reported high in-hospital mortality (44.7 %) in 38 patients, whereas first-day mortality reached 21.1 %. Similar findings were reported by Mollazadeh et al. [12] who observed 50 % mortality.

Although in-transit thrombus is an infrequent complication in the setting of acute PE, it represents a potentially fatal entity in which the best therapeutic approach is still controversial. Since it has a more severe clinical presentation, therapeutic measures and decisions should be different and more extreme. The current evidence we have is coming from case reports, registries, or small studies including different treatment as heparin, surgical embolectomy, percutaneous embolectomy, or thrombolysis [13, 14] (Table 8.2). Considering that evidence is weak current clinical guidelines [15, 16] do not recommend a specific treatment, leaving physicians confused in a therapeutic dilemma to decide the best treatment option.

Table 8.2 Studies show results with different treatments

Author (year)	Number of patients (evaluation)	Treatment		Death *n* (%)
Torbiki et al. (1995–1996)	42 (14 days)	Thrombolysis	24	5 (20.8)
		Heparin	17	4 (23.5)
		Surgery/techniques interventional	4	1 (25)
	42 (3 months)	Thrombolysis	24	7 (29.2)
		Heparin	17	5 (29.4)
		Surgery/techniques interventional	4	1 (25)
Chartier et al. (1986–1998)	30	Surgery	17	8 (47)
		Thrombolysis	9	2 (22)
		Heparin	8	5 (62.5)
		Techniques interventional	4	2 (50)
Mollazadeh et al. (2004–2006)	12	Thrombolysis	3	1 (33.3)
		Heparin	5	4 (80)
		Techniques interventional	4	1 (25)
Mohan et al. (2003–2008)	19	Heparin + OAC	12	0 (0)
		Thrombolysis	4	1 (25)
		Surgery	3	1 (33.3)
Pierre-Justin (1997–1999)	12	Thrombolysis	7	1 (14.2)
		Heparin	5	3 (60)
Chapoutot et al. (1985–1993)	14 (12 treated)	Without treatment	2	2 (100)
		Heparin	2	1 (50)
		Thrombolysis	2	0 (0)
		Surgery	8	1 (12.5)

Thrombolysis: Which Logical Reasoning Sustains Thrombolytic Use?

Thrombolysis is a systemic treatment with a specific capacity to dissolve thrombi: thrombus located in pulmonary arteries or even in the deep venous system circulation also thrombus in-transit [10]. This therapeutic approach is accessible to the majority of the centers; it can be started bed-side with a rapid effect. Although FDA approved drugs for PE treatment, a specific position related with in-transit thrombus is not mentioned (Table 8.3).

Treatment benefit among PE patients has been proved, but major bleeding is the main limiting risk. Konstantinides et al. [17] reported a major bleeding risk of 11.1 % among 169 patients: 21.9 % in thrombolytic treated versus 7.8 % in heparin treated, although intracranial bleeding was scarce, only 2 patients in each group: 1.2 % and 0.4 %, respectively. A review of the literature from 1966 to 1998 , in which different drugs and doses were evaluated, showed that benefit is higher and faster with thrombolytic treatment; but also the bleeding risk, compared with heparin monotherapy; these results are even more important when a small but significant risk of intracranial bleeding was observed [18].

Table 8.3 FDA approved thrombolytic treatment to PE

Drug[a]	Dose	Approved date
Streptokinase	250,000 U/30 min follow by 100,000 U/h in 24 h	1977
Urokinase	4400 U/kg in 10 min follow by 4400 U/kg/h in 12–24 h	1978
rt-PA	100 mg in 2 h	1990

[a]Intravenous infusion; *rt-PA* recombinant human plasminogen activator, *h* hour

A more recent report [19], that included new thrombolytic drugs showed a 9.24 % major bleeding risk with thrombolysis compared with 3.42 % when only anticoagulation was used, intracranial bleeding occurred in 1.46 % versus 0.19 %, respectively. Those evidences forced experts to insist about relative and absolute contraindications when thrombolytic treatment is proposed.

Talking about in-transit thrombus there are some crucial questions: what happens with the thrombus after thrombolytic treatment is started, and how long does this lesion last and when does it disappear? Small studies address this question, like the published by Ferrari et al. [20]. They reported 343 patients admitted with PE, 18 of them (5.3 %) diagnosed with in-transit thrombus, 16 patients were treated with thrombolysis (recombinant human plasminogen activator (rt-PA) 10 mg in bolus and 90 mg in continuous infusion for 2 h) and follow-up with echocardiogram showing 50 % thrombus resolution in <2 h after infusion, 50 % showed resolution at 12 h and the other half by 24 h, all patients were alive at 24 h and also at 30 days.

Greco et al. [21] analyzed thrombus behavior by echocardiogram during rt-PA infusion in seven patients with in-transit thrombus; they noted clot lysis between 45 and 60 min after the start of treatment. Lysis occurred with a progressive fragmentation in small particles that migrate from the heart cavities to pulmonary circulation to finally disappear. After 2 h of infusion all echocardiographic parameters showed significant improvement. During treatment and hospitalization no adverse events were noted, there was no PE recurrence, major bleeding, or death.

In-Transit Thrombus Trapped in Patent Foramen Ovale

This is an event caused by a thrombus that remains trapped through patent foramen ovale, adding the risk of paradoxical embolism [22]. In 1930 the first case of "paradoxical embolism" was diagnosed and the risk of systemic or cerebral embolism was considered [23]. Diagnosis criteria for paradoxical embolism are: history of venous thrombosis or PE, abnormal right to left heart communication, clinical, angiographic, or pathological evidence of systemic embolism, and favorable pressure gradient to promote right to left heart communication [22, 24].

Two studies, published by Meacham et al. [24] in 1998, and Myers et al. [22] in 2014, with 30 and 174 cases, respectively, describe 24-h mortality of 11.5 % and 30-day mortality of 18.4 %, respectively. Most patients were treated immediately but 55 % had systemic embolism. Surgical treatment was performed in 103 patients

Table 8.4 Thrombolytic regimens used for in-transit thrombus

Author	Thrombolysis (*n*)	Deaths	Regimen
Chartier et al.	9	2	rtPA (60–100 mg in 2 h)
Mollazadeh et al.	3	1	SK 250,000 U/10 min and 100,000/h for 12 h
Mohan et al.	4	1	250,000 U SK IV bolus infusion followed by 30 m 100,000 U/h 12–24 h or 15 mg bolus IV rtPA in 10 m followed by 85 mg in 2 h (total 100 mg)
Pierre-Justin et al.	7	1	rtPA bolus 10 mg, 40 mg for 2 h and 50 mg for 5 h not more than 100 mg total
Chapoutot et al.	2	0	20 mg rtPA bolus and bolus IU Urokinase 4400+2000 IU/h for 24 h

(62.4 %), thrombolysis in 19 (11.5 %), and anticoagulation in only 46 (26.1 %). Twenty-four hour mortality was 10.6 %, 26.3 %, and 25.6 %, respectively. Despite these reports, therapeutic debate remains, since in these severely ill, complex, and heterogeneous patients, individualized treatment is always needed. Hospital resources and also clinical experience are mandatory to choose the best options [22].

Evidence-based guides are difficult to implement since this is a rare condition and even the largest reports like Myers et al. [22], tend to be slanted and show heterogeneous patients without standardized treatments (Table 8.4). Previous evidence reported that although patent foramen ovale prevalence was high (26 %) [25], paradoxical embolism was rare. However, current evidence suggest higher patent foramen ovale and paradoxical embolism incidence [26]. In acute PE associated to patent foramen ovale the ischemic stroke prevalence, and the "gold standard" diagnosis method, remain unknown.

A prospective monocentric study in 41 consecutive PE intermediate-risk patients was conducted to evaluate patent foramen ovale and ischemic stroke prevalence, and to identify, which transesophageal- or transthoracic-echocardiography is the best diagnostic method in this context. Brain magnetic resonance imaging was used to confirm clinically obvious strokes or to diagnose subclinical ones [26].

Contrast transesophageal echocardiography revealed patent foramen ovale in 56.1 %, whereas contrast transthoracic echocardiography showed so in only 19.5 % ($P<0.001$). Of note, all patent foramen ovale observed with transthoracic echocardiography were also diagnosed by transesophageal echocardiography. Ischemic stroke occurred in 17.1 % and was always associated with patent foramen ovale and large shunt. Transesophageal echocardiography revealed that patent foramen ovale was associated with atrial septal aneurysm in 71 % in patients with recent ischemic stroke and 32.4 % in nonrecent ischemic stroke [26].

Recent ischemic stroke patients (seven) had new neurologic signs at admission (28.6 %), electrocardiogram with right ventricular strain (100 %), troponin 0.39 (0.07–0.59), and brain natriuretic peptide type-B expression 500 (223–708) pg/dL compared with nonrecent ischemic stroke patients (34) new neurologic signs at admission (0), electrocardiogram with right ventricular strain (82.4 %), troponin 0.16 (0.06–0.56), and brain natriuretic peptide type-B expression 434 (250–662) pg/dL [26].

In this study the patients with intermediate-risk PE presented a high incidence of paradoxical embolism. This study could be the first to show such a high incidence (17.7 %) of paradoxical embolism in submassive PE. Because patent foramen ovale and related ischemic strokes was frequent in intermediate-risk PE, transesophageal echocardiography is much more efficient than transthoracic echocardiography for patent foramen ovale diagnosis. Considering the high risk of intracranial bleeding with thrombolysis in PE, which may be partly due to hemorrhagic transformation of subclinical strokes, the screening patent foramen ovale with transesophageal echocardiography TEE should be considered in intermediate-risk PE when thrombolytic treatment is discussed [26].

Considering venous thromboembolism endothelial dysfunction, complex thrombus mechanisms, the broad thrombus distribution (venous system, pulmonary arteries and in-transit), high incidence of patent foramen ovale, with paradoxical cerebral embolism and possible also systemic, as well as right and left ventricular myocarditis [2], PE could be considered as complex and systemic disease.

Although surgical and percutaneous procedures are out of the scope of this book, for in-transit thrombus complexity both therapeutic approaches will be analyzed.

Surgical Embolectomy

Has been recommended in PE patients with absolute thrombolysis contraindication, as well as in those suffering in-transit thrombus and paradoxical embolism [15, 16]. Leacche et al. [27] reported surgical success in 47 PE with right ventricular with thrombolysis contraindications and medical treatment failure.

Early mortality was reported on only 6 %, and a high experienced surgical team helped with a preoperative transesophageal echocardiogram-performed surgery. Preoperative transesophageal echocardiogram, allowed a more defined intracardiac image, foramen ovale patency, or septal defects. In some cases, an epicardial echocardiogram helped surgeons to establish exact thrombus location to guide cannulation. Surgery was performed on normothermia without cardioplegia with longitudinal or transverse main pulmonary arteriotomy, although a right pulmonary artery arteriotomy between ascendant aorta and superior vena cava was occasionally performed. Thrombi were removed under direct visualization using a gallbladder stone forceps. No Fogarty catheter was used to avoid pulmonary artery lesions. Inferior vena cava filters were also implanted.

Multidisciplinary approach resulted in favorable outcomes along with a 24/7 availability team, a fast and precise diagnosis, and an always-ready operating room. Obviously, few centers have enough resources to perform these cardiothoracic surgeries to allow imitate this methodology [27]. Moreover, since shock raises mortality 3–7 times and most of fatalities occurred in the first hour ("*golden hour*") [28, 29]. Other potential complications are related to anesthesia, and also a prolonged surgery related to the increased difficulty to remove thrombi when they reach sites beyond central arteries.

Percutaneous Embolectomy

It is another potential therapeutic approach that can be performed during pulmonary angiography. Potential complications are related to the tendency of catheters to fragment thrombus instead of removing it. Particles produced can compromise pulmonary circulation even more, resulting in a dangerous and acute pulmonary hypertension [30].

Previous evidence shows fast and suitable diagnostic and therapeutic strategies are needed in this uncommon but severe disease. Treatment including heparin, thrombolysis, and/or surgical embolectomy should search for less complications and improving survival. Current guides are mainly based on expert recommendations and case reports with limited scientific evidence. Future trials should be oriented in comparing different treatments to establish the best options for individualized patients.

Thrombolysis advantages include availability, fast and systemic effect, but this approach has the intrinsic risk of bleeding. Careful patient selection and strict surveillance can decrease this complication. This recommendation is particularly important in the case of in-transit thrombus, where the additional risk of embolism is present, particularly for thrombus trapped inside a foramen ovale that can complicate with systemic embolism. Those risks should be taken into account during treatment selection [31].

Multidisciplinary team formation is essential to get the best results regarding mortality and complications. Team experience can only be reached by treating patients in large centers, and reporting results obtained. Joining forces of different centers should enable improve our knowledge of this interesting and challenging disease.

Thrombolysis in Pregnancy

Venous thromboembolism has been related with high maternal morbidity and mortality during pregnancy and peripartum. The absolute incidence of pregnancy associated with venous thromboembolism has been reported as 1 in 1000 to 1 in 2000 deliveries. Additionally, pregnancy carries a fivefold venous thromboembolism risk, and this risk higher in postpartum than to antepartum period [32].

Clinical presentation of PE in pregnancy is extremely variable [32], after third trimester progressive physiologic cardiopulmonary and systemic hemodynamic change emerges; so clinical suspicion and diagnosis approach is a challenge. Diagnosis of PE in pregnant women is out of the scope of this chapter, however an excellent review is available [32].

In normal pregnancy a hypercoagulable state develops, with the overexpression of pro-coagulants as factors VII VIII, X, von Willebrand factor and fibrinogen, and a decrease in anticoagulant proteins (protein C and S) [33]. Besides, plasminogen activator inhibitor type 1 levels are fivefold increased suggesting fibrinolysis inhibition; plasminogen activator inhibitor type 2 produced by the placenta increases exponentially up to the third trimester. This hypercoagulability state could increase in the postpartum and prevail during a considerable period of time, with a range from 4 to 8 weeks after childbirth or even longer [32]. Other mechanisms could have important participation, as increased venous capacitance, venous outflow decreased, and vein mechanical obstruction by the uterus; as well as decreased mobility and an increased vascular injury. Another important risk factor is represented by the history of venous thromboembolism events [32].

If these mechanisms are the only responsible for venous thromboembolism in pregnancy is an open question. As have been previously published the recognition of congenital or acquired thrombophilia in women with PE is mandatory. These risk factors have been identified in up to 50 % in women experiencing at least one thromboembolism episode during pregnancy or in the postpartum period. The congenital or acquired thrombophilia identified in both situations are not different than observed in general population as protein C and S and anti-thrombin III deficiency, factor V Leiden mutation (G1691A), and prothrombin gene mutation (G20210A) [34].

The cornerstone of pharmacological treatment in venous thromboembolism is anticoagulation and thrombolysis depending on clinical instability or not. Anticoagulation alone constitutes a challenge in daily clinical practice due to hemorrhagic and teratogenic complications for mother and fetus. Thrombolysis plus intravenous anticoagulation is considered as high-risk treatment in this clinical situation [35]. Both options are considered as high-risk treatment in pregnancy and possibly harmful for mother and fetus.

Venous thromboembolism has been identified as important cause of maternal death in several countries, it is the second cause of maternal death in the Netherlands and the most important cause of maternal death in the United Kingdom [35], and thrombolysis has been considered in the therapeutic approach in PE with clinical instability and pregnancy. As well as other specific scenarios, as in-transit thrombus, in pregnancy the evidence to use thrombolysis is scarce, weak, and depending on small case series or case reports.

In nonpregnant patients thrombolysis improve clinical instability, ventricular dysfunction, and acute pulmonary arterial hypertension with acceptable bleeding complications incidence. However, in pregnant women anticoagulation alone or thrombolysis plus heparin could be associated with bleeding complications and serious consequences.

The most commonly used thrombolytic agents are rt-PA, streptokinase and tenecteplase-tissue-type plasminogen activator. Rt-PA is not allergenic, can be administered in short-infusion and being a large polypeptide, it does not cross the placenta barrier. Streptokinase is also a large molecule derived from group C streptococci, and it does not cross the placenta in amounts significant enough to induce fetal coagulopathy. Tenecteplase-tissue-type plasminogen activator has not been tested in well-controlled studies in human pregnancy. Although tenecteplase could be given during pregnancy when benefit outweighs risk, there is no clinical evidence [35].

From 2009 to 2011, 78 pregnant women with PE and clinical instability has been published [32, 35–39]. Streptokinase was effective and safe in 36 women, one-third of them with massive PE, with an 8 % incidence of bleeding, mainly consisting of no complicated genital tract bleedings [36]. In other 28 cases thrombolysis was successful in 90 % with complications of 11 % and a 7 % mortality. Fetus mortality was high (23 %) however, thrombolysis was responsible for only two fetal fatalities. None of the live born children suffered a permanent deficit [37]. The most widely thrombolytic regimen was rt-PA, and also streptokinase and urokinase were used in less proportion. No differences among thrombolytics were identified. In 2009 another case, with extensive literature review was published [35]. Patient was a 34-year-old primigravida female, presented at 25 weeks gestation with PE and clinical instability, who received streptokinase as a bolus of 250,000 U followed by a continuous infusion of 100,000 U/h during 24 h followed by a weight-adjusted dose of low-molecular-weight heparin. Patient developed large subcutaneous hematomas, on site of the skin injuries, and collapsed, requiring two units of red blood cell transfusion. In this review 12 cases were included. In Table 8.5, it is possible to identify the thrombolytic used, demographic characteristics and complications. This series has higher incidence of bleeding complications compared with previous reported cases.

Recently, another three cases of massive PE, treated with streptokinase and rt-PA, with a positive course for mothers and babies were published [38]. Fasullo et al. [39] reported one case of thrombolysis in a woman with clinical instability, cardiogenic shock, and severe respiratory failure; 2 h after standard rt-PA regimen patient improved her clinical condition. In this study, previously to thrombolysis a preserved fetal heartbeat, regular placental, and normal liquid presence without bleeding suggested fetus viability. The authors consider that in all pregnant women with PE and clinical instability, these parameters suggesting viability or not could assist in deciding the thrombolysis use.

Our experience with thrombolysis in PE includes 130 PE with right ventricular dysfunction submitted to thrombolysis [40–44]; other 131 has been described in the Chap. 7; additionally other 30 patients were submitted to tenecteplase-tissue-type plasminogen activator (Chap. 7). Among all of them (289) PE patients submitted to different thrombolytic regimens, one patient was a pregnant woman with clinical instability. She was 26-years-old, previously healthy, radiology fellow with 6-month normal pregnancy, who suddenly developed severe respiratory failure and clinical instability (blood pressure 80/40 mmHg). Electrocardiogram showed right ventricular overload and a transthoracic echocardiogram proved right ventricular dysfunction and severe pulmonary arterial hypertension. V/Q lung scan showed right lung exclusion. Because of the clinical instability One-Hour alteplase infusion was used, with unfractionated heparin as adjunctive treatment. Patient had clinical, electrocardiographic, V/Q lung scan and echocardiographic improvement and was discharged in good clinical condition. Three months later had in normal delivery she gave birth to a male newborn weighting 3.400 kg. Ten years later, both of them are in good health (data not published)

Finally, considering that evidence is coming from small series and case reports, the safety and effectiveness of thrombolysis in PE pregnant women with clinical instability remains unknown. Considering this weak evidence, it is possible to establish that in the setting of PE and pregnancy, thrombolysis has the same indications as in non-pregnant women: the clinical instability. In addition, it is important to emphasize that a trend exists to publish only successful cases.

Table 8.5 Pulmonary embolism treatment during pregnancy

Author (year)	Treatment	Total dose	Gestational week	Outcome mother	Outcome child	Preterm delivery	Bleeding complications
Ahearn (2002)	rt-Pa	100 mg	12	Good	Good	No	No
Baudo (1990)	rt-Pa	100 mg	35	Good	Death at 14th day	Yes (20 h)	No
Flossdorf (1990)	rt-Pa	43 mg	31	Good	Good	Yes (48 h)	Yes, minor
Patel (2003)	rt-Pa	100 mg	20	Good	Good	No	No
Yap (2002)	rt-Pa	100 mg	30	Good	Good	No	No
Trukhacheva (2005)	rt-Pa	100 mg	23	Good	Good	No	No
Fagher (1990)	SK	1,100,000 U	28	Good	Good	Yes (10 h)	Yes, major
McTaggart (1977)	SK	290,000 U	34	Good	Death 0–8 h	Yes (18 days)	Yes, minor
Hall (1972)	SK	1,800,000 U	32	Good	Good	Yes (0 h)	Yes, major
Mazeika (1994)	SK	140,000 U	25	Good	Good	No	Yes, major
Te Raa (2009)	SK	2,650,000 U	25	Good	Good	No	Yes, major
Kramer (1995)	UK	4400 U/kg	21	Good	Good	No	No
Delclos (1986)	UK	57,200 U/kg	28	Good	Good	No	Yes, minor

rt-*PA* recombinant human tissue plasminogen activator, *SK* streptokinase, *UK* urokinase. Raa et al. Thrombosis Research 2009; 124:1–5, with permission

Factor-Specific Oral Anticoagulants

Safety and efficacy assessments have been completed for the factor-specific oral anticoagulants (FSOA) previously referred to as novel oral anticoagulants. For some patients, FSOA, which act by directly inhibiting factor IIa or factor Xa, may provide safer, more convenient alternatives to warfarin. Their advantages include ease of use, reduced monitoring requirements, and lower bleeding risk than traditional therapy [45].

Clinical trials have established non-inferiority of FSOA to warfarin for the prevention of recurrent venous thromboembolism. These trials have demonstrated that FSOA exhibit similar or lower bleeding rates, particularly intracranial bleeding rates compared with warfarin. Anticoagulation therapy with FSOA may allow early discharge or outpatient management options for low-risk patients with deep venous thrombosis and PE.

Because of all advantages provided by these drugs, an interesting and open question is: could FSOA have a role in the setting of PE submitted to thrombolysis? In order to answer this question, we performed a systematic review.

We conducted a PubMed (National Library of Medicine, Bethesda, MD) search with the subject headings "thrombolytic therapy," "thrombolysis," "fibrinolytic therapy," "new oral anticoagulants," "factor-specific oral anticoagulants," "target-specific oral anticoagulants," "rivaroxaban," "dabigatran," "apixaban," "edoxaban," and "pulmonary embolism" to identify reports of PE in female patients who received treatment with FSOA. We limited our search to English literature. Data on the type and total dose of thrombolytic agent, FSOA, and bleeding complications were extracted. From January 2009 to January 2015, only two reports matched with the keywords. The first was an experimental study and was excluded. We identified 98 consecutive patients with symptomatic PE treated by a combination of "safe dose thrombolysis" and rivaroxaban [46].

From January 2012 to January 2013, 98 consecutive patients with symptomatic PE were treated by a combination of "safe dose thrombolysis" and rivaroxaban. At present time rivaroxaban has been approved in the United States for the treatment of venous thromboembolism, so in this study rivaroxaban was off-label for most of the duration of the study.

All patients had ≥3 new signs and symptoms: chest pain, tachypnea (resting respiratory rate ≥22/min), tachycardia (resting heart rate ≥90/min), dyspnea, oxygen desaturation (resting $PO_2 < 95$ %), or elevated jugular venous pressure (≥10 cm H_2O). The onset of symptoms occurred within a mean of 7 ± 3 days (range, 1 day–6 weeks). Diagnosis of PE was made by an objective testing with a computed tomographic pulmonary angiogram (CTA) in 86 patients and ventilation/perfusion radioisotope imaging in 12 [46].

Moderate and severe PE were defined in terms of PE extension and clinical instability, respectively. Echocardiogram was performed prior to thrombolysis in 90 patients and within 36 h post-thrombolysis in 95 and at 6 months after discharge. Serum brain natriuretic peptide type-B, D-dimer, and troponin I was measured before "safe dose thrombolysis" in most patients. Right ventricular enlargement was defined as a right ventricle/left ventricle ratio of >0.9. Pulmonary arterial hypertension was defined as: pulmonary arterial systolic pressure ≥40 mmHg. Patients were evaluated at least daily while in-hospital, within 3 weeks of discharge, and every 6 months thereafter. The mean follow-up was 12 ± 2 months [46].

All patients received unfractionated heparin given at 70 U/kg as bolus, but not to exceed 6000 U, with subsequent dose adjustment to keep the activated partial thromboplastin time at 60–100 s for 24 h. While rt-PA was being infused and for 3 h thereafter, the maintenance dose of heparin was kept at 8–10 U/kg/h, not to exceed 1000 U/h. It was subsequently adjusted to reach the target PTT at 60–100 s. No heparin bolus was given for PTT adjustment. After 24 h of infusion, heparin was stopped.

The "safe dose thrombolysis" was 50 mg of rt-PA, given as a 10-mg bolus by an intravenous push within 1 min, followed by infusion of the remaining 40 mg within 2 h. Heparin was the only parenteral anticoagulant administered. Patients received rivaroxaban at doses of 15 or 20 mg daily, 2 h after termination of heparin infusion depending on creatinine clearance (>30 L/min 20 mg and with a creatinine clearance of 15–30 L/min received 15 mg daily).

Among 92 patients, 84 had moderate PE and 14 severe PE, of whom 8 were hypotensive. The majority was female (52 %), younger (56 ± 10) with overweight (BMI 28 ± 3); unprovoked PE in 55 %, with active cancer 15 % and history of cancer 6 %; concomitant deep venous thrombosis in 53 %, D-dimer elevation in 100 %, troponin expression in 61 % and brain natriuretic peptide type-B in 74 %. In terms of echocardiographic findings: right ventricular dilatation in 49 % and right ventricular hypokinesis in 23 %. All patients received ≥1 month treatment with rivaroxaban. There were 18 patients who had to change to warfarin (with bridging with enoxaparin) later, due to myalgia in one and for insurance reasons in 17 [46].

Indefinite anticoagulation was considered in 64 % patients. The 20-mg daily dose of rivaroxaban was given in 94 patients. All patients completed a minimum of 4 months of anticoagulation, and 2 were lost to follow-up. At a mean follow-up of 12 ± 2 months, 78 % of the patients were on anticoagulation. Nine patients were on aspirin, and another three were on aspirin and clopidogrel. The median duration of treatment with rivaroxaban for the 18 patients who switched to warfarin was 49 days (range, 32–62 days), whereas it was 392 days (range, 242–485 days) for the remaining patients [46].

In terms of safety and efficacy outcomes, there was no in-hospital mortality and major or minor bleeding. Later minor hemorrhages were related with enoxaparin 2 months after discharge and with rivaroxaban and amiodarone use. No in-hospital PE recurrent events occurred, and in the follow-up two patients developed deep venous thrombosis and one PE, these patients were under warfarin treatment with subtherapeutic INR ranges. No one of the patients on rivaroxaban developed VTE [46]. In-hospital duration: In 78 patients in whom hospital admission was primarily due to PE and who had received SDT and rivaroxaban early on admission, the duration of hospitalization was 1.9 ± 0.2 days.

Until our knowledge this could be the first evidence relating PE and thrombolysis with FSOA. In spite of the favorable results, it is important to emphasize that patients had low-risk for bleeding complications and a modified unfractionated heparin dosage as adjunctive treatment was used. In this study rivaroxaban dose was considered for atrial fibrillation management; nevertheless, rivaroxaban regimen is more intensive in deep venous thrombosis patients (20 mg b.i.d for 7 days and then 20 mg od); the authors rationale were, the absence of previous experience with rivaroxaban associated to thrombolysis and common sense to use lower dose when rT-PA is given. Despite the results, more information is mandatory to use rivaroxaban or other FSOA as adjunctive treatment. Physicians also have to be in warning when a patient under FSOA treatment arrives to emergency departments with PE and thrombolysis indication.

References

1. Kronik G. The European Cooperative Study on the clinical significance of right heart thrombi, European Working Group on Echocardiography. Eur Heart J. 1989;10:1046–59.
2. Begieneman MVP, Van de Goot FRW, Van der Bilt IAC, Vonk Noordegraaf C, Spreeuwenberg MD, Paulus WJ, Van Hinsbergh VWM, Visser FC, Niessen HWM. Pulmonary embolism causes endomyocarditis in the human heart. Heart. 2008;94:450–6.
3. Goldhaber SZ. Echocardiography in the management of pulmonary embolism. Ann Intern Med. 2002;136:691–700.
4. Ogren M, Bergqvist D, Eriksson H, Lindblad B, Sternby NH. Prevalence and risk of pulmonary embolism in patients with intracardiac thrombosis: a population-based study of 23796 consecutive autopsies. Eur Heart J. 2005;26:1108–14.
5. Goldhaber SZ, Visani L, De Rosa M. Acute pulmonary embolism: clinical outcomes in the International Cooperative Pulmonary Embolism Registry (ICOPER). Lancet. 1999;353:1386–9.
6. Torbicki A, Galié N, Covezzoli A, Rossi E, De la Rosa M, Golldhaber SZ. Right heart thrombi in pulmonary embolism: results from the International Cooperative Pulmonary Registry (ICOPER). J Am Coll Cardiol. 2003;41:2245–51.
7. Chapoutot L, Nazeyrollas P, Metz D, Maes D, Maillier B, Jennesseaux C, Elaerts J. Floating right heart thrombi and pulmonary embolism: diagnosis, outcome and therapeutic management. Cardiology. 1996;87:169–74.
8. Labovitz AJ, Noble VE, Bierig M, Goldstein SA, Jones R, Kort S, Porter TR, Spencer KT, Tayal VS, Wei K. Focused cardiac ultrasound in the emergent setting: a consensus statement of the American Society of Echocardiography and American College of Emergency Physicians. J Am Soc Echocardiogr. 2010;23:1225–30.
9. Pierre-Justin P, Pierard L. Management of mobile right heart thrombi: a prospective series. Int J Cardiol. 2005;99:381–8.
10. Chartier L, Bera J, Delomez M, Asseman P, Beregi JP, Bauchart JJ, Warembourg H, Théry C. Free-floating thrombi in the right heart: diagnosis, management, and prognostic indexes in 38 consecutive patients. Circulation. 1999;99:2779–83.
11. Mohan B, Chhhabra S, Gulati A, Mittal C, Mohan G, Tandon R, Kumbkarni S, Aslam N, Soodnk NK, Wander GS. Clinical and echocardiographic diagnosis, follow-up and management of right sided cardiac thrombi. Indian Heart J. 2013;65:529–35.
12. Mollazadeh R, Ostovan MA, Abdi Ardekani AR. Right cardiac thrombus in transit among patients with pulmonary thromboemboli. Clin Cardiol. 2009;32:E27–31.
13. Casazza F, Bongarzoni A, Centonze F, Morpurgo M. Prevalence and prognostic significance of right-sided cardiac mobile thrombi in acute massive pulmonary embolism. Am J Cardiol. 1997;79:1433–5.
14. Rose PS, Punjabi NM, Pearse DB. Treatment of right heart thromboemboli. Chest. 2002;121:806–14.

15. Konstantinides SV, Torbicki A, Agnelli G, Danchin N, Fitzmaurice D, Galie N, Gibbs JSR, Huisman MV, Humbert M, Kucher N, Lang I, Lankeit M, Lekakis J, Maack C, Mayer E, Meneveau N, Perrier A, Pruszczyk P, Rasmussen LH, Schindler TH, Svitil P, Noordegraaf AV, Zamorano JL, Zompatori M. 2014 ESC guidelines on the diagnosis and management of acute pulmonary embolism. The Task Force for the Diagnosis and Management of Acute Pulmonary Embolism of the European Society of Cardiology (ESC). Eur Heart J. 2014;35:3033–80. doi:10.1093/eurheartj/ehu283.
16. Jaff MR, McMurtry MS, Archer SL, Cushman M, Goldenberg NA, Goldhaber SZ, Jenkins JS, Kline JA, Michaels AD, Thistlethwaite P, Vedantham S, White RJ, Zierler BK, On behalf of the American Heart Association Council on Cardiopulmonary, Critical Care, Perioperative and Resuscitation, Council on Peripheral Vascular Disease, and Council on Arteriosclerosis, Thrombosis and Vascular Biology. Management of massive and submassive pulmonary embolism, iliofemoral deep vein thrombosis, and chronic thromboembolic pulmonary hypertension: a scientific statement from the American Heart Association. Circulation. 2011;123:1788–830. doi:10.1161/CIR.0b013e318214914f.
17. Konstantinides S, Geibel A, Olschewski M, Heinrich F, Grosser K, Rauber K, Iversen S, Redecker M, Kienast J, Just H, Kasper W. Association between thrombolytic treatment and the prognosis of hemodynamically stable patients with major pulmonary embolism: results of a multicenter registry. Circulation. 1997;96:882–8.
18. Arcasoy SM, Kreit JW. Thrombolytic therapy of pulmonary embolism. Chest. 1999;115: 1695–707.
19. Chatterjee S, Chakraborty A, Weinberg I, Kadakia M, Wilensky RL, Sardar P, Kumbhani DJ, Mukherjee D, Jaff MR, Giri J. Thrombolysis for pulmonary embolism and risk of all-cause mortality, major bleeding, and intracranial hemorrhage a meta-analysis. JAMA. 2014;311: 2414–21.
20. Ferrari E, Benhamou M, Berthier F, Baudouy M. Mobile thrombi of the right heart in pulmonary embolism: delayed disappearance after thrombolytic therapy. Chest. 2005;121:1051–3.
21. Greco F, Bisignani G, Serafini O, Guzzo D, Stingone A, Plastina F. Successful treatment of right heart thromboemboli with IV recombinant tissue-type plasminogen activator during continuous echocardiographic monitoring: a case series report. Chest. 1999;116:78–82.
22. Myers PO, Bounameaux H, Panos A, Lerch R, Kalangos A. Impending paradoxical embolism: systematic review of prognostic factors and treatment. Chest. 2010;137:164–70.
23. Thomppson T, Evans W. Paradoxical embolism. QJM. 1930;23:135–50.
24. Meacham III RR, Headley AS, Bronze MS, Lewis JB, Rester MM. Impending paradoxical embolism. Arch Intern Med. 1998;158:438–48.
25. Meier B, Lock JE. Contemporary management of patent foramen ovale. Circulation. 2003;107:5–9.
26. Doyen D, Castellani M, Moceri P, Chiche O, Lazdunski R, Bertora D, Cerboni P, Chaussade C, Ferrari E. Patent foramen ovale and stroke in intermediate-risk pulmonary embolism. Chest. 2014;146:967–73.
27. Leacche M, Unic D, Goldhaber SZ, Rawn JD, Aranki SF, Couper GS, Mihaljevic T, Rizzo RJ, Cohn LH, Aklog L, Byrne JG. Modern surgical treatment of massive pulmonary embolism: results in 47 consecutive patients after rapid diagnosis and aggressive surgical approach. J Thorac Cardiovasc Surg. 2005;129:1018–23.
28. Major WK, Embolism P. Review of a pathophysiologic approach to the golden hour of hemodynamically significant pulmonary embolism. Chest. 2002;121:877–905.
29. PIOPED Investigators. Value of the ventilation/perfusion scan in acute pulmonary embolism: results of the prospective investigation of pulmonary embolism diagnosis (PIOPED). JAMA. 1990;263:2753–9.
30. Kuo WT, Gould MK, Louie JD, Rosenberg JK, Sze DY, Hofmann LV. Catheter directed therapy for the treatment of massive pulmonary embolism: systematic review and meta-analysis of modern techniques. J Vasc Interv Radiol. 2009;20:1431–40.
31. The ATLANTIS. ECASS, and NINDS rt-PA Study Group Investigators Association of outcome with early stroke treatment: pooled analysis of ATLANTIS, ECASS, and NINDS rt-PA stroke trials. Lancet. 2004;363:768–74.

32. Conti E, Zezza L, Ralli E, Comito C, Sada L, Passerini J, Caserta D, Rubattu S, Autore C, Moscarini M, Volpe M. Pulmonary embolism pregnancy. J Thromb Thrombolysis. 2013. doi:10.1007/s11239-013-0941-9.
33. Eichinger S, Weltermann A, Philipp K. Prospective evaluation of hemostatic system activation and thrombin potential in healthy pregnant women with and without factor V Leiden. Thromb Haemost. 1999;82:1232–6.
34. Heit JA, Kobbervig CE, James AH. Trends in the incidence of venous thromboembolism during pregnancy or postpartum: a 30-year population-based study. Ann Intern Med. 2005;143:697–706.
35. Te Raa DG, Ribbert LSM, Snijder RJ, Biesma DH. Treatment options in massive pulmonary embolism during pregnancy. A case-report and review of literature. Thromb Res. 2009; 124:1–5.
36. Turrentine MA, Braems G, Ramirez MM. Use of thrombolytics for the treatment of thromboembolic disease during pregnancy. Obstet Gynecol Surv. 1995;50:534–41.
37. Leonhardt G, Gaul C, Nietsch HH. Thrombolytic therapy in pregnancy. J Thromb Thrombolysis. 2006;21:271–6.
38. Holden EL, Ranu H, Sheth A. Thrombolysis for massive pulmonary embolism in pregnancy—a report of three cases and follow up over a two year period. Thromb Res. 2011;127:58–9.
39. Fasullo S, Maringhini G, Terrazzino G. Thrombolysis for massive pulmonary embolism in pregnancy: a case report. Int J Emerg Med. 2011;4:69–74.
40. Jerjes-Sánchez C, Ramírez RA, Arriaga NR, Pimentel MG. Dosis altas e infusión rápida de estreptoquinasa para el tratamiento de tromboembolia pulmonar masiva. Arch Inst Cardiol Mex. 1993;63:227–34.
41. Jerjes-Sanchez C, Gutierrez-Fajardo P, Ramirez-Rivera A, Garcia ML, Hernández CHG. Infarto agudo del ventrículo derecho secundario a tromboembolia pulmonar masiva. Arch Inst Cardiol Mex. 1995;65:65–73.
42. Jerjes-Sanchez C, Ramirez-Rivera A, Garcia ML, Arriaga-Nava R, Valencia-Sanchez S, Rosado-Buzzo A, Pierzo JA, Rosas ME. Streptokinase and heparin versus heparin alone in massive pulmonary embolism: a randomized controlled trial. J Thromb Thrombolysis. 1995;2:67–9.
43. Jerjes-Sanchez C, Ramirez-Rivera A, Arriaga-Nava R, Iglesias-Gonzalez S, Gutierrez P, Ibarra-Perez C, Martinez A, Valencia S, Rosado-Buzzo A, Pierzo JA, Rosas E. High dose and short-term streptokinase infusion in patients with pulmonary embolism. Prospective with seven-year follow-up trial. J Thromb Thrombolysis. 2001;12:237–47.
44. Jerjes-Sanchez C, Villarreal-Umaña S, Ramirez-Rivera A, Garcia-Sosa A, Canseco LM, Archondo T, Reyes E, Garza A, Arriaga R, Castillo F, Jasso O, Garcia H, Bermudez M, Hernández JM, Garcia J, Martinez P, Rangel F, Gutierrez J, Comparan A. Improving adjunctive treatment in pulmonary embolism and fibrinolytic therapy. The role of enoxaparin and weight-adjusted unfractionated heparin. J Thromb Thrombolysis. 2009;27:154–62.
45. Pollack CV. The use of oral anticoagulants for the treatment of venous thromboembolic events in an ED. Am J Emerg Med. 2014;32:1526–33.
46. Sharifi M, Bay C, Schwartz F, Skrocki L. Safe-dose thrombolysis plus rivaroxaban for moderate and severe pulmonary embolism. Clin Cardiol. 2014;37:78–82.

Index

C. Jerjes-Sánchez, *Thrombolysis in Pulmonary Embolism*,
DOI 10.1007/978-3-319-19707-4

MIX
Papier aus verantwortungsvollen Quellen
Paper from responsible sources
FSC® C105338

If you have any concerns about our products,
you can contact us on
ProductSafety@springernature.com

In case Publisher is established outside the EU,
the EU authorized representative is:
Springer Nature Customer Service Center GmbH
Europaplatz 3, 69115 Heidelberg, Germany

Printed by Libri Plureos GmbH
in Hamburg, Germany